MW00814214

National Symposium on Family Issues

Series Editors: Alan Booth and Susan M. McHale

For other titles published in this series, go to
www.springer.com/series/8381

Alan Booth • Susan M. McHale
Nancy S. Landale
Editors

Biosocial Foundations of Family Processes

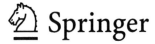 Springer

Editors
Alan Booth
Distinguished Professor of Sociology
Human Development & Demography
The Pennsylvania State University
University Park, PA
USA
axb24@psu.edu

Nancy S. Landale
Director
Population Research Institute
Professor of Sociology and Demography
The Pennsylvania State University
University Park, PA
USA
landale@pop.psu.edu

Susan M. McHale
Director
Social Science Research Institute
Professor of Human Development
The Pennsylvania State University
University Park, PA
USA
x2u@psu.edu

ISBN 978-1-4419-7360-3   e-ISBN 978-1-4419-7361-0
DOI 10.1007/978-1-4419-7361-0
Springer New York Dordrecht Heidelberg London

Printed on acid-free paper

Springer is part of Springer Science+Business Media (www.springer.com)

Preface

Conceptual shifts and technological breakthroughs have placed new emphasis on the importance of combining nature and nurture to understand family processes and problems. The link between biology and behavior is no longer regarded as a simple, unidirectional, cause and effect process. Today's researchers emphasize bidirectional relations between physiological processes and behavior, processes that operate in the context of previous experience and the demands of a multilayered ecology. Biological factors mediate and moderate behavioral adaptation to a range of environmental challenges. At the same time, environmental challenges and behavioral responses affect biological processes. Family relationships are at the intersection of many biological and environmental influences.

The contributions to *Biosocial Foundations of Family Processes* are based on papers presented at the 17th Annual Penn State Symposium on Family Issues in October 2009, Biosocial Research Contributions to Understanding Family Processes and Problems. The goal of this volume is to stimulate conversation among scholars who construct and use biosocial models, as well as among those who want to know more about biosocial processes. Researchers interested in both biological and social/environmental influences on behavior, health, and development are represented among the volume's contributing authors, including researchers whose work emphasizes behavioral endocrinology, behavior genetics, neuroscience, evolutionary psychology, sociology, demography, anthropology, and psychology.

This edited volume is the culmination of 2 days of stimulating presentations and discussions of biosocial research as it relates to family processes. Chapter authors consider physiological and social environmental influences on parenting and early childhood development, followed by adolescent adjustment and family formation. Finally, family resources, genes, and child well-being are examined.

Each of the four parts in this volume includes a chapter by a lead author, followed by shorter chapters by discussants. Care has been taken to bring together perspectives from diverse disciplines in each part. The volume concludes with an integrative commentary.

The volume begins with four chapters devoted to parenting. The first chapter is a comprehensive psychobiological overview of the mechanisms regulating the onset, maintenance, and development of mothering written by psychologists Viara Mileva-Seitz, Institute of Medical Sciences and Psychology, University of Toronto, and Alison Fleming of the University of Toronto, Mississauga. This is followed by a comparable analysis of paternal behavior authored by behavioral ecologists Anne Storey and Carolyn Walsh, of Memorial University at Newfoundland. Author Susan Calkins, a developmental psychologist at University of North Carolina Greensboro, then focuses on early offspring physical regulation, which is linked to later behavioral regulation, and the influence of caregiver behavior on such regulation. In the fourth chapter, developmental psychologist Jay Belsky, of Birbeck University in London, calls attention to the importance of taking into account individual susceptibility to adverse environments when studying the influence of parents and children on one another.

The next four chapters focus on the physiological and social factors that influence development and adjustment in adolescence. The first chapter describes how the interplay of genetic and environmental factors is linked to family relationships in ways that affect adolescent outcomes. Developmental psychologist Jenae Neiderhiser of Penn State describes the way in which rapid advances in molecular genetics add to our knowledge. In the second chapter, Alexandra Burt, clinical psychologist and behavior geneticist at Michigan State, shows how gene-environment outcomes vary extensively by the type of outcomes such as physical aggression vs. rule breaking. In the next chapter, psychologist Sheri Berenbaum of Penn State provides a detailed analysis of the ways in which puberty shapes psychological function and social responses on the part of the adolescent and others in ways that affect adolescent development and adjustment. In the fourth chapter, clinical psychologist Sally Powers of University of Massachusetts Amherst, examines the question of why many devastating mental illnesses have their onset during adolescence.

The four chapters that constitute part three center on the physiological and social factors that influence mate selection, family formation, and fertility. In the first chapter, University of New Mexico anthropologist Steven Gangestad shares his expertise in evolutionary psychology in a discussion of the development of contemporary patterns of family formation and fertility. In the next chapter, Brian D'Onofrio of the Department of Psychological and Brain Sciences at Indiana University, and his colleagues at Karolinska Institutet of Sweden, describe how social neuroscience research, quasi-experimental research, and behavior genetic analysis might influence and be influenced by evolutionary explanations of fertility. In the following chapter psychologist David Schmitt of Bradley University, details how harsh environments lead to very different reproductive strategies than do cultures with less stress and more resources. In the final chapter, sociologist Philip Morgan of Duke offers an alternative to Gangestad's explanation for major shifts in family fertility.

Part four of the volume focuses on family resources, genes, and child well-being. The lead chapter by sociologist Guang Guo of University of North Carolina, considers the role molecular genetics may play in understanding family influences on child well-being. In the second chapter, anthropologist Mark Flinn of University of Columbia, Missouri examines the links between neuroendocrinology and children's complex socio-cognitive adaptation to family life. Next, Pilyoung Kim of the National

Institute of Mental Health and Gary Evans, professor of human development at Cornell University review a large number of studies indicating that children's environmental risk factors interact with genes that predict a wide range of behavioral problems. The authors examine the biological mechanisms that account for the gene-environment interactions. Concluding this section is sociologist Dalton Conley of New York University. He points out that much contemporary research on gene–phenotype associations is carried out without fully taking into account exogenous sources of environmental variation. His chapter constitutes a useful set of guidelines for those planning or conducting behavioral genetic research.

The final chapter is an integrative commentary by Jennifer Buher Kane and Chun-Bun Lam, graduate students at Penn State in Sociology and Human Development and Family Studies, respectively. This interdisciplinary team summarizes major themes and suggests next steps for research.

Acknowledgments

The editors are grateful to the many organizations at Penn State that sponsored the 2009 Symposium on Family Issues and this resulting volume, including the Population Research Institute; the Children, Youth, and Families Consortium; the Prevention Research Center; the Women's Studies Program; and the departments of Sociology, Labor Studies and Employment Relations, Human Development and Family Studies, Anthropology, and Psychology. The editors also gratefully acknowledge essential core financial support in the form of a 5-year grant from the National Institute of Child Health and Human Development (NICHD), as well as guidance and advice from Christine Bachrach (Office of Behavioral and Social Sciences Research, National Institutes of Health), Rebecca Clark, Rosalind King, and Peggy McCardle of NICHD. The ongoing support of all these partners has enabled us to attract excellent scholars from a range of backgrounds and disciplines – the sort of group on whom the quality and integrity of the series depends.

A lively, interdisciplinary team of scholars from across the Penn State community meets with us annually to generate symposia topics and plans and is available throughout the year for brainstorming and problem solving. We appreciate their enthusiasm, intellectual support, and creative ideas. In the course of selecting speakers, symposium organizers consult with a wide range of people at other universities, at NICHD, and at other organizations so the most qualified people are identified and contacted about participating. We also sincerely thank Elizabeth Skowron, H. Harrington (Bo) Cleveland, David Puts, and Valarie King for presiding over symposium sessions.

The many details that go into planning a symposium and producing a volume cannot be overestimated. In this regard, we are especially grateful for the assistance of our administrative staff, including Tara Murray and Sherry Yocum. Finally, we could not have accomplished this work without Carolyn Scott, whose organizational skills, commitment, and attention to the many details that go into organizing a good conference and edited book series make it possible for us to focus on the ideas.

Alan Booth
Susan McHale
Nancy Landale

Contents

Contributors

Jay Belsky, Ph.D.
Institute for the Study of Children, Families and Social Issues, Birkbeck College,
University of London, London, UK
j.belsky@bbk.ac.uk

Sheri A. Berenbaum, Ph.D.
Department of Psychology, The Pennsylvania State University,
University Park, PA, USA
sberenbaun@psu.edu

S. Alexandra Burt, Ph.D.
Department of Psychology, Michigan State University, East Lansing, MI, USA
burts@msu.edu

Susan D. Calkins, Ph.D.
Department of Psychology, The University of North Carolina,
Greensboro, NC, USA
sdcalkin@uncg.edu

Dalton Conley, Ph.D.
Department of Sociology, New York University, New York, NY, USA
dc66@nyu.edu

Brian M. D'Onofrio, Ph.D.
Department of Psychology, Indiana University, Bloomington, IN, USA
bmdonofr@indiana.edu

Gary W. Evans, Ph.D.
Department of Design and Environmental Analysis, Cornell University,
Ithaca, NY, USA

Alison S. Fleming, Ph.D.
Department of Psychology, University of Toronto, Ontario, Canada
alison.fleming@utoronto.ca

Mark V. Flinn, Ph.D.
Department of Anthropology, University of Missouri, Columbia, MO, USA
FlinnM@missouri.edu

Steven W. Gangestad, Ph.D.
Department of Psychology, University of New Mexico, Albuquerque, NM, USA
sgangest@unm.edu

Guang Guo, Ph.D.
Department of Sociology, University of North Carolina, Chapel Hill, NC, USA
guang_guo@unc.edu

Jennifer B. Kane
Department of Sociology, The Pennsylvania State University,
University Park, PA, USA
jbuher@pop.psu.edu

Pilyoung Kim, Ph.D.
Emotion and Development Branch, National Institute of Mental Health,
Bethesda, MD, USA
pilyoung.kim@nih.gov

Chun Bun Lam
Department of Human Development and Family Studies,
The Pennsylvania State University, University Park, PA, USA

Niklas Langstrom, M.D., Ph.D.
Department of Child and Adolescent Psychiatry,
Karolinska Institutet in Stockholm, Sweden

Paul Lichtenstein, Ph.D.
Department of Medical Epidemiology and Biostatistics,
Karolinska Institutet in Stockholm, Sweden

S. Philip Morgan, Ph.D.
Department of Sociology, Duke University, Durham, NC, USA
pmorgan@soc.duke.edu

Jenae M. Neiderhiser, Ph.D.
Department of Psychology, The Pennsylvania State University,
University Park, PA, USA
jenaemn@psu.edu

Sally I. Powers, Ph.D.
Department of Psychology and Neuroscience and Behavior Program,
University of Massachusetts at Amherst, MA, USA
powers@psych.umass.edu

David P. Schmitt, Ph.D.
Department of Psychology, Bradley University, Peoria, IL, USA
dps@bradley.edu

Viara Mileva-Seitz, Ph.D.
Institute of Medical Science (IMS), University of Toronto, Ontario, Canada
Viara.mileva@utoronto.ca

Anne Storey, Ph.D.
Department of Psychology, Memorial University of Newfoundland, St. John's,
Newfoundland and Labrador, Canada
astorey@mun.ca

Carolyn Walsh, Ph.D.
Department of Psychology, Memorial University of Newfoundland, St. John's,
Newfoundland and Labrador, Canada

Part I
Parenting and Early Childhood Behavior and Development

Chapter 1
How Mothers Are Born: A Psychobiological Analysis of Mothering

Viara Mileva-Seitz and Alison S. Fleming

Abstract A quick scan of how mothers engage with their infants and how they feel about it indicates just how variable mothering is – some mothers talk to their infants, while others sing, stroke and cuddle, and disattend, and, sadly, will neglect or be harsh with them. Although "responsive" maternal behavior enhances the fitness of the mother by ensuring the survival and reproductive efficacy of the offspring, this broad "phenotype" is not a unitary construct, controlled by a single endocrine or brain system, but instead comprises multiple behavioral systems, each with its own neural, endocrine, and behavioral profile. The quality of mothering shown by a new mother depends on her experiences with infants while growing up, her stress level, her affective state, her attention and executive function, how her perceptual systems are tuned, the salience to her of infants and infant-related cues, and how rewarding she finds her interactions with her infant. These behavioral systems are affected by circulating hormones and are mediated by an equally complex set of brain systems with their own neurochemistries and sensitivities. These systems in turn have developed as a function of mothers' genetics and early experiences in the family of origin. Using both animals and humans as models for one another, this chapter explores this array of interacting factors that contribute to mothers' responses to their young infants.

Introduction

Given the enormous complexity of mothering, it is quite extraordinary that mammalian mothers are generally so adept at raising their offspring. Explaining this by invoking concepts of instinct or innateness is taking the assertion to a different

V. Mileva-Seitz (✉)
Institute of Medical Science (IMS), University of Toronto, Ontario, Canada
e-mail: Viara.mileva@utoronto.ca

A.S. Fleming
Department of Psychology, University of Toronto, Ontario, Canada
e-mail: alison.fleming@utoronto.ca

A. Booth et al. (eds.), *Biosocial Foundations of Family Processes*,
National Symposium on Family Issues, DOI 10.1007/978-1-4419-7361-0_1,
© Springer Science+Business Media, LLC 2011

analytic level, one related to concepts of evolution, natural selection, and "fitness." However, explanations at the level of individual development and proximate mechanism can also be invoked. The focus of this chapter is a description and analysis of this complexity. The behavior of new mothers toward their offspring shows both marked similarities and considerable differences within cultures, across cultures, and certainly across species. The obvious similarities among mammalian species that show mothering include nursing and a posture designed to enhance the neonates' access to the teat, some form of communication system between mother and offspring to indicate "needs" of both, a way of transporting offspring, especially if they are altricial or immature at birth, and some form of maternal "protective" defense of offspring. Most mothers also keep their offspring clean by grooming and provide a home base or "nest site" either in the environment or on their bodies where the young can sleep. In addition to performing these functions, human mothers also normally develop feelings of nurturance and warmth (or "love") toward the baby, anxiety in response to distress or unexpected separations from the baby, and grief with his/her loss or death (see Corter & Fleming, 2002; Fleming & Li, 2002; Gonzalez, Atkinson, & Fleming, 2009); see also edited volumes by Bridges (2008) and Bornstein (2002).

The differences among species in the typography, timing, and duration of the behaviors, their developmental trajectory, and the range of proximal causal mechanisms are vast. The differences emerge as a function of the developmental maturity of the young. In most mammalian species, the young are altricial, often born with their eyes and ears closed and with immature nervous systems; these young require extensive care and are very dependent for early survival. Other species are much more mature, or precocial, at birth and are more independent early on (as with ungulates where the young stand within minutes of birth and ambulate behind the mother within days) (Numan, Fleming, & Levy, 2006). Humans are mostly altricial: although they can see and hear at birth, they require a long period of care before they can fend for themselves (some would say this takes two decades or more!!!). Arguably more intriguing – or less well understood – than cross-species differences are individual differences within a species.

In humans, there are both cross-cultural similarities and differences in mothering behaviors. Among the modal similarities are included nursing (Leiderman & Leiderman, 1977), singing (Trehub, Unyk, & Trainor, 1993), and contingent responding to infant distress (Ainsworth, Bell, & Stayton, 1974; Corter & Fleming, 2002; Pederson et al., 1990). However, in the absence of explicit practice, first-time mothers exhibit a range of different responses to their infants: some look at them directly while others gaze avert (Brazelton, 1972); some keep their babies unclothed and stroke their bodies; others swaddle them instead (see Corter & Fleming, 2002). Some talk or sing to their babies; others do not (Tronick, 1987). Some sleep with their babies, while others put their babies in a cot next to them or in their own rooms (see Thoman, 2006). Babies are also transported in different ways – some on the front of the body, others on the back; some on cradle boards and others still, in a vehicle.

More subtly, within a culture mothers show large variations in the post-partum development of nurturant feelings, from minutes to months (Leifer, 1980;

Moss & Jones, 1977; Robson, 1967; Robson & Kumar, 1980; Trevathan, 1983) and once "attached" or emotionally committed, in the intensity with which they exhibit different caregiving behaviors. More extremely, some are motivated to provide warmth, shelter, and food to the infant, while others neglect or even abuse their infants (see Corter & Fleming, 2002; Hrdy, 2005, 2009).

In this chapter, we describe the proximal mechanisms regulating the onset, maintenance, and development of mothering, comparing and contrasting two altricial mammals, rat and human, with quite different ecologic constraints and evolutionary histories. Rats are nocturnal, litter-bearers, very immature at birth, rapid developing, short-lived, and have relatively thin nonvariegated cortices reflecting simplicity of cognitive function. In contrast, humans, as we know are diurnal, bearer of singletons or, more rarely, multiples, have a long period of prepubertal development, are long-lived, and have an extensive neocortex and cognitive life (see Numan et al., 2006). The primary goal of this chapter is to unpack the complexity of mothering in rats and humans in terms of the behavioral systems that contribute to individual differences in effective mothering and their distinct and overlapping hormonal, neural, and neurochemical mechanisms. Given the psychobiological approach to mothering that we adopt and the audience for whom this chapter is intended, we emphasize cross-species similarities in organizational principles rather than phenomenologies and mechanisms associated with the obvious differences.

The Thesis

Mothering is not a structure; it is not a reflex; it is not unidimensional. To engage in mothering behavior, mothers have to be sensitive to infant cues and select those cues for processing, utilizing multiple sensory and perceptual modalities; the cues must be attractive and salient for the mother, recruiting reward and approach systems. Mothers must be emotionally prepared and positively motivated to engage socially with the infant, depending on systems regulating affect. They must selectively attend to the offspring in the context of competing stimuli, enacted through systems that regulate attention, and they must be restrained and consistent in their responsiveness, depending on systems that regulate impulsivity. Finally, mothers gain through experiences, acquired both early in life and with young as juveniles and in adulthood. These experiences are acquired, consolidated, and stored as motor or sensory memories and are based on extensive brain plasticity.

In short, to mother appropriately requires the action of multiple behavioral systems in the domains of sensation, perception, affect, reward, attention and executive function, impulsivity, and learning. And then, of course, there is the motor system without which no behavior could occur. This chapter discusses each of these behavioral systems as they apply to rat and human mothers, both descriptively, in terms of the phenomenology and in terms of their underlying hormonal, neural, neurochemical, and genetic regulation. It also discusses some developmental studies that provide clues about how early experiences of being mothered – or not – influence the development of mothering and contributing behavioral and physiological systems. This chapter is not intended to be exhaustive in its scholarship. Instead, it depends heavily on the work our laboratory has done, while attempting to integrate our work with closely related work in the field. Given how extensive the "mothering" field has become, we apologize in advance if we have failed to cite some of the more seminal studies. We are likely to omit many of our own as well.

Psychology of Mothering

Hormonal Background to the Psychology of Mothering

The influence of pregnancy hormones (those normally elevated during pregnancy) on maternal behavior has long been a topic of interest and research, but primarily in relation to nonhuman species. Extensive research in rats and other mammals has shown that the hormonal milieu of pregnancy and parturition (high levels of oxytocin, prolactin, and estradiol, with a decline of progesterone) provides a hormonal basis for maternal behavior (Bridges, 1990, 2008; Insel, 1990; Numan et al., 2006; Pryce, Martin, & Skuse, 1995; Rosenblatt, Olufowobi, & Siegel, 1998 Rosenblatt, Mayor, & Giordano, 1988) (see Fig. 1.1a for changes in estrogen, progesterone, and prolactin across pregnancy; oxytocin not shown). In rats, this same hormonal profile also increases mothers' attraction to infant cues, enhances the reinforcing value of pups, and results in marked changes in mothers' affective state (Numan & Insel, 2003; Numan et al., 2006). A similar hormonal effect may also be present in human mothers, although the actual estrogen and progesterone profile in humans differs somewhat from the rat and some other mammals (Fleming, Ruble, Krieger, & Wong, 1997; see Fig. 1.1b for changes in estrogen and progesterone across pregnancy; prolactin and oxytocin not shown). In pregnant women feelings of attachment to the fetus grow during the pregnancy, unrelated to changing levels of pregnancy hormones. However, Fleming, Ruble, et al. (1997) found that mothers who experienced greater attachment to their new babies after the birth underwent an increase from early to late pregnancy in their estradiol/progesterone ratio, whereas those with low attachment experienced a decrease in the estradiol/progesterone ratio over this same time period. Interestingly, this hormonal profile shift was also associated with mothers' affective state; mothers with a greater shift in the E to P ratio across pregnancy also experienced greater postpartum well-being. Although well-being and attachment feelings were both related to hormones and to one another, further analyses indicated that hormones are related to attachment both indirectly, by altering mothers' affect, and directly. Hormones and well-being together explain 40–50% of the variance in mothers' attachment (Fleming, Ruble, et al., 1997).

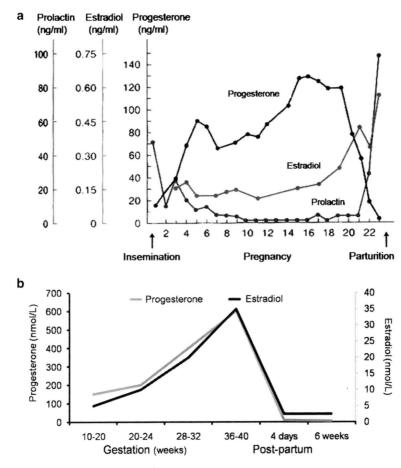

Fig. 1.1 Hormonal profile during gestation and parturition in humans (**a**) and rats (**b**). (Adapted from Rosenblatt, Mayer, & Giordano, 1988 (A); and Fleming, Ruble, Krieger & Wong, 1997 (B)).

In addition to pregnancy hormones, postpartum hormones from the hypothalamic–pituitary–adrenal (HPA) axis may also play a role in mothers' response to their newborns. The HPA axis has been studied extensively in relation to reactivity to social, behavioral, and psychological stimuli (Cacioppo et al., 1998; Dettling, Gunnar, & Donzella, 1999; Kirschbaum, Wust, & Hellhammer, 1992; McEwen, De Kloet, & Rostene, 1986; Smyth et al., 1998; Stansbury & Gunnar, 1994). Fleming and colleagues (Corter & Fleming, 1990; Fleming, Steiner, & Anderson, 1987) examined cortisol in relation to maternal behavior in the early postpartum period when cortisol levels are relatively high and mothers' emotional status is labile. The latter studies indicate that higher cortisol levels on days 3 and 4 postpartum were significantly and strongly associated with maternal approach behaviors, positive maternal attitudes, or more vocally active infants.

Sensory/Perceptual Regulation

Rat pups and human infants represent a constellation of olfactory, auditory, and visual cues that orient, arouse, and direct mothers' attention. These cues are of special salience to mothers, compared with nonmothers. This salience can occur prior to extensive contact with the young, under the influence of the parturitional hormones, but is definitely enhanced by actual experiences interacting with the young (Fleming et al., 1993; Fleming, Steiner, & Corter, 1997; Orpen & Fleming, 1987; Schaal & Porter, 1991).

An example of stimulus salience in the olfactory domain is presented in a study in which new postpartum rat dams (mothers) and same-aged nonmother virgin females were compared for duration of sniffing of woodchips used as nesting material by a lactating female and her pups, and of woodchips used as nesting material by a nonlactating female. New mothers showed a clear preference for the lactating/ pup nest material, whereas the nonlactating female showed no preference, indicating that the odors associated with lactation and pups are positive and salient to the postpartum animal (Fleming, Cheung, Myhal, & Kessler, 1989). That this preference was *not* primarily the result of the actual experience of the odor of lactation and pups is indicated by a follow-up study showing that a similar preference for the lactating/pup odors was found among virgin animals who had received hormonal priming that mimics the hormonal changes associated with later pregnancy and parturition that are normally experienced in the new parturient mother (Fleming et al., 1989).

Using an analogous procedure, similar results were found among populations of human mothers. Fleming et al. (1993) asked groups of mothers of 2-day-olds, 1-month-olds, and female and male nonparent controls to rate the pleasantness of a variety of infant-related and noninfant odorants. Odors consisted of 2- to 3-day-old infant t-shirts (worn for 8–12 h), infant urine, infant feces, adult axillary odors, spice, and cheese. The primary findings show that new mothers give higher hedonic ratings to the infant t-shirts than do nonmothers, while not differing in response to other stimuli. Mothers who give positive ratings experienced, on the one hand, a shorter postpartum interval to the first extended contact and nursing of their infants and, on the other hand, a heightened maternal responsiveness, measured both behaviorally and by self-report. Based on these findings, it seems that new mothers show heightened attraction to the general body odors of infants, but this attraction varies as a function of early postpartum contact and experiences interacting with young.

In addition to experience, the postpartum hormone cortisol influences responses to newborn baby odors (Fleming, Steiner, et al., 1997). In general, associations between cortisol and hedonics are found only in primiparous mothers: higher levels of cortisol predicted higher ratings of infants' t-shirt body odors and urine but were unrelated to control odorants (Fleming, Steiner, et al., 1997). Maternal report of greater prior experience with infants also predicted higher ratings. These patterns suggest that both cortisol and experience are tied to attraction to infant odors and further suggest that prior experience could mask hormonal effects on attraction since they were seen only in first-time mothers. In addition, there was a positive correlation between cortisol levels and the success at recognizing one's own infant, but only for multiparous mothers (Gonzalez, Jenkins, Steiner, & Fleming, 2009).

Mother rats are also selectively responsive to their offspring's vocalizations, which when presented in combination with pup olfactory cues elicits selective orientation and approach. The same is true for hormonally primed nonmothers by not for non-hormonally primed animals (Farrell & Alberts, 2002). Human mothers are also very responsive to infant vocalizations, especially their cries (Stallings, Fleming, Corter, Worthman, & Steiner, 2001). Mothers, but not nonmothers, experience elevated levels of sympathy and alertness in response to cries of babies but not in response to white noise. Moreover, as with odor responsiveness, the extent of sympathy experienced by mothers uniquely is related both to mothers' cortisol levels and to her heart rate (Stallings et al., 2001). Mothers with higher circulating levels of cortisol and higher baseline heart rates (prior to stimulus presentation) tend to respond more sympathetically when they hear the infant cries (Stallings et al., 2001). The positive association between cortisol levels and sympathetic responses is consistent with our earlier findings of a positive association between cortisol and positive responses to infants and infant odors in new mothers (Fleming, Steiner, et al., 1997). In the Stallings et al. (2001) study, mothers with higher baseline cortisol levels also showed greater sympathy to pain cries and less sympathy to hunger cries than did mothers with lower cortisol. Furthermore, mothers with higher baseline cortisol levels also had higher baseline heart-rate responses, and both physiological measures showed a similar relation to sympathetic feelings. In contrast to the patterns of individual differences, there was little evidence of differential infant stimulus effects. That is, there were no differences in either hormones or heart rate in responses to cries vs. odors. In fact, hormones underwent very little change with either stimulus. Thus, individual differences in maternal physiology, perhaps as part of personality differences, seem to play a major part in affective responses to infant stimuli.

Finally, unlike most animals that have been studied soon after birth, humans are strongly visual animals and mothers are adept at recognizing the face of their own newborn from a set of infant pictures (Kaitz, Good, Rokem, & Eidelman, 1988; Kaitz, Rokem, & Eidelman, 1988). A study by Wiesenfeld and Klorman (1978) demonstrated physiological arousal effects for parents at the sight of their own baby crying or smiling; heart rate (HR) first decelerated and then accelerated as parents viewed silent videotapes of their 5-month-old infants. Leavitt and Donovan (1979) found that mothers of 3-month-old infants responded with HR acceleration when the gaze of an unfamiliar infant was directed toward them but did not display this arousal pattern when the infant was looking away. At the behavioral level, the infant's gaze appears to evoke mother's gaze (Messer & Vietze, 1984) and thus lead to "en face" behavior between the two, which Klaus, Trause, and Kennell (1975) have described as species-typical maternal behavior. These and other studies (Butterfield, Emde, Svejda, & Naiman, 1982; Stern, 1974; Trevathan, 1987) indicate that infant visual stimuli are powerful stimuli for the elicitation of maternal behavior and are clearly important in the sequence of interaction between infant and mother.

Taken together, these results suggest that like a number of other species in which infant odor attraction contributes to mothers' early attachment to their offspring (Levy, 2008) and mothers are sensitive to the distress vocalizations of their infants, human mothers find infant-related odors to be attractive and cries to be salient. These perceptions are affect-laden and related to hormones and enhanced by experience. They also have motivational properties (Bridges, 2008; Fleming, Gonzalez, Afonso, & Lovic, 2008).

Affect and Attention

Once mothers have become maternal or become "attached" to their infants, the ways in which they interact with their infants also show significant individual differences, and these differences reflect differences in mothers' mood, attentional capacity, impulsivity, and ability to learn about their infants and about mothering.

The postpartum period is a period of huge endocrine upheaval. The hormonal shifts that occur at this time are among the greatest in any time in a female's life. Although, as we have seen, the specific hormones may vary, in both rats and humans they act not only to alter perception; they also function to modulate mothers' affect, which in turn influences behavior. In rats, this affective change takes the form of a change along the activity and fear dimensions. In humans, it is along the depression dimension.

When placed into an open-field apparatus used to assess activity and "anxiety," new mother rats and hormonally primed rats exhibit hyperactivity and reduced neophobia in response to a novel object (Fleming et al., 1989; Fleming & Luebke, 1981) in comparison to virgin nonmothers, as reflected in the proportion of activity spent in the center as opposed to the periphery of the field and time spent sniffing a novel object. Similar effects are found using other measures of anxiety (the elevated plus maze) (Neumann, Wigger, Liebsch, Holsboer, & Landgraf, 1998). Under the influence of the parturitional hormones, new mothers are less neophobic and, hence, less avoidant of pups than are nonmothers (Fleming & Luebke, 1981). Drugs or manipulations that reduce the neophobia in virgins also have the effect of facilitating maternal responding to foster pups in virgin animals that are normally not maternally responsive to pups (Hansen, Ferreira, & Selart, 1985; Mayer, 1983).

Among humans, the most notable change that a new mother undergoes with the birth of a baby is in her mood. A high proportion of mothers experience what has come to be known as the "postpartum blues" and also heightened lability within the first postpartum week (ca. 26–85%, depending on the diagnostic criteria; Bright, 1994; Gold, 2002; O'Hara, Zekoski, Philipps, & Wright, 1990); a small but substantial percent of women also experience more severe dysphoria and postpartum depression (PPD) that extends past the first few weeks, although it usually remits by 5 months postpartum (Cooper & Murray, 1995; Cox, Connor, & Kendell, 1982; Cox, Murray, & Chapman, 1993; Gold, 2002; Stowe & Nemeroff, 1995). The symptom profile of PPD resembles that of a major depressive episode experienced at other times in life, including fatigue, negative affect, negative thoughts, suicidal ideation, and low self-esteem (Beck, 2002; Gold, 2002; Seyfried & Marcus, 2003; Wisner & Stowe, 1997), but it is unique in its timing, always involving at least the mother–baby dyad and in most cases an entire family unit.

Although it is widely believed that these mood changes are hormonally mediated, there is considerable debate in the literature as to the causes of this clinical condition (e.g., Ross, Sellers, Gilbert Evans, & Romach, 2004; Steiner, 1998). What is clear, however, is that dysphoric women often have difficulty interacting with their infants. Although depressed mothers do not report feeling less attached to their infants (Fleming, Ruble, Flett, & Shaul, 1988), and in fact may show considerable warmth and interest (Stein et al., 1991), depressed mothers respond less sensitively and more negatively to their infants than do nondepressed mothers (Cohn, Campbell, Matias, & Hopkins, 1990; Field, Healy, Goldstein, & Guthertz, 1990; Fleming et al., 1988; Murray, Fiori-Cowley, Hooper, & Cooper, 1996; Stanley, Murray, & Stein, 2004). At 2 months postpartum, their speech contains more negative affect, and in play interactions they exhibit fewer responses to the infant's behavior (Murray et al., 1996). During face-to-face interactions with their infants, depressed mothers are also more prone to exhibit controlling, intrusive, and overstimulating behavior, or withdrawal, passivity, and disengagement (Cohn et al., 1990; Field et al., 1990; Lovejoy, Graczyk, O'Hare, & Neuman, 2000; Malphurs, Raag, Field, Pickens, & Pelaez-Nougeras, 1996). Moreover, when observed interacting with their infants they tend to spend less time than nondepressed mothers engaging in behaviors that "match" the behaviors of their infants and more negative states were matched (Field et al., 1990). Similarly, other studies have found that the depressed dyad presents fewer vocalizations and fewer visual communications; at 6 months postpartum, they use less affective and less informative speech, and their overall level of tactile interaction behavior is lower (Fleming et al., 1988; Herrera, Reissland, & Shepherd, 2004; Righetti-Veltema, Conne-Perreard, Bousquet, & Manzano, 2002).

Although the literature indicates that depression itself also predisposes people to problems with attention, to date no studies relate PPD to inattention in new mothers. There are also no studies on attentional or impulsivity changes associated with parturition in rats; preliminary studies in humans do not show that new mothers are more generally attentive, using the Cambridge Neuropsychological Test Automated Battery (CANTAB) (Sahakian et al., 1988), than are nonmothers (Chico, Ali, Eaton, Gonzalez, & Fleming, in preparation). However, there is considerable evidence that general (nonspecific) attention (and perhaps impulsivity) is related to quality of mothering (Gonzalez, Jenkins, Steiner, & Fleming, submitted). In animal studies, mother rats who show reduced selective attention using an animal version of an attention test normally administered to human subjects (the Wisconsin card sorting task) and reduced sensorimotor gating (an "automatic" startle-attention task, prepulse inhibition test) also show reduced crouching behavior and licking of the young (Lovic & Fleming, 2004). Tests of motor impulsivity similarly indicate a strong inverse relation between motor impulsivity and mothering behaviors (Lovic et al., 2010), suggesting that these general behavioral systems must be working

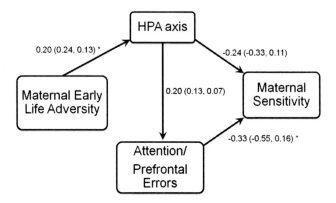

Fig. 1.2 Path diagram of model relationships between maternal early life adversity, hypothalamic-pituitary-adrenal (HPA) axis and lateral prefrontal cortex (LPFC) function (measured by cortisol area under the curve and CANTAB extra-dimensional (ED) shifting score, respectively), and maternal sensitivity towards infant during a 30 min video-recorded interaction at 3–5 months postpartum. Numbers represent standardized coefficients (unstandardized coefficients and standard errors, respectively, in brackets). $*p < 0.05$ (modified from Gonzalez et al., in preparation)

optimally for adequate maternal behavior to occur. In humans, as well, we now know that attention is related to sensitive mothering.

In a series of studies, (Gonzalez, Jenkins, Steiner, Atkinso, and Fleming 2009, Gonzalez, Atkinso, & Fleming, 2009) found that 6 months postpartum mothers who experienced earlier neglect or adversity in family of origin were less sensitive to their infants than those living with both parents in a noncontentious environment, a relation mediated by also being less attentive in computer-based tests of selective attention (Fig. 1.2). Of interest is that, again, the hormone cortisol is implicated in this relation. In humans, studies also show that other so-called prefrontal functions are also associated with mothering. In an fMRI study, Leibenluft, Gobbini, Harrison, and Haxby (2004) found that the simple viewing of one's own child evoked a unique pattern of neural activation in mothers that reflected maternal attachment and was associated with those regions of the brain (i.e., amygdala [AMY], posterior superior temporal sulcus, prefrontal regions) that were involved with representing the mental state of others. It may be that mothers who are characterized as having good "theory of mind" and empathy in general are more sensitive in their interactions with their infants (Hrdy, 2009).

Reward

It is often difficult to ascertain how rewarding the young are to the new mother. However, when deprived of young for a period, new rat mothers will bar press in an operant box adapted to deliver pups with each bar press (Lee, Clancy, & Fleming, 2000). Nonmothers will not. Also, rat mothers develop conditioned place preference for chambers that have been associated with pups, whereas nonmothers tend to avoid those chambers (Magnusson & Fleming, 1995), suggesting a difference between the two kinds of animals in the rewarding properties of pups. More impressively the, work by Morrell and colleagues (Mattson, Williams, Rosenblatt, & Morrell, 2001; Seip & Morrell, 2007; see Pereira, Seip, & Morrell, 2008) shows that when given a choice between a chamber that has been associated with pups and one associated with cocaine, soon after parturition new mothers will prefer the pup-associated chambers, whereas later in the postpartum period, as weaning is occurring, the preference shifts to the cocaine-associated chamber (Mattson et al., 2001; Seip & Morrell, 2007). The reward value of young has not been studied in the same way in humans, but there is no question that with experience new mothers spend increasing amounts of time talking about infants, often at the expense of apparent interest in the partner – an effect that reverses itself toward the end of the first postpartum year, possibly in preparation for the initiation of a new maternity cycle!

Young must have rewarding properties to help sustain maternal motivation and responsiveness and to insure long-term maintenance of interest in young. A substantial literature shows that new mothers learn about their offspring and they do this relatively easily. In a series of studies on the maternal experience effect, Bridges (1975) as well as Fleming and her colleagues (see Fleming & Li, 2002) have explored the situational and sensory factors contributing to this learning. Summarizing an extensive behavioral literature, it is clear that as little as half an hour of interactive contact with young after their birth is adequate to sustain some level of maternal responsiveness for many days, in the absence of the continued presence of pups. The nature of the experience is, however, important. If, during the interactions, the mother cannot smell the young (Fleming, Gavarth, & Sarker, 1992; Mayer & Rosenblatt, 1977) or cannot experience somatosensory input on the ventrum after an anesthetic is applied, this responsiveness is sustained less well (Jakubowski & Terkel, 1986; Stern, 1983). Moreover, simple exposure to pup-related odors, or visual and auditory cues, is not adequate to sustain the responsiveness to pups (Morgan, Fleming, & Stern, 1992). Apparently for robust learning to occur, mothers must actively interact with the pups and receive sensory input during that interaction (Morgan, Watchus, Milgram, & Fleming, 1999). A similar situation occurs in many other mammalian species, especially in ungulates where individual recognition of individual offspring (unlike rats which recognize litters but not individuals in a litter) is essential to prevent the ewe from rejecting the young altogether. In the case of these species, the learning is clearly olfactory based and is rapid and enduring (see Numan et al., 2006).

In humans, individual recognition of the infants' odors as well as the infants cries and the tactile characteristics of the hand also occur (see Corter & Fleming, 2002; Kaitz, Good, Rokem, & Eidelman, 1987; Kaitz, Lapidot, Bronner, & Eidelman, 1992; Porter, Cernoch, & McLaughlin, 1983). Recognition is based on experience with the infant and also occurs in the first few days of the infant's life (see Corter & Fleming, 2002). In addition to this kind of sensory learning among humans, experience interacting with the infant at birth and after birth enhances the mothers' feelings of competence and self-esteem, which affects her subsequent interactions with her baby (e.g., Thompson, Walker, & Crain, 1981). In fact, there is an extensive disputed literature on early postpartum learning by the mother, where researchers in the 1970s claimed that human mothers also have a critical period in which to interact with the baby in order for appropriate attachment to occur (e.g., Klaus and Kennell, 1976). This claim has continued to be debated, with some recent indications that aspects of maternal behavior and infant development may in fact be correlated with an early postpartum period of contact between infant and mother (Bystrova et al., 2009); however, other studies have indicated no adverse effects on mother's attachment of separation from the baby at this time (see Moore, Anderson, & Bergman, 2007).

The role of hormones in the early postpartum learning, while clearly demonstrated in sheep (Numan et al., 2006) and possibly even in rats (Numan et al., 2006), seems not to be the case in humans – as far as we know.

Taken together, behavioral studies suggest that the onset of mothering at parturition and its expression during the early postpartum period depend on appropriate activation or functioning of systems that we believe are essential for mothering, including systems associated with perception, affect, attention, reward, and learning. Changes in all these systems occur at the time of birth. Where we have explored it, they are enhanced or modulated by the parturitional and postpartum hormones, established either experimentally as in the rat model or through a correlational approach in humans.

The Physiology of Mothering

Neuroanatomy of Maternal Behavior

Through extensive work produced by a number of laboratories, the neural circuitry underlying the onset and expression of maternal behavior in rats is well delineated. In summary, there seem to be three primary systems that intersect and that are activated by pups and by hormones in the maternal rat.

Perceptual System Intersecting with the Emotion System

As shown in Fig. 1.3, one system that mediates olfactory processing and activation of "emotion" involves the olfactory bulbs, the lateral olfactory tract, and projection sites within the AMY (see Fleming & Li, 2002; Numan et al., 2006). This system is an excitatory system and dependent on the hormonal condition of the animal, it either inhibits the expression of maternal behavior or enhances it. Hence, lesions of all structures within this system in virgin animals shorten the time it takes for virgins to express maternal behavior when they are given foster pups (Fleming, Vaccarino, Tambosso, & Chee, 1979); in other words, lesions of this system disinhibit the behavior. The interpretation of these results is that lesions of the olfactory

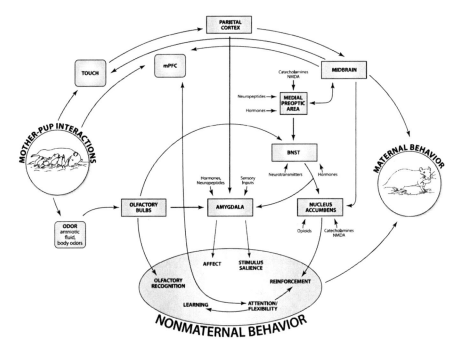

Fig. 1.3 Functional neuroanatomy mediating maternal and related behaviors in mammals. Neuroanatomical structures include olfactory bulbs, amygdala, nucleus accumbens, bed nucleus of the stria terminalis (BNST), medial preoptic area (MPOA), ventromedial hypothalamus (VMH), midbrain, and parietal cortex. Relevant neurochemistry includes the catecholamines, NE, and dopamine, the neuropeptides, and the opioids (adapted from Fleming, O'Day, & Kraemer, 1999; and Fleming & Gonzalez, 2009)

system, by removing the sense of smell, remove olfactory information from the pups that is novel and hence fear-inducing, which explains why normally virgin animals withdraw from pups and avoid them (Fleming & Luebke, 1981). Lesioning within the AMY removes cells that actually mediate the fear and emotion and thereby reduces the fear and avoidant behavior, allowing approach to occur; once animals are in close proximity to pups, other sensory systems come into play to promote mothering behavior (Fleming, Vaccarino, & Luebke, 1980). The assumption is that the hormones of parturition exert their effects on the perceptual and fear systems by inhibiting this generalized neophobia that characterizes non postpartum female rats (see references in Fleming & Li, 2002).

The Final Common Path for Maternal Behavior

The second system that constitutes the "final common path" for the expression of the behavior includes the medial preoptic area/ventral bed nucleus of the stria terminalis (MPOA/vBNST) and its downstream projections into the midbrain [ventral tegmental area (VTA)] and hindbrain [periaqueductal gray (PAG)] and sensory, limbic, and cortical systems that project into the MPOA/-vBNST. The MPOA contains receptors for all the hormones involved in the activation of maternal behavior, including receptors for estradiol, progesterone, prolactin, oxytocin, vasopressin, and opioids (Numan & Insel, 2003; Numan et al., 2006). Lesions to the MPOA eliminate most maternal behaviors in the postpartum rat, and electrical or hormonal stimulation of this group of neurons activates or facilitates maternal behavior in nonmaternal animals (Bridges, 2008; Numan et al., 2006).

Afferents to the MPOA from Systems Mediating Reward, Emotion, Attention and Memory

Neurons projecting into the MPOA are involved in many of the other behavioral changes described above, including changes in mothers' affect [AMY orbitofrontal, prefrontal (mPFC) and anterior cingulate cortices (ACC)], sensitivity to stimulus salience [(AMY) and to reward striatum/nucleus accumbens (NAC)] as well as attention (NAC, mPFC), and memory (NAC, mPFC). Some of these brain sites also contain hormone receptors (AMY, mPFC) and may be the sites where the periparturitional hormones act to change behavior at the time of parturition (Numan et al., 2006). The relatively complicated neuroanatomy of maternal behavior is based predominantly on work with rats, voles, sheep, and primates (Bridges, 2008; Numan et al., 2006). Taken together, these cross-species studies indicate a striking similarity in the neuroanatomy that underlies mothering.

Work on neural bases of maternal behavior in humans is derived primarily from approximately ten fMRI studies where mothers, nonmothers, and sometimes fathers are presented with either pictures of their own infants or same-aged unfamiliar infants (Bartels & Zeki, 2004; Leibenluft et al., 2004; Nitschke et al., 2004), recorded infant cries (Lorberbaum et al., 2002; Seifritz et al., 2003), or videotapes of infants (Ranote et al., 2004). All studies demonstrate that many of the same hypothalamic, limbic, and cortical sites important for emotional or social (face) processing or for regulation of maternal behavior in other mammals are implicated in response to infant stimuli. Although promising, these fMRI studies are still few in number, often with small sample sizes and great variation in methodology, including age of infant/child tested, use of own vs. other infant/child as experimental stimuli, use of control stimuli, and stimulus matching-standardization procedures.

We have been investigating the neural response to positive and negative infant faces in non-PPD mothers at approximately 3 months postpartum (see Barrett et al., 2010). Analyses of face ratings in our current fMRI study (data from 18/23 moms) revealed that in response to own compared to other positive infant faces, mothers reported feeling significantly more alert, calm, delighted and interested as well as experiencing a greater "need to respond." Interestingly, no significant differences were found for the negative faces. We have also found that, compared with viewing other positive infant faces, viewing own positive infant faces was associated with increased brain activation in the anterior cingulate cortex and regions of the medial prefrontal cortex (PFC). Our behavioral and neuroanatomical results suggest that viewing own positive infant faces was more salient for mothers and resulted in greater activity in reward/emotion and possibly, mothering-related brain regions.

Neurochemistry of Maternal Behavior

The importance of the MPOA, NAC, and mPFC in the expression of maternal behavior, pup reward, emotion, and attention points to the importance of a number of neurotransmitter systems that promote communication among these sites and that are important for the motivation and expression of maternal behavior. Although there are a number of relevant neuropeptides and neurotransmitters (serotonin, dopamine, glutamate, GABA, oxytocin, etc.), here we discuss one primary one on which we have worked extensively. This is the dopamine system.

Dopamine is a neurotransmitter that is synthesized in the VTA and is released through projections into the dorsal striatum (nigrostriatal system), the ventral striatum or NAC and AMY (mesolimbic dopamine system), or the cingulate cortex and medial and orbitofrontal prefrontal cortices (mesocortical dopamine systems). The systems of most interest in the present context are the mesolimbic and mesocortical systems, which function in the mediation of reward, stimulus salience, and attention (Berridge & Robinson, 1998). In terms of dopaminergic effects on maternal behavior, there is now substantial literature showing that dopamine receptors in the NAC are activated by pups; systemically administered DA receptor antagonists disrupt pup approach and retrieval in mother rats (Hansen et al., 1985; Li, Budin, Fleming, & Kapur, 2005; Li, Davidson, Budin, Kapur, & Fleming, 2004; Numan et al., 2005; Parada, King, Li, & Fleming, 2008) and when infused directly into the NAC, they block both retrieval responses (Li & Fleming, 2003a, 2003b; Numan et al., 2005; Stern & Keer, 1999) and consolidation of experiences with the offspring acquired by the mother postpartum (Li & Fleming, 2003a, 2003b). Conversely, infusion of DA receptor (DRD1) agonists into the NAC enhances maternal behavior (Numan et al., 2005).

In a follow-up series of studies in our laboratory, Afonso and colleagues (Afonso, Grella, Chatterjee, & Fleming, 2008; Afonso, King, Chatterjee, & Fleming, 2009) have explored the pattern of dopamine release within the NAC in response to pups and food in new recently parturient mothers, in females that are not postpartum but are maternally experienced, in virgin females, in virgin females administered parturitional hormones, and in females that were reared without their own mothers. New mothers show a robust sustained dopamine response to pups whereas virgin nonmothers do not; both show an acute response to food. Hormonal experience contributes to this mother effect since if virgins are administered the hormones by means of silastic capsules and are presented with pups, they too show a robust dopamine response to pups, even if they are not yet maternally interactive with them (Afonso et al., 2009). However, although hormones augment dopamine responsiveness they are not necessary to the dopamine response, since multiparous animals that are not postpartum, but are cycling, when given pups, also show elevated dopamine in response to pups (Afonso et al., 2008). In this case, however, the dopamine response is more acute and less sustained.

The additive effects of experiences being maternal has also been demonstrated, where multiparous animals reinduced to be maternal through sensitization or continuous exposure to pups show a greater dopamine response to pups than do multiparous animals not recently exposed to pups; both show higher DA responses than do virgin animals induced to be maternal through pup exposure (Afonso et al., 2008). However, all maternal groups have higher extracellular DA levels than do inexperienced virgins. Although on first glance the results appear somewhat complicated, if one equates dopamine release in this context with reward (and that is, of course, a disputable assumption!), then these studies suggest that both the hormones associated with parturition and prior experiences interacting with pups confer on the pups reinforcing properties, and animals experience pups as rewarding stimuli. If one were to prioritize experiences in terms of the rewarding value of pups (using DA here as that measure), it appears that effects are additive: pups are most rewarding to the female who has been exposed to both hormones and experience, followed by experience alone or by hormones alone. However, if mothers are raised without mothers but on an artificial feeding regimen, their later maternal behavior is disrupted as is their preference for pup cues. Moreover, in this situation DA is still released in response to pups but to a considerably reduced extent (Afonso, Burton, Nabakov, & Flerming, in preparation).

Maternal Genetics

Animal models clearly provide evidence for biological and neuroendocrine substrates behind the regulation of maternal behavior. A logical question is whether these substrates and subsequent behaviors have a genetic component. In mice, knockouts in genes relating to endocrine function (oxytocin, CRF – e.g., Gammie, Bethea, & Stevenson, 2007; Pedersen, Vadlamudi, Boccia, & Amico, 2006), as well as strains with disrupted serotonergic signaling (Lerch-Haner, Frierson, Crawford, Beck, & Deneris, 2008), show disruptions in maternal behavior. Using microarrays to determine the pattern of gene expression during the exhibition of maternal behavior, we have found that many categories of genes are expressed at parturition. These include genes associated with general metabolism, brain plasticity, steroid hormones, multiple enzyme systems, and selected neurotransmitters. However, of particular interest in the present context are the dopamine and serotonin genes as well as genes associated with endocrine changes of parturition. Preliminary analyses indicate that within the medial preoptic area (MPOA), a number of genes for dopamine receptors show differential expression between virgin and postpartum animals and between groups exposed to pups and those not exposed (Kent et al., in preparation). Using gene expression microarrays to screen for transcripts of a variety of dopamine-related genes, Akbari et al. (in preparation) found that in comparison to non pup-exposed groups, postpartum and virgin maternal animals showed a greater expression of some of the dopamine receptors and the dopamine transporter (DAT) gene. Expression levels for some of these dopamine-related genes were also correlated with hedonic behaviors, especially between DRD4 and sucrose intake and pup retrieval.

In another program of research on rats where we are exploring single neucleotide polymorphisms (SNPs) in selected candidate genes, we have found that at least one dopamine gene, the dopamine 2 receptor (*DRD2*) gene is polymorphic (with three variants or "triallelic") at a particular locus on the gene. Moreover, we are finding that the density of dopamine receptors in the NAC is affected by one particular variant of the *DRD2* gene (Belay et al., 2010) and an interaction is occurring between this gene and early environment in the density of D2 receptor binding in the accumbens region. Animals with one of the *DRD2* genotypes, if raised in a deprived environment, show lower dopamine receptor density than those raised in a normal environment. Environment has no impact on receptor density in the NAC in animals carrying the alternate genotype (Lovic et al., 2010). Whether these gene by environment interactive effects on dopamine physiology translate into effects specifically on maternal reward, hedonics, and mothering in the rat, we do not yet know.

However, thanks to advances made by the Human Genome Project, we are beginning to understand *some* of the genetics that underlie *some* of the psychological mediators or modulators of mothering. That some aspects of maternal behavior (e.g., warmth, positivity, physical affection, and control) are heritable was first indicated by twin studies (e.g., Harlaar et al., 2008; Neiderhiser et al., 2004). Recent molecular genetic work examining the dopamine, serotonin, and oxytocin systems also suggests that maternal genotype may predict maternal behaviors. For example, variation in the dopamine transporter (*DAT1*) gene is associated with differences in the frequency of maternal verbal commands (Lee et al., 2008), whereas catechol-*O*-methyltransferase (*COMT*) and DA receptor 4 (*DRD4*) alleles associated with less efficient transmission predict decreased maternal sensitivity in mothers with high levels of self-reported daily hassles (van Ijzendoorn, Bakermans-Kranenburg, & Mesman, 2008). Also, mothers with less efficient alleles in the serotonin transporter (*5HTT*) and oxytocin receptor (*OXTR*) genes are less sensitive in their interactions with their infants (Bakermans-Kranenburg & van Ijzendoorn, 2008).

A multi-systems approach to mothering can partially illuminate these findings, as well as target additional candidate genes by considering systems involved in maternal affect, attention, and cognitive function, all of which are involved in mothering.

Genetics and Maternal Affect

Low levels of serotonin and dopamine are indirectly linked with depression (Ruhe, Mason, & Schene, 2007), and variants in the *5HTT*, *COMT*, and monoamine-oxidase A (*MAOA*) genes appear to be particularly important predictors of depression risk. One of the most widely known gene by environment (G × E) effects is the interaction between stress – particularly early adversity (Brown & Harris, 2008) – and the S-allele of the *5HTT* promoter polymorphism (*5HTTLPR*), which is predictive of greater depressive symptoms (Caspi et al., 2003). Our findings do not show the same interactive effects on maternal behavior, but they do show a main independent effect of *5HTTLPR* genotype on maternal sensitivity and the frequency with which mothers look away from their infants during an interaction at 6 months postpartum (Mileva-Seitz et al., in preparation) (Fig. 1.4).

Genetics and Maternal Attention

As indicated above, there is evidence that attentional mechanisms in humans are central to maternal sensitivity (Gonzalez, Steiner, & Fleming, in preparation), and the logical question which is yet to be addressed is whether genetic predictors of human attentional characteristics are also associated with differences in maternal sensitivity.

The DA system helps regulate executive functions and attention, but molecular genetic studies have focused primarily on disorders like attention deficit/hyperactivity disorder (ADHD) and much less on normal variation of dopamine function in nonclinical adult populations. For example, the *DRD4* ExonIII 7-repeat polymorphism is an established predictor of ADHD in children, and it is associated with brain morphological differences in ADHD adults (Monuteaux et al., 2008). Polymorphisms in the dopamine transporter (*DAT1*) and *COMT* genes are associated with differences in cognitive function, as well as prefrontal activation (e.g., Caldu et al., 2007). Thus, genetic differences that predict cognitive and attentional differences might also be associated with maternal behavior differences.

In adults, the *5HTTPR* polymorphism also interacts with adverse life events on ADHD severity (Muller et al., 2008). It is not clear if these polymorphisms are associated with attention or executive function in nonclinical populations, and this has never been assessed in mothers.

Genetics and Hedonics/Reward

New mothers develop an attraction to infant cues and these become rewarding. It is well established from animal literature that the dopamine system is involved with regulating maternal hedonics and maternal behavior, and that dopamine transmission outside of a normal range is associated with deficits in the initiation and consolidation of maternal behavior (Numan et al., 2005, 2006; Parada et al., 2008). The dopamine system is an integral component of reward processing, but most of the molecular genetics studies have examined genetic predictors of neuropsychopathologies in the reward system, including impulsivity, addiction, and gambling. In a study of genetic variation on nonpathological reward system function, Dreher, Kohn, Kolachana, Weinberger, and Berman (2009) found that

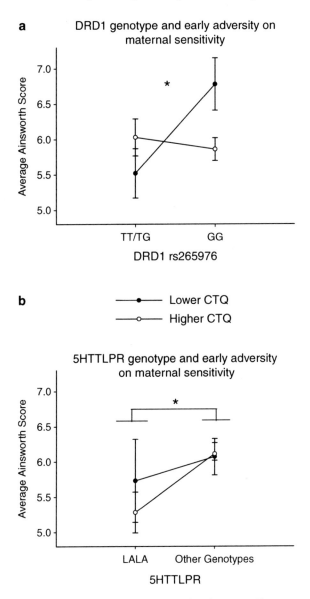

Fig. 1.4 DRD1 (rs265967) and 5HTTLPR genotype and environment effects on average maternal sensitivity score (Ainsworth Maternal Sensitivity Scales, Ainsworth 1974), assessed during a 30-minute mother-infant interaction at 6 months postpartum. For this and subsequent figure, the environmental variable is a retrospective report of early childhood neglect and abuse, as assessed by the Childhood Trauma Questionnaire (CTQ), and dichotomized using a 25th percentile cut-off. "Lower CTQ" sample represents mothers under the 25th percentile, or having low reported levels of early abuse and neglect. (**a**) DRD1 genotype interacts with early adversity to predict maternal sensitivity; (**b**) 5HTTLPR genotype alone predicts differences in maternal sensitivity, without any significant G × E effects. *$p < 0.05$

polymorphisms in two DA-system genes, *DAT1* and *COMT*, were associated with interindividual differences in activation of brain regions involved in reward processing and anticipation, including the ventral striatum and PFC.

Genetics and Hormones

There is evidence that maternal hedonics and sensitivity is related to both cortisol (positively in the early postpartum period; see Corter & Fleming, 1990, 2002; Fleming et al., 1987; Fleming, Steiner, et al., 1997) and depression (Fleming, Steiner, & Gonzalez, in preparation). Predictably, depressed persons have higher cortisol (Gillespie & Nemeroff, 2005). Serotonin system gene polymorphisms (especially *5HTTLPR*) moderate the role of stress in the development of depression. One such interaction might be through the role of the polymorphism val/met (*MAOA* VNTR) in HPA-axis reactivity to psychological and endocrine challenges (Gotlib, Joormann, Minor, & Hallmayer, 2008; Jabbi, Korf, Ormel, Kema, & den Boer, 2008). Another study reports that *5HTTLPR* is associated with elevated waking cortisol in girls as young as 9 years of age (Chen, Joormann, Hallmayer, & Gotlib, 2009). If this polymorphism is associated with life-long cortisol profiles, then it might also be important for maternal behavior, in both depressed and nondepressed mothers. It is unclear if genetic variation associated with these underlying differences in mood and endocrine profile is associated with maternal behavior in a predictable way.

We are currently investigating genetic variation in dopamine (DA) and serotonin (5HT) genes in new mothers, as part of a larger study on maternal adversity, vulnerability, and neurodevelopment (MAVAN). The study follows a longitudinal sample of 250 women, recruited at pregnancy and followed until at least 4 years postpartum. We have targeted several DA candidate genes for our association analyses, and preliminary findings indicate that there are some gene–environment effects on the outcome of maternal sensitivity, as measured by the Ainsworth Maternal Sensitivity Scales (Ainsworth, Bell, & Stayton, 1971; Ainsworth et al., 1974) (Fig. 1.4a). Specifically, a DA receptor 1 (*DRD1*) polymorphism, rs265976, appears to interact with early life adversity, as measured by the Childhood Trauma Questionnaire (CTQ; Bernstein et al., 1994, 2003) to predict level of maternal sensitivity. Mothers who are homozygous for the "G" allele at this locus of *DRD1* and who have had a low level of early adversity are more sensitive to their infants during a 30-min mother–infant interaction at 6 months postpartum (Fig. 1.4a). This polymorphism is part of a haplotype (combination of alleles at multiple loci which are usually transferred together) containing three other polymorphisms along the *DRD1* gene, and we are continuing our analysis to determine if there are similar associations between haplotypes and maternal behavior that we are seeing with the single polymorphism.

Although the DRD1 receptor is widespread in the human brain, it appears to be particularly abundant in the PFC, striatum, and NAC (Jackson & Westlind-Danielsson, 1994; Missale, Nash, Robinson, Jaber, & Caron, 1998), regions which we know are involved in maternal behavior regulation. In addition, in rat mothers, DRD1 – along with DRD2 – receptors appear to be involved in maternal memory (Parada et al., 2008), and disruptions by antagonists or agonists in the DA system which result in abnormal levels of DA in the maternal circuit also result in disrupted maternal behavior (e.g., Byrnes, Rigero, & Bridges, 2002; Hansen, Harthon, Wallin, Lofberg, & Svensson, 1991; Numan et al., 2006).

Within the serotonin system, which is involved in social behaviors and mood, we began with the *5HTT* gene, and asked whether variation in this gene might be associated with differences in maternal behavior. Serotonergic neurons extend from the raphe nucleus of the brain stem into many regions of the brain including the NAC and reward systems. 5HTT has a role in the termination of serotonergic signaling. The *5HTTLPR* polymorphism is one of the major polymorphisms on this gene, and it has received much attention for its putative role in the etiology of depression (e.g., Caspi et al., 2003; Risch et al., 2009). The "short" (S) allele at this locus is associated with lower expression of 5HTT mRNA in vitro (Hu et al., 2006), as well as lower 5HTT binding potential in certain human brain regions (Praschak-Rieder et al., 2007). In this way it may serve as an indicator of 5HT turnover, which has in turn been associated with difference in levels of social aggression in humans (e.g., Siever, 2008).

In rhesus macaques, an analogous polymorphism (rh5HTTLPR) has been linked with differences in 5HT metabolites in the cerebrospinal fluid (Cleveland, Westergaard, Trenkle, & Higley, 2004), which further underlines its role in serotonergic turnover. Interestingly, the relationship between this polymorphism and adult 5HT metabolite levels appears to be mediated by early environment; the S allele predicts lower levels of metabolites in peer-raised (early adversity) but not in mother-raised monkeys (see Suomi, 2006). Environment alone also appears to predict differences in serotonergic transmission: peer-raised monkeys have significantly lower 5HTT binding potential (Ichise et al., 2006). Additional studies suggest that monkey maternal behavior may be related to levels of 5HT metabolites, although the direction of this relationship seems unclear (Cleveland et al., 2004; Maestripieri et al., 2006). Nonetheless, these studies highlight the importance of considering both genotype and environment in assessments of subsequent behavior.

Our findings suggest that there are gene-independent effects of *5HTTLPR* genotype on maternal sensitivity; mothers who carry two copies of the LA allele (the A variant of the long "L" allele) are significantly less sensitive to their 6-month-old infants during a free-play interaction (Fig. 1.4b). These mothers also look away from their infants far more frequently (Fig. 1.5); looking away is also correlated negatively with sensitivity. In addition, there are effects of the early environment (childhood abuse, neglect, parental bonding, etc.) on aspects of maternal behavior including tactile interaction. Finally, we are finding that there are interactions between the 5HTTLPR genotype and early adversity on maternal vocal interaction with the infant.

By considering genetic factors in analyses that previously relied on other independent variables, we might be able to find effects we have previously discounted.

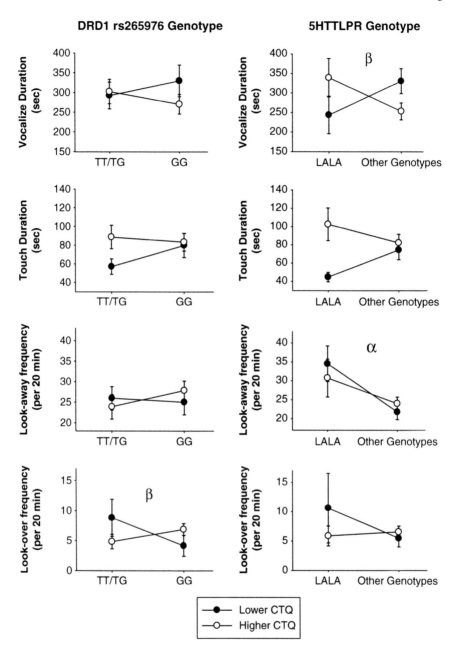

Fig. 1.5 DRD1 (rs265976) and 5HTTLPR genotype and environment effects on maternal behavior during a 20-min segment of recorded mother-infant interaction at 6 months postpartum. 5HTTLPR genotype alone predicts frequency of maternal look-away from baby; α = genotype-only effect; β = G × E interaction; $p < 0.05$

This is particularly true where G × E effects might explain differences in maternal behavior that were not obvious by examining simply environmental effects. For example, as in our case, early adversity may predict that mothers are less vocal when interacting with their infants, but only if the mothers are of a particular genotype. If they have the alternate genotype, early adversity might actually predict increased vocalization and when considered as a function of environment alone, the effect seems to disappear (Fig. 1.4).

Conclusion

Although maternal behavior is crucial for humans and most mammalian species, its onset, maintenance, and variation across and within species is complex and not fully understood. Particularly in humans, this complexity cannot be explained easily and unimodally. Certainly, hormonal, experiential, environmental, sociocultural, and personality factors are involved. Add to that genetic effects, interactions between genes and environment, and perhaps epigenetic modulation – a facet we have not addressed here – and it becomes clear that we are only beginning to understand the underpinnings of this fundamental aspect to mammalian survival.

We have a number of messages we hope to convey in this chapter. First and foremost, we believe that it is helpful to explore cross-species similarities and differences in order at the least to ask biologically relevant questions concerning the etiology of mothering in humans. Second, the analysis of mothering requires an understanding of the regulation of multiple behavioral systems including aspects of perception, emotion, attention, memory, and sensory-motor control. The level of functioning of these systems and their biases impact on mothers' motivation to mother and her success in mothering. Since we know, for example, that attentional, motivational, and hormonal/physiological neurocognitive components have different and perhaps competing influences on maternal behavior, then we might do better to devise ways of assessing components of observed maternal behavior that are related to each of these underlying components in turn. A videotaped mother–infant interaction coded with an attentional framework in mind might look quite different from one coded with a motivation-related coding schema. Finally, to discuss mothering in humans within a psychobiological context, as we have done here, departs from the usual way of looking at human mothering. By invoking biology, we are in no way eschewing freedom of choice and women's right to decide about their mothering. It does not mean that somehow mothering is "determined" by biology. Understanding behavior in terms of its psychobiology in fact *permits* us to understand what factors may be brought into play when choices *are* made and when infants are born. The new work on genetics and on gene by environmental interactions is a case in point.

Here we have emphasized the similarities between rat and human mothers, in terms of many of the putative proximal regulatory mechanisms. We find that humans, like rats, experience reliable hormonal changes with parturition, which are similar across species. We find that humans, like rats, become attentive to infant cues and become attracted to them with a minimum of interaction with the young. In rats, these changes in hedonic responses are produced by hormones; in humans, they are associated with hormones, albeit different ones! We find in both rats and humans that the quality of mothering is associated with functioning of other behavioral systems. In both, mothering is associated with mothers' affective or mood state; by mothers' attention and other measures of executive function; and by mothers' ability to acquire and retain information, that is, by their plasticity. That these relations are mediated by the same mechanisms in rat and human mothers, in their entirety, is unlikely. That they share some mechanisms in common is likely. We have delineated the neuroanatomy and neurochemistry of mothering in rats, with an emphasis on the mesolimbic and dopamine systems. Recent genetic and fMRI studies suggest a similarity between systems that are activated in rat and human mothers by their offspring. Clearly in humans, other systems relating to earlier experiences, planfulness, executive functions, theory of mind, and cognitions also come into play. The study of many of these very human characteristics and their neurobiology in relation to human mothering is still in its infancy and will provide grist for the mill for many generations of students.

Among the areas that will prove productive are studies relating genetics to epigenetics, using animal models. While there is an emerging literature on epigenetic modulation of maternal behavior as a function of early experience in rats (e.g., Champagne et al., 2008), relating the animal's genotype and environmental influences to the molecular mechanisms regulating activation of the "maternal" genes has not been done. We would also like to see more studies combining fMRI and other more refined measures of brain activation, in an attempt to reveal the functional neuroanatomy and physiology of human maternal behavior. Finally, there is a huge need to apply research about the role of early adversity and early experiences – and the mediating role of physiological or psychological mechanisms – on later mothering, particularly in high-risk populations, including teenaged mothers or depressed and schizophrenic populations. Related to this is the need to assess rehabilitation and remediation programs for problematic mothering, perhaps targeting problems that might be population-specific. For example, depressed mothers might show patterns of mothering deficits different from those in teenaged nondepressed mothers, and universal remediation approaches might not be appropriate.

References

Afonso, V. M., Burton, C., Nabakov, & Flerming, A. S. (in preparation). Effect of early isolation rearing on dopamine releases to pup- and food-stimuli.
Afonso, V. M., Grella, S. L., Chatterjee, D., & Fleming, A. S. (2008). Previous maternal experience affects accumbal dopaminergic responses to pup-stimuli. *Brain Research, 1198*, 115–123.
Afonso, V. M., King, S., Chatterjee, D., & Fleming, A. S. (2009). Hormones that increase maternal responsiveness affect accumbal dopaminergic responses to pup- and food-stimuli in the female rat. *Hormones and Behavior, 56*(1), 11–23.

Ainsworth, M., Bell, S., & Stayton, D. (1971). Individual differences in strange situations behavior of one year olds. In H. Schaffer (Ed.), *The origins of human social relations.* New York: Academic.

Ainsworth, M., Bell, S., & Stayton, D. (1974). Infant-mother attachment and social development: socialization of reciprocal responsiveness to signals. In M. Richards (Ed.), *The integration of a child into a social world* (pp. 99–135). Cambridge: Cambridge University Press.

Akbari, E., Shams, S., Westwood, T., Kent, C., Sokolowski, M., & Fleming, A. S. (2010). Effects of pup stimulation on gene expression in the MPOA and amygdala of postpartum & virgin females: A microarray study. Manuscript in preparation.

Bakermans-Kranenburg, M. J., & van Ijzendoorn, M. H. (2008). Oxytocin receptor (OXTR) and serotonin transporter (5-HTT) genes associated with observed parenting. *Social Cognitive and Affective Neuroscience, 3*(2), 128–134.

Barrett, J., Wonch, K. E., Hall, G., Gonzalez, A., Ali, N., Steiner, M., et al. (2010). Consistency of early care in family of origin influences brain response to infant stimuli in reward & affect brain regions. Manuscript submitted for publication.

Bartels, A., & Zeki, S. (2004). The neural correlates of maternal and romantic love. *NeuroImage, 21*(3), 1155–1166.

Beck, C. T. (2002). Postpartum depression: A metasynthesis. *Qualitative Health Research, 12*(4), 453.

Belay, H., Burton, C., Lovic, L., Meaney, M., Sokolowski, M., & Fleming, A. S. (2010). Effects of dopamine receptor gene polymorphisms and of early isolation rearing on HPA axis and behavior in rats. Manuscript submitted for publication.

Bernstein, D., Fink, L., Handelsman, L., Foote, J., Lovejoy, M., Wenzel, K., et al. (1994). Initial reliability and validity of a new retrospective measure of child abuse and neglect. *American Journal of Psychiatry, 151*(8), 1132.

Bernstein, D. P., Stein, J. A., Newcomb, M. D., Walker, E., Pogge, D., Ahluvalia, T., et al. (2003). Development and validation of a brief screening version of the childhood trauma questionnaire. *Child Abuse & Neglect, 27*(2), 169–190.

Berridge, K. C., & Robinson, T. E. (1998). What is the role of dopamine in reward: Hedonic impact, reward learning, or incentive salience? *Brain Research Reviews, 28,* 309–369.

Bornstein, M. H. (Ed.). (2002). *Handbook of parenting: Biology and ecology of parenting.* Hillsdale: Lawrence Erlbaum Associates.

Brazelton, T. B. (1972). Implications of infant development among the Mayan Indians of Mexico. *Human Development, 15*(2), 90–111.

Bridges, R. S. (1975). Long-term effects of pregnancy and parturition upon maternal responsiveness in the rat. *Physiology & Behavior, 14*(3), 245–249.

Bridges, R. S. (1990). Endocrine regulation of parental behavior in rodents. In N. A. Krasnegor & R. S. Bridges (Eds.), *Mammalian parenting: Biochemical, neurobiological, and behavioral determinants* (pp. 93–117). New York: Oxford University Press.

Bridges, R. S. (Ed.). (2008). *Neurobiology of the parental brain.* San Diego: Academic.

Bright, D. A. (1994). Postpartum mental disorders. *American Family Physician, 50*(3), 595–598.

Brown, G. W., & Harris, T. O. (2008). Depression and the serotonin transporter 5-HTTLPR polymorphism: A review and a hypothesis concerning gene-environment interaction. *Journal of Affective Disorders, 111*(1), 1–12.

Butterfield, P., Emde, R., Svejda, M., & Naiman, S. (1982). Silver nitrate and the eyes of the newborn: Effects on parental responsiveness during infant social interaction. In R. Emde & R. Harmon (Eds.), *The development of attachment and affiliative systems* (pp. 95–108). New York: Plenum.

Byrnes, E. M., Rigero, B. A., & Bridges, R. S. (2002). Dopamine antagonists during parturition disrupt maternal care and the retention of maternal behavior in rats. *Pharmacology, Biochemistry, and Behavior, 73,* 869–875.

Bystrova, K., Ivanova, V., Edhborg, M., Matthiesen, A. S., Ransjo-Arvidson, A. B., Mukhamedrakhimov, R., et al. (2009). Early contact versus separation: Effects on mother-infant interaction one year later. *Birth, 36*(2), 97–109.

Cacioppo, J. T., Berntson, G. G., Malarkey, W. B., Kiecolt-Glaser, J. K., Sheridan, J. F., Poehlmann, K. M., et al. (1998). Autonomic, neuroendocrine, and immune responses to psychological stress: The reactivity hypothesis. *Annals of the New York Academy of Sciences, 840,* 664–673.

Caldu, X., Vendrell, P., Bartres-Faz, D., Clemente, I., Bargallo, N., Jurado, M. A., et al. (2007). Impact of the COMT Val108/158 met and DAT genotypes on prefrontal function in healthy subjects. *NeuroImage, 37*(4), 1437–1444.

Caspi, A., Sugden, K., Moffitt, T. E., Taylor, A., Craig, I. W., Harrington, H., et al. (2003). Influence of life stress on depression: Moderation by a polymorphism in the 5-HTT gene. *Science, 301*(5631), 386–389.

Champagne, D. L., Bagot, R. C., van Hasselt, F., Ramakers, G., Meaney, M. J., de Kloet, E. R., et al. (2008). Maternal care and hippocampal plasticity: Evidence for experience-dependent structural plasticity, altered synaptic functioning, and differential responsiveness to glucocorticoids and stress. *Journal of Neuroscience, 28*, 6037–6045.

Chen, M. C., Joormann, J., Hallmayer, J., & Gotlib, I. H. (2009). Serotonin transporter polymorphism predicts waking cortisol in young girls. *Psychoneuroendocrinology, 34*(5), 681–686.

Chico, E., Ali, N., Eaton, H., Gonzalez, A., & Fleming, A. S. (in preparation). Executive function and mothering in teenage mothers.

Cleveland, A., Westergaard, G. C., Trenkle, M. K., & Higley, J. D. (2004). Physiological predictors of reproductive outcome and mother-infant behaviors in captive rhesus macaque females (macaca mulatta). *Neuropsychopharmacology: Official Publication of the American College of Neuropsychopharmacology, 29*(5), 901–910.

Cohn, J. F., Campbell, S. B., Matias, R., & Hopkins, J. (1990). Face-to-face interactions of postpartum depressed and nondepressed mother-infant pairs at 2 months. *Developmental Psychology, 26*(1), 15–23.

Cooper, P., & Murray, L. (1995). Course and recurrence of postnatal depression. evidence for the specificity of the diagnostic concept. *The British Journal of Psychiatry, 166*(2), 191–195.

Corter, C. M., & Fleming, A. S. (1990). Maternal responsiveness in humans: Emotional, cognitive, and biological factors. *Advances in the Study of Behavior, 19*, 83–136.

Corter, C. M., & Fleming, A. S. (2002). Psychobiology of maternal behavior in human beings. In M. H. Bornstein (Ed.), *Handbook of parenting: Biology and ecology of parenting* (pp. 141–182). Hillsdale: Lawrence Erlbaum Associates.

Cox, J. L., Connor, Y., & Kendell, R. E. (1982). Prospective study of the psychiatric disorders of childbirth. *The British Journal of Psychiatry: The Journal of Mental Science, 140*, 111–117.

Cox, J. L., Murray, D., & Chapman, G. (1993). A controlled study of the onset, duration and prevalence of postnatal depression. *The British Journal of Psychiatry: The Journal of Mental Science, 163*, 27–31.

Dettling, A. C., Gunnar, M. R., & Donzella, B. (1999). Cortisol levels of young children in full-day childcare centers: Relations with age and temperament. *Psychoneuroendocrinology, 24*(5), 519–536.

Dreher, J. C., Kohn, P., Kolachana, B., Weinberger, D. R., & Berman, K. F. (2009). Variation in dopamine genes influences responsivity of the human reward system. *Proceedings of the National Academy of Sciences of the United States of America, 106*(2), 617–622.

Farrell, W. J., & Alberts, J. R. (2002). Maternal responsiveness to infant Norway rat (rattus norvegicus) ultrasonic vocalizations during the maternal behavior cycle and after steroid and experiential induction regimens. *Journal of Comparative Psychology, 116*(3), 286–296.

Field, T., Healy, B. T., Goldstein, S., & Guthertz, M. (1990). Behavior-state matching and synchrony in mother-infant interactions of nondepressed versus depressed dyads. *Developmental Psychology, 26*(1), 7–14.

Fleming, A. S., Cheung, U., Myhal, N., & Kessler, Z. (1989). Effects of maternal hormones on "timidity" and attraction to pup-related odors in female rats. *Physiology & Behavior, 46*(3), 449–453.

Fleming, A. S., Corter, C., Franks, P., Surbey, M., Schneider, B., & Steiner, M. (1993). Postpartum factors related to mother's attraction to newborn infant odors. *Developmental Psychobiology, 26*(2), 115–132.

Fleming, A. S., Gavarth, K., & Sarker, J. (1992). Effects of transections to the vomeronasal nerves or to the main olfactory bulbs on the initiation and long-term retention of maternal behavior in primiparous rats. *Behavioral and Neural Biology, 57*(3), 177–188.

Fleming, A. S., & Gonzalez, A. (2009). Neurobiology of human maternal care. In P. T. Ellison & P. B. Gray (Eds.), *Endocrinology of social relationships* (pp. 294–318). Cambridge: Harvard University Press.

Fleming, A. S., Gonzalez, A., Afonso, V. M., & Lovic, V. (2008). Plasticity in the maternal neural circuit: experience, dopamine, and mothering. In R. S. Bridges (Ed.), *Neurobiology of the parental brain* (pp. 519–536). New York: Academic.

Fleming, A. S., & Li, M. (2002). Psychobiology of maternal behavior and its early determinants in nonhuman animals. In M. H. Bornstein (Ed.), *Handbook of parenting: Biology and ecology of parenting* (Vol. 2, pp. 141–182). Hillsdale: Lawrence Erlbaum Associates.

Fleming, A. S., & Luebke, C. (1981). Timidity prevents the virgin female rat from being a good mother: Emotionality differences between nulliparous and parturient females. *Physiology & Behavior, 27*(5), 863–868.

Fleming, A. S., O'Day, D. & Kraemer, G. (1999). Neurobiology of Mother-infant Interactions: Experience and central nervous system plasticity across development. *Neuroscience and Biobehavioral Reviews, 23*(5), 673–685.

Fleming, A. S., Ruble, D., Krieger, H., & Wong, P. Y. (1997). Hormonal and experiential correlates of maternal responsiveness during pregnancy and the puerperium in human mothers. *Hormones and Behavior, 31*(2), 145–158.

Fleming, A. S., Ruble, D. N., Flett, G. L., & Shaul, D. L. (1988). Postpartum adjustment in first-time mothers: Relations between mood, maternal attitudes, and mother–infant interactions. *Developmental Psychology, 24*(1), 71–81.

Fleming, A. S., Steiner, M., & Anderson, V. (1987). Hormonal and attitudinal correlates of maternal behavior during the early postpartum period in first-time mothers. *Journal of Reproductive and Infant Psychology, 5*(4), 193–205.

Fleming, A. S., Steiner, M., & Corter, C. (1997). Cortisol, hedonics, and maternal responsiveness in human mothers. *Hormones and Behavior, 32*(2), 85–98.

Fleming, A. S., Vaccarino, F., & Luebke, C. (1980). Amygdaloid inhibition of maternal behavior in the nulliparous female rat. *Physiology & Behavior, 25*(5), 731–743.

Fleming, A., Vaccarino, F., Tambosso, L., & Chee, P. (1979). Vomeronasal and olfactory system modulation of maternal behavior in the rat. *Science, 203*(4378), 372–374.

Gammie, S. C., Bethea, E. D., & Stevenson, S. A. (2007). Altered maternal profiles in corticotrophin-releasing factor receptor 1 deficient mice. *BMC Neuroscience, 8*, 17.

Gillespie, C., & Nemeroff, C. (2005). Early life stress and depression. *Current Psychiatry, 4*(10), 15–30.

Gold, L. H. (2002). Postpartum disorders in primary care: Diagnosis and treatment. *Primary Care, 29*(1), 27–41.

Gonzalez, A., Atkinson, L., & Fleming, A. S. (2009). Attachment and the comparative psychobiology of mothering. In M. D. Haan & M. R. Gunnar (Eds.), *Handbook of developmental social neuroscience* (pp. 225–245). New York: Guilford Press.

Gonzalez, A., Jenkins, J. M., Steiner, M., & Fleming, A. S. (2009). The relation between early life adversity, cortisol awakening response and diurnal salivary cortisol levels in postpartum women. *Psychoneuroendocrinology, 34*(1), 76–86.

Gonzalez, A., Jenkins, J. M., Steiner, M., & Fleming, A. S. (submitted). Neuropsychology and physiology: Intervening variables between maternal early adversity and parenting.

Gotlib, I. H., Joormann, J., Minor, K. L., & Hallmayer, J. (2008). HPA axis reactivity: A mechanism underlying the associations among 5-HTTLPR, stress, and depression. *Biological Psychiatry, 63*(9), 847–851.

Hansen, S., Ferreira, A., & Selart, M. E. (1985). Behavioral similarities between mother rats and benzodiazepine-treated non-maternal animals. *Psychopharmacology, 86*(3), 344–347.

Hansen, S., Harthon, C., Wallin, E., Lofberg, L., & Svensson, K. (1991). The effects of 6-OHDA-induced dopamine depletions in the ventral and dorsal striatum on maternal and sexual behavior in the female rat. *Pharmacology, Biochemistry and Behavior, 39*, 71–77.

Harlaar, N., Santtila, P., Bjorklund, J., Alanko, K., Jern, P., Varjonen, M., et al. (2008). Retrospective reports of parental physical affection and parenting style: A study of Finnish twins. *Journal of Family Psychology: Journal of the Division of Family Psychology of the American Psychological Association (Division 43), 22*(4), 605–613.

Herrera, E., Reissland, N., & Shepherd, J. (2004). Maternal touch and maternal child-directed speech: Effects of depressed mood in the postnatal period. *Journal of Affective Disorders, 81*(1), 29–39.

Hrdy, S. B. (2005). Evolutionary context of human development: the cooperative breeding model. In C. S. Carter & L. Anhert (Eds.), *Attachment and bonding: A new synthesis*. Cambridge: MIT Press.

Hrdy, S. B. (2009). *Mothers and others: The evolutionary origins of mutual understanding*. Cambridge: Harvard University Press.

Hu, X. Z., Lipsky, R. H., Zhu, G., Akhtar, L. A., Taubman, J., Greenberg, B. D., et al. (2006). Serotonin transporter promoter gain-of-function genotypes are linked to obsessive-compulsive disorder. *American Journal of Human Genetics, 78*(5), 815–826.

Ichise, M., Vines, D. C., Gura, T., Anderson, G. M., Suomi, S. J., Higley, J. D., et al. (2006). Effects of early life stress on [11C]DASB positron emission tomography imaging of serotonin transporters in adolescent peer- and mother-reared rhesus monkeys. *The Journal of Neuroscience: The Official Journal of the Society for Neuroscience, 26*(17), 4638–4643.

Insel, T. (1990). Oxytocin and maternal behavior. In N. A. Krasnegor & R. S. Bridges (Eds.), *Mammalian parenting: Biochemical, neurobiological, and behavioral determinants* (pp. 260–280). New York: Oxford University Press.

Jabbi, M., Korf, J., Ormel, J., Kema, I. P., & den Boer, J. A. (2008). Investigating the molecular basis of major depressive disorder etiology: A functional convergent genetic approach. *Annals of the New York Academy of Sciences, 1148*, 42–56.

Jackson, D. M., & Westlind-Danielsson, A. (1994). Dopamine receptors: Molecular biology, biochemistry and behavioral aspects. *Pharmacology & Therapeutics, 64*, 291–370.

Jakubowski, M., & Terkel, J. (1986). Establishment and maintenance of maternal responsiveness in postpartum wistar rats. *Animal Behavior, 34*(1), 256–262.

Kaitz, M., Good, A., Rokem, A. M., & Eidelman, A. I. (1988). Mothers' and fathers' recognition of their newborns' photographs during the postpartum period. *Journal of Developmental and Behavioral Pediatrics, 9*(4), 223–226.

Kaitz, M., Lapidot, P., Bronner, R., & Eidelman, A. I. (1992). Parturient women can recognize their infants by touch. *Developmental Psychology, 28*(1), 35–39.

Kaitz, M., Rokem, A. M., & Eidelman, A. I. (1988). Infants' face-recognition by primiparous and multiparous women. *Perceptual and Motor Skills, 67*(2), 495–502.

Kaitz, M., Good, A., Rokem, A. M., & Eidelman, A. I. (1987). Mothers' recognition of their newborns by olfactory cues. *Developmental Psychobiology, 20*(6), 587–91.

Kirschbaum, C., Wust, S., & Hellhammer, D. (1992). Consistent sex differences in cortisol responses to psychological stress. *Psychosomatic Medicine, 54*(6), 648–657.

Klaus, M., Trause, M., & Kennell, J. (1975). Does human maternal behavior after birth show a characteristic pattern?: Parent-infant interaction. *CIBA Foundation Symposium, 33*, 69–85.

Klaus, M. H., & Kennell, J. H. (1976). *Maternal-infant bonding*. St. Louis: Mosby.

Leavitt, L. A., & Donovan, W. L. (1979). Perceived infant temperament, locus of control, and maternal physiological response to infant gaze. *Journal of Research in Personality, 13*(3), 267–278.

Lee, A., Clancy, S., & Fleming, A. S. (2000). Mother rats bar-press for pups: Effects of lesions of the mpoa and limbic sites on maternal behavior and operant responding for pup-reinforcement. *Behavioral Brain Research, 100*(1–2), 15–31.

Lee, S. S., Chronis-Tuscano, A., Keenan, K., Pelham, W. E., Loney, J., Van Hulle, C. A., et al. (2008). Association of maternal dopamine transporter genotype with negative parenting: Evidence for gene x environment interaction with child disruptive behavior. *Molecular Psychiatry*, in press. Epub ahead of print retrieved November 5, 2009, from http://www.ncbi.nlm.nih.gov/pubmed/18779819.

Leibenluft, E., Gobbini, M. I., Harrison, T., & Haxby, J. V. (2004). Mothers' neural activation in response to pictures of their children and other children. *Biological Psychiatry, 56*(4), 225–232.

Leiderman, P. H., & Leiderman, G. F. (1977). Economic change and infant care in an East African agricultural community. In P. H. Leoderman, S. R. Tulkin, & A. Rosenfeld (Eds.), *Culture and infancy: Variations in the human experience* (pp. 405–438). New York: Academic.

Leifer, M. (1980). *Psychological effects of motherhood: A study of first pregnancy*. New York: Praeger.

Lerch-Haner, J. K., Frierson, D., Crawford, L. K., Beck, S. G., & Deneris, E. S. (2008). Serotonergic transcriptional programming determines maternal behavior and offspring survival. *Nature Neuroscience, 11*(9), 1001–1003.

Levy, F. (2008). Neural substrates involved in the onset of maternal responsiveness and selectivity in sheep. In R. S. Bridges (Ed.), *Neurobiology of the parental brain* (pp. 23–38). New York: Academic.

Li, M., Budin, R., Fleming, A. S., & Kapur, S. (2005). Effects of chronic typical and atypical antipsychotic drug treatment on maternal behavior in rats. *Schizophrenia Research, 75*(2–3), 325–336.

Li, M., Davidson, P., Budin, R., Kapur, S., & Fleming, A. S. (2004). Effects of typical and atypical antipsychotic drugs on maternal behavior in postpartum female rats. *Schizophrenia Research, 70*(1), 69–80.

Li, M., & Fleming, A. S. (2003a). Differential involvement of nucleus accumbens shell and core subregions in maternal memory in postpartum female rats. *Behavioral Neuroscience, 117*(3), 426–445.

Li, M., & Fleming, A. S. (2003b). The nucleus accumbens shell is critical for normal expression of pup-retrieval in postpartum female rats. *Behavioral Brain Research, 145*(1–2), 99–111.

Lorberbaum, J. P., Newman, J. D., Horwitz, A. R., Dubno, J. R., Lydiard, R. B., Hamner, M. B., et al. (2002). A potential role for thalamocingulate circuitry in human maternal behavior. *Biological Psychiatry, 51*(6), 431–445.

Lovejoy, M. C., Graczyk, P. A., O'Hare, E., & Neuman, G. (2000). Maternal depression and parenting behavior: A meta-analytic review. *Clinical Psychology Review, 20*(5), 561–592.

Lovic, V., & Fleming, A. S. (2004). Artificially-reared female rats show reduced prepulse inhibition and deficits in the attentional set shifting task – reversal of effects with maternal-like licking stimulation. *Behavioral Brain Research, 148*(1–2), 209–219.

Lovic, V., Keer, D., Fletcher, P., & Fleming, A. S. (2010). Dissociative effects of early-life maternal separation and social isolation through artificial rearing on different forms of impulsivity. Manuscript submitted for publication.

Maestripieri, D., Higley, J. D., Lindell, S. G., Newman, T. K., McCormack, K., & Sanchez, M. M. (2006). Early maternal rejection affects the development of monoaminergic systems and adult abusive parenting in rhesus macaques. *Behavioral Neuroscience, 120*, 1017–1024.

Magnusson, J. E., & Fleming, A. S. (1995). Rat pups are reinforcing to the maternal rat: Role of sensory cues. *Psychobiology, 23*(1), 69–75.

Malphurs, J. E., Raag, T., Field, T., Pickens, J., & Pelaez-Nogueras, M. (1996). Touch by intrusive and withdrawn mothers with depressive symptoms. *Early Development and Parenting, 5*(2), 111–115.

Mattson, B. J., Williams, S., Rosenblatt, J. S., & Morrell, J. I. (2001). Comparison of two positive reinforcing stimuli: Pups and cocaine throughout the postpartum period. *Behavioral Neuroscience, 115*(3), 683–694.

Mayer, A. D. (1983). The ontogeny of maternal behavior in rodents. In R. W. Elwood (Ed.), *Parental behavior of rodents* (pp. 1–20). Chichester: Wiley.

Mayer, A. D., & Rosenblatt, J. S. (1977). Effects of intranasal zinc sulfate on open field and maternal behavior in female rats. *Physiology & Behavior, 18*(1), 101–109.

McEwen, B. S., De Kloet, E. R., & Rostene, W. (1986). Adrenal steroid receptors and actions in the nervous system. *Physiological Reviews, 66*(4), 1121–1188.

Messer, D. J., & Vietze, P. M. (1984). Timing and transitions in mother's infant gaze. *Infant Behavior & Development, 7*(2), 167–181.

Mileva-Seitz, V. M., Kennedy, J., Atkinson, L., Levitan, R., Sokolowski, M., & Fleming, A. (in preparation). 5HTT genotype associated with maternal behavior in human mothers.

Missale, C., Nash, S. R., Robinson, S. W., Jaber, M., & Caron, M. G. (1998). Dopamine receptors: From structure to function. *Physiological Reviews, 78*(1), 189–225.

Monuteaux, M. C., Seidman, L. J., Faraone, S. V., Makris, N., Spencer, T., Valera, E., et al. (2008). A preliminary study of dopamine D4 receptor genotype and structural brain alterations in adults with ADHD. *American Journal of Medical Genetics. Part B, Neuropsychiatric Genetics: The Official Publication of the International Society of Psychiatric Genetics147B*(8), 1436–1441.

Moore, E. R., Anderson, G. C., & Bergman, N. (2007). Early skin-to-skin contact for mothers and their healthy newborn infants. *Cochrane Database of Systematic Reviews (Online), 3*(3), CD003519.

Morgan, H. D., Fleming, A. S., & Stern, J. M. (1992). Somatosensory control of the onset and retention of maternal responsiveness in primiparous Sprague-dawley rats. *Physiology & Behavior, 51*(3), 549–555.

Morgan, H. D., Watchus, J. A., Milgram, N. W., & Fleming, A. S. (1999). The long lasting effects of electrical simulation of the medial preoptic area and medial amygdala on maternal behavior in female rats. *Behavioral Brain Research, 99*(1), 61–73.

Moss, H. A., & Jones, S. J. (1977). Relations between maternal attitudes and maternal behavior as a function of social class. In P. H. Leiderman, S. R. Tulkin, & A. Rosenfeld (Eds.), *Culture and infancy*. New York: Academic.

Muller, D. J., Mandelli, L., Serretti, A., DeYoung, C. G., De Luca, V., Sicard, T., et al. (2008). Serotonin transporter gene and adverse life events in adult ADHD. *American Journal of Medical Genetics. Part B, Neuropsychiatric Genetics: The Official Publication of the International Society of Psychiatric Genetics, 147B*(8), 1461–1469.

Murray, L., Fiori-Cowley, A., Hooper, R., & Cooper, P. (1996). The impact of postnatal depression and associated adversity on early mother-infant interactions and later infant outcome. *Child Development, 67*(5), 2512–2526.

Neiderhiser, J. M., Reiss, D., Pedersen, N. L., Lichtenstein, P., Spotts, E. L., Hansson, K., et al. (2004). Genetic and environmental influences on mothering of adolescents: A comparison of two samples. *Developmental Psychology, 40*(3), 335–351.

Neumann, I. D., Wigger, A., Liebsch, G., Holsboer, F., & Landgraf, R. (1998). Increased basal activity of the hypothalamo-pituitary-adrenal axis during pregnancy in rats bred for high anxiety-related behavior. *Psychoneuroendocrinology, 23*(5), 449–463.

Nitschke, J. B., Nelson, E. E., Rusch, B. D., Fox, A. S., Oakes, T. R., & Davidson, R. J. (2004). Orbitofrontal cortex tracks positive mood in mothers viewing pictures of their newborn infants. *NeuroImage, 21*(2), 583–592.

Numan, M., Fleming, A. S., & Levy, F. (2006). Maternal behavior. In J. D. Neill (Ed.), *Knobil and Neill's physiology of reproduction* (pp. 1921–1993). San Diego: Elsevier.

Numan, M., & Insel, T. R. (2003). *The neurobiology of parental behavior*. New York: Springer.

Numan, M., Numan, M. J., Pliakou, N., Stolzenberg, D. S., Mullins, O. J., Murphy, J. M., et al. (2005). The effects of D1 or D2 dopamine receptor antagonism in the medial preoptic area, ventral pallidum, or nucleus accumbens on the maternal retrieval response and other aspects of maternal behavior in rats. *Behavioral Neuroscience, 119*(6), 1588–1604.

O'Hara, M. W., Zekoski, E. M., Philipps, L. H., & Wright, E. J. (1990). Controlled prospective study of postpartum mood disorders: Comparison of childbearing and nonchildbearing women. *Journal of Abnormal Psychology, 99*(1), 3–15.

Orpen, B. G., & Fleming, A. S. (1987). Experience with pups sustains maternal responding in postpartum rats. *Physiology & Behavior, 40*(1), 47–54.

Parada, M., King, S., Li, M., & Fleming, A. S. (2008). The roles of accumbal dopamine D1 and D2 receptors in maternal memory in rats. *Behavioral Neuroscience, 122*(2), 368–376.

Pedersen, C. A., Vadlamudi, S. V., Boccia, M. L., & Amico, J. A. (2006). Maternal behavior deficits in nulliparous oxytocin knockout mice. *Genes, Brain, and Behavior, 5*(3), 274–281.

Pederson, D. R., Moran, G., Sitko, C., Campbell, K., Ghesquire, K., & Acton, H. (1990). Maternal sensitivity and the security of infant-mother attachment: A Q-sort study. *Child Development, 61*(6), 1974–1983.

Pereira, M., Seip, K. M., & Morrell, J. I. (2008). Maternal motivation and its neural substrate across the postpartum period. In R. S. Bridges (Ed.), *Neurobiology of the parental brain*. New York: Academic.

Porter, R. H., Cernoch, J. M., & McLaughlin, F. J. (1983). Maternal recognition of neonates through olfactory cues. *Physiology & Behavior, 30*(1), 151–154.

Praschak-Rieder, N., Kennedy, J., Wilson, A. A., Hussey, D., Boovariwala, A., Willeit, M., et al. (2007). Novel 5-HTTLPR allele associates with higher serotonin transporter binding in putamen: A [(11)C] DASB positron emission tomography study. *Biological Psychiatry, 62*(4), 327–331.

Pryce, C. R., Martin, R. D., & Skuse, D. (1995). *Motherhood in human and nonhuman primates: Biosocial determinants.* New York: Karger.

Ranote, S., Elliott, R., Abel, K. M., Mitchell, R., Deakin, J. F., & Appleby, L. (2004). The neural basis of maternal responsiveness to infants: An fMRI study. *Neuroreport, 15*(11), 1825–1829.

Righetti-Veltema, M., Conne-Perreard, E., Bousquet, A., & Manzano, J. (2002). Postpartum depression and mother-infant relationship at 3 months old. *Journal of Affective Disorders, 70*(3), 291–306.

Risch, N., Herrell, R., Lehner, T., Liang, K. Y., Eaves, L., Hoh, J., et al. (2009). Interaction between the serotonin transporter gene (5-HTTLPR), stressful life events, and risk of depression: A meta-analysis. *JAMA: The Journal of the American Medical Association, 301*(23), 2462–2471.

Robson, K. M., & Kumar, R. (1980). Delayed onset of maternal affection after childbirth. *The British Journal of Psychiatry: The Journal of Mental Science, 136*, 347–353.

Robson, K. S. (1967). The role of eye-to-eye contact in maternal-infant attachment. *Journal of Child Psychology and Psychiatry, and Allied Disciplines, 8*(1), 13–25.

Rosenblatt, J. S., Mayer, A. D., & Giordano, A. L. (1988). Hormonal basis during pregnancy for the onset of maternal behavior in the rat. *Psychoneuroendocrinology, 13*, 29–46.

Rosenblatt, J. S., Olufowobi, A., & Siegel, H. I. (1998). Effects of pregnancy hormones on maternal responsiveness, responsiveness to estrogen stimulation of maternal behavior, and the lordosis response to estrogen stimulation. *Hormones and Behavior, 33*(2), 104–114.

Ross, L. E., Sellers, E. M., Gilbert Evans, S. E., & Romach, M. K. (2004). Mood changes during pregnancy and the postpartum period: Development of a biopsychosocial model. *Acta Psychiatrica Scandinavica, 109*(6), 457–466.

Ruhe, H. G., Mason, N. S., & Schene, A. H. (2007). Mood is indirectly related to serotonin, norepinephrine and dopamine levels in humans: A meta-analysis of monoamine depletion studies. *Molecular Psychiatry, 12*(4), 331–359.

Sahakian, B. J., Morris, R. G., Evenden, J. L., Heald, A., Levy, R., Philpot, M., et al. (1988). A comparative study of visuospatial memory and learning in Alzheimer-type dementia and Parkinson's disease. *Brain: A Journal of Neurology, 111*(Pt 3), 695–718.

Schaal, B., & Porter, R. (1991). Microsmatic humans revisited: The generation and perception of chemical signals. *Advances in the Study of Behavior, 20*, 135–199.

Seifritz, E., Esposito, F., Neuhoff, J. G., Luthi, A., Mustovic, H., Dammann, G., et al. (2003). Differential sex-independent amygdala response to infant crying and laughing in parents versus nonparents. *Biological Psychiatry, 54*(12), 1367–1375.

Seip, K. M., & Morrell, J. I. (2007). Increasing the incentive salience of cocaine challenges preference for pup- over cocaine-associated stimuli during early postpartum: Place preference and locomotor analyses in the lactating female rat. *Psychopharmacology, 194*(3), 309–319.

Seyfried, L. S., & Marcus, S. M. (2003). Postpartum mood disorders. *International Review of Psychiatry, 15*(3), 231–242.

Siever, L. J. (2008). Neurobiology of aggression and violence. *The American Journal of Psychiatry, 165*(4), 429–442.

Smyth, J., Ockenfels, M. C., Porter, L., Kirschbaum, C., Hellhammer, D. H., & Stone, A. A. (1998). Stressors and mood measured on a momentary basis are associated with salivary cortisol secretion. *Psychoneuroendocrinology, 23*(4), 353–370.

Stallings, J., Fleming, A. S., Corter, C., Worthman, C., & Steiner, M. (2001). The effects of infant cries and odors on sympathy, cortisol, and autonomic responses in new mothers and nonpostpartum women. *Parenting, 1*(1&2), 71–100.

Stanley, C., Murray, L., & Stein, A. (2004). The effect of postnatal depression on mother-infant interaction, infant response to the still-face perturbation, and performance on an instrumental learning task. *Development and Psychopathology, 16*(1), 1–18.

Stansbury, K., & Gunnar, M. R. (1994). Adrenocortical activity and emotion regulation. *Monographs of the Society for Research in Child Development, 59*(2–3), 108–134.

Stein, A., Gath, D. H., Bucher, J., Bond, A., Day, A., & Cooper, P. J. (1991). The relationship between post-natal depression and mother-child interaction. *The British Journal of Psychiatry: The Journal of Mental Science, 158*, 46–52.

Steiner, M. (1998). Perinatal mood disorders: Position paper. *Psychopharmacology Bulletin, 34*(3), 301–306.

Stern, D. (1974). Mother and infant at play: The dyadic interaction involving facial, vocal and gaze behaviors. In M. L. Rosenblum (Ed.), *The effects of the infant on its caregiver* (pp. 187–213). New York: Wiley.

Stern, J. M. (1983). Maternal behavior priming in virgin and caesarean-delivered long-evans rats: Effects of brief contact or continuous exteroceptive pup stimulation. *Physiology & Behavior, 31*(6), 757–763.

Stern, J. M., & Keer, S. E. (1999). Maternal motivation of lactating rats is disrupted by low dosages of haloperidol. *Behavioral Brain Research, 99*(2), 231–239.

Stowe, Z. N., & Nemeroff, C. B. (1995). Women at risk for postpartum-onset major depression. *American Journal of Obstetrics and Gynecology, 173*(2), 639–645.

Suomi, S. J. (2006). Risk, resilience, and gene x environment interactions in rhesus monkeys. *Annals of the New York Academy of Sciences, 1094*, 52–62.

Thoman, E. B. (2006). Co-sleeping, an ancient practice: Issues of the past and present, and possibilities for the future. *Sleep Medicine Reviews,* 10(6), 407 417.

Thompson, E. T., Walker, L. O., & Crain, H. C. (1981). *Effects of parity and time on maternal attitudes in the neonatal period.* Unpublished manuscript, University of Texas at Austin, Austin.

Trehub, S. E., Unyk, A. M., & Trainor, L. J. (1993). Maternal singing in cross-cultural perspective. *Infant Behavior & Development, 16*(3), 285–295.

Trevathan, W. R. (1983). Maternal "en face" orientation during the first hour after birth. *The American Journal of Orthopsychiatry, 53*(1), 92–99.

Trevathan, W. R. (1987). *Human birth: An evolutionary perspective.* Hawthorne: Aldine DeGruyter.

Tronick, E. Z. (1987). *An interdisciplinary view of human intuitive parenting behaviors and their role in interactions with infants.* Paper presented at the meetings of the Society for Research in Child Development, Baltimore.

van Ijzendoorn, M. H., Bakermans-Kranenburg, M. J., & Mesman, J. (2008). Dopamine system genes associated with parenting in the context of daily hassles. *Genes, Brain, and Behavior, 7*(4), 403–410.

Wiesenfeld, A. R., & Klorman, R. (1978). The mother's psychophysiological reactions to contrasting affective expressions by her own and an unfamiliar infant. *Developmental Psychology,* 14(3), 294–304.

Wisner, K. L., & Stowe, Z. N. (1997). Psychobiology of postpartum mood disorders. *Seminars in Reproductive Endocrinology,* 15(1), 77–89.

Chapter 2
How Fathers Evolve: A Functional Analysis of Fathering Behavior

Anne Storey and Carolyn Walsh

Abstract In mammals, paternal care is rarer and more variable in its proximate mechanisms of development and underlying neural mechanisms than is maternal care. Here, we discuss how species differences in these proximate mechanisms reflect ecological pressures that have been selected for biparental care and argue that paternal care is more fixed (i.e., shaped less by social experiences) in those species where it is most important for infant survival. A second theme is that glucocorticoids such as cortisol and corticosterone are associated with both positive (more responsive to infant cues, more domestic work) and negative aspects of parenting (find parenting more difficult) in human fathers, findings that mirror research on maternal behavior. Finally, we discuss an animal model with obligatory biparental care, a seabird, the common murre (*Uria aalge*) – and show, as in humans, that elevated corticosterone is associated with both positive and negative aspects of parental responses, depending on environmental (foraging) context. We conclude that biparental care contributes to flexibility in reproductive strategies that allow organisms to extend their seasonal or geographic breeding ranges.

Questions about parenting behavior can be examined from at least four different perspectives (as in Tinbergen, 1963). We share this view with Mileva and Fleming (see Chap. 1), based in part on the common training that Fleming and Storey received from the Institute of Animal Behavior and have shared with students and colleagues. These four perspectives include studies of mechanism and development at the individual level, which has been Fleming's focus, and studies of why and how the behavior evolved, which has been our emphasis. Studies of mechanism include all components discussed by Mileva and Fleming, including how sensory stimuli from the young initiate the hormonal and neural responses that trigger parental behavior. Mileva and Fleming's overview of the mechanisms underlying maternal behavior covered the field beautifully, summarizing the seminal contributions of

A. Storey (✉)
Department of Psychology, Memorial University of Newfoundland, St. John's,
Newfoundland and Labrador, Canada
e-mail: astorey@mun.ca

A. Booth et al. (eds.), *Biosocial Foundations of Family Processes*,
National Symposium on Family Issues, DOI 10.1007/978-1-4419-7361-0_2,
© Springer Science+Business Media, LLC 2011

Fleming and her colleagues. In fact, the work by Fleming and colleagues in this area is so comprehensive that there are no gaps.

For this reason, we develop a comparison here with the much smaller literature on the other parent, the father. We are interested in evolutionary/functional questions such as why there are species and individual differences in fathers' involvement in the care of offspring. We explore how selection for flexibility in the expression of paternal care under different social and environmental conditions has shaped its development and neural mechanisms. In connection with fathers, we develop two other themes from the Mileva and Fleming chapter: the role of glucocorticoids (cortisol and corticosterone), hormones linked to both positive and negative aspects of parenting, and the use of an animal model to understand the ecological context in which biparental care evolves.

Function and Evolution of Mammalian Paternal Care

Paternal care is rare in mammals; in fact, it is seen in less than 10% of species (Kleiman & Malcolm, 1981). Mammalian paternal care has been is less common than maternal care due to differences in selective pressures during evolution: males can increase their reproductive success by caring for offspring and/or by mating with other females. Given the specialized reproductive physiology, female mammals can rarely increase their reproductive success by initiating a new pregnancy if the cost is to invest less in specialized their current dependent offspring. Paternal care in mammals has evolved separately and independently in a number of lineages where care by two parents has been selected by difficult environmental conditions. Limited comparative evidence in mammals supports this contention; for two pairs of closely related rodent species, paternal care has evolved in the member of each pair living with the harsher ecological conditions (Schradin & Pillay, 2004; Wynne-Edwards, 1995).

Paternal care should only be selected if it promotes higher male reproductive success than not providing care. Paternal care increases survival of young in California mice (*Peromyscus californicus*; Gubernick, Wright, & Brown, 1993), bat-eared foxes (*Otocyon megalotis*; Wright, 2006), dwarf hamsters (*Phodopus cambelli*; Wynne-Edwards & Lisk, 1989), and humans (Hewlett, 1992; Hurtado & Hill, 1992). Other potential fitness measures linked to mammalian paternal care include higher offspring growth rates (Alvergne, Faurie, & Raymond, 2009; Huber, Millesi, & Dittami, 2002; Schradin & Pillay, 2004; Storey & Snow, 1987), protection of juveniles in group conflicts (Buchan, Alberts, Silk, & Altmann, 2003; Carpentier, Van Horn, Altmann, & Alberts, 2008), and the development of behavioral coping styles (Jia, Tai, An, Zhang, & Broders, 2009).

Parental investment theory suggests that males should be selected to recognize and differentially invest in their own offspring. There is some support for this prediction in mammals: male savannah baboons (*Papio cynocephalus*) differentially intervene in conflicts on behalf of the juvenile offspring whose mothers they had previously associated with (Buchan, Alberts, Silk, & Altmann, 2003).

Further, Sengelese men differentially invest in offspring with facial and odor similarities to themselves (Alvergne, Faurie, & Raymond, 2009). These studies suggest that both familiarity and phenotype matching influence paternal investment decisions. Despite these examples, however, paternal certainty often does not correlate with the extent of paternal investment within a species. One important reason for this predictive failure is that males may take care of young to enhance their chances of future matings with the mothers (Woodroffe & Vincent, 1994). Males may also care for unrelated young because the cost of a recognition error (i.e., not caring for related young) may be too high.

Social Experience and the Development of Paternal Responsiveness

Mammalian paternal behavior is characterized by considerable variation at individual (Gubernick, Schneider, & Jeannotte, 1994; Parker & Lee, 2001) and population levels (Roberts, Williams, Wang, & Carter, 1998; comparison of Oliveras & Novak, 1986 and Storey, Bradbury, & Joyce, 1994). Human paternal care is also highly variable (Barry & Paxson, 1971; Belsky, Steinberg, & Draper, 1991). This variability, which reflects genetic variation and the effects of social experiences, is presumably maintained so that individuals can respond optimally to various mating and parental opportunities.

Although Mileva and Fleming outline how traumatic events can diminish maternal responsiveness, mammalian mothers generally require less social experience to behave parentally than mammalian fathers. For example, parentally, naïve male meadow voles (*Microtus pennsylvanicus*) differ in their responses to pups (ranging from being infanticidal to caretaking; Parker & Lee, 2001; Storey & Joyce, 1995), but after siring pups and living with the pregnant female, males were no longer infanticidal and many spent significant amounts of time in the nest with pups (Storey & Joyce, 1995; Storey & Walsh, 1994). Female meadow voles, on the other hand, required no postweaning social experience to act maternally with their first litters. Paternal behavior was also enhanced in meadows voles by having the father present in early development (Storey & Joyce, 1995) or by being cross-fostered and reared by pairs of a more paternal vole species, the prairie vole (*Microtus ochrogaster* McGuire, 1988). Female meadow voles also vary in whether they allow males to acquire pup experience (Oliveras & Novak, 1986; Storey, Bradbury, & Joyce, 1994). Thus, variability in how parentally-experienced males respond to pups and in whether females allow males to acquire particular social experiences.

This variability has resulted in the evolution of a system with maximum flexibility, such that males and their partners can maximize reproductive success in different ways depending on different conditions (Storey, Delahunty, McKay, Walsh & Wilhelm, 2006). This flexibility may be important in a species where females and pups cohabit with males during the colder parts of the breeding season (Madison, Fitzgerald, & McShea, 1984) but live away from males when it is warmer.

In contrast to meadow voles and most other paternal mammals, males of two very highly paternal rodent species do not need particular social interactions as adults in order to provide care for young (Djungarian hamsters, *P. campbelli*; Jones & Wynne-Edwards, 2001; prairie voles, *M. ochrogaster;* Roberts, Williams, Wang, & Carter, 1998). As we document in the next section, the critical neuroendocrine events in these two species occur just after birth (Cushing & Wynne-Edwards, 2006), not in adulthood. Further, unlike other paternal mammals (e.g., Roberts, Jenkins, Lawler, Wegner, & Newman, 2001), reduction of prolactin levels does not interfere with paternal behavior in male Djungarian hamsters (Brooks, Vella, & Wynne-Edwards, 2005). Together, these findings suggest that when paternal care is critical for pup survival (as documented in Wynne-Edwards & Lisk, 1989), the underlying neuroendocrine mechanisms may evolve to lose socially induced flexibility and become fixed earlier in development.

In humans, paternal experience changes how males respond hormonally to infant cues. We measured prolactin reactivity, that is, how much prolactin levels increased in response to infant stimuli, as they would, for example, when a mother nurses her baby. Expectant first-time mothers exposed to infant stimuli (infant cries and videos of family-center births) showed an increase in prolactin before the birth of their first babies. In contrast, the same men tested near the births of their first two children did not show a prolactin increase until after the birth of their second babies (Delahunty, McKay, Noseworthy, & Storey, 2007; see also Fleming, Corter, Stallings, & Steiner, 2002). Prolactin increases were more likely to occur when men had not recently held their babies, suggesting that changes in patterns of infant contact with the arrival of the second child may have also played a role in the pro-lactin increases after the second births (Delahunty, McKay, Noseworthy, & Storey, 2007). Similarly, among nonparents, women responded more to infant cries in an fMRI study than men, but there were no differences between mothers and fathers (Seifritz et al., 2003). These findings mirror those in the animal literature: most paternal species of mammals require some social stimulation to become paternal.

Physiological Mechanism of Paternal Behavior

One implication of the difference between mothers and fathers was highlighted in the Mileva and Fleming chapter. They discussed the final common path for maternal behavior and outlined several hormonal changes common to pregnant and parturient mammals. In contrast, there has been both less attention and less success in finding a common neural and hormonal pathway for paternal behavior. Results to date appear to be largely species-specific, findings that support the idea that paternal care has evolved separately in scattered lineages throughout mammals.

The most detailed work on the neurohormonal mechanisms of paternal behavior has occurred in the monophyletic group Rodentia, especially within the Family Muridae, which includes rats, mice, voles, lemmings, gerbils, and hamsters (Iwaniuk, 2005). The variation in social organization and affiliative behavior within genera, such as *Microtus* (voles) and *Phodopus* (hamsters), have allowed for interesting interspecific comparisons of paternal behavior and its associated neural mechanisms. Much of this research indicates that estrogen receptor alpha (ERα) patterns in brain regions known to mediate social (including maternal) behavior, such as the medial amygdala (MeA) and the bed nucleus of the stria terminalis (BNST), are related to differences in affiliative and paternal behavior (e.g., review in Cushing & Kramer, 2005; Han & De Vries, 2003; Cushing, Perry, Musatov, Ogawa, & Papademetriou, 2008). For example, the prairie vole, *M. ochragaster*, and the pine vole, *M. pinetorum*, are both monogamous and biparental, with males showing high levels of pup care. The congeneric meadow vole, *M. pennsylvanicus*, and montane vole, *M. montanus*, in contrast, are polygynous in American populations with males showing little or no care of offspring (see Young, Liu & Wang, 2008). Similar comparisons can be made between two congeneric hamsters, *P. campbelli*, the biparental Djungarian hamster, and *P. sungorus*, the nonparental Siberian hamster. In these voles and hamsters, patterns of ERα expression correlate with social organization, such that males, but not females, of socially monogamous and biparental species exhibit lower levels of ERα-immunoreactivity in the MeA and BNST than less parental species (or less social populations of the same species; Cushing et al., 2004; Cushing & Wynne-Edwards, 2006). Also, in biparental species only, ERα-immunoreactivity is sexually dimorphic, with males showing lower receptor levels than females (Cushing & Wynne-Edwards, 2006).

It has been proposed that a sexually dimorphic pattern of ERα may explain the demonstration of female-like behaviors in males, such as the direct care of offspring (Cushing et al., 2004). Since males have higher steroid hormone and aromatase (an enzyme converting testosterone to estrogen) activity during early development, the time during which sex-specific behavior is organized, they are exposed to relatively more estrogen than females. If males and females have the same numbers of ERα, then males will be more affected by estrogen, leading to masculinized behavior. If males have fewer ERα, they will be less affected by estrogen during development, thereby reducing/removing masculinizing effects and leading to more female-like behavior patterns. Prairie voles show persisting sexually dimorphic patterns of ERα patterns between days 8 and 21 of age in various hypothalamic nuclei, the BNST, and the MeA (Yamamoto, Carter, & Cushing, 2006).

Indeed, the influence of steroid hormones (testosterone, estrogen) and neuropeptides (oxytocin, vasopression) may be critically important for organizing the neural machinery during early development which sets the typical parameters for the amount of prosocial and paternal behavior that can be expressed. Kramer, Perry, Golbin, & Cushing (2009) demonstrated that reducing the steroid exposure of male prairie voles during the second postnatal week negatively affected juvenile alloparental care, suggesting a role for endogenous hormones in organizing male parental behavior. Similarly, biparental Djungarian hamsters exposed to an aromatase inhibitor around weaning showed decreases in paternal care, while those exposed at later ages did not (Timonin & Wynne-Edwards, 2008).

Steroid hormones are also implicated in activating adult behavior in several species. In adult parental males, a reduction in testosterone at the time of offspring birth is generally seen (hamsters, Reburn & Wynne-Edwards, 1999; gerbils, Brown, Murdoch, Murphy, & Moger, 1995; Clark & Galef, 1999; humans, Storey, Walsh, Quinton, & Wynne-Edwards, 2000; Berg & Wynne-Edwards, 2001; Gray, Kathlenberg, Barrett, Lipson, & Ellison, 2002; Fleming, Corter, Stallings, & Steiner, 2002). However, in the biparental California mouse (*Peromyscus californicus*), testosterone, converted to estradiol, is required for males to show parental care (Trainor & Marler, 2002). Interestingly, this is a species in which males need reproductive experience (copulation and cohabitating with a mate and pups) before showing robust paternal care (Gubernick, Schneider, & Jeannotte, 1994). Recent work has shown that the medial preoptic area (MPOA) of the hypothalamus and the BNST, areas important for maternal care, are activated by pup cues in male California mice when they become fathers (de Jong, Chauke, Harris, & Saltzman, 2009). Similarly, paternally behaving Volcano mice *Neotomodon alstoni* also exhibit high testosterone, suggesting a mechanism for paternal care that may be similar to the California mouse (Luis et al., 2009). To date, patterns of ERα have not been examined in these species.

It seems likely that the neural pathways for paternal behavior, at least in the murid rodents, are evolutionarily conserved to some extent. In species with obligate biparental care, such as the prairie vole and Djungarian hamster, it may be that the neural mechanism to permit paternal responsiveness is extremely robust and relatively impermeable to environmental influences that could dramatically alter patterns of male behavior. Such a scenario may occur if this machinery is configured during early development (e.g., by establishing patterns of low ERα) and then "turned on" appropriately in adulthood. The existence of male juvenile alloparental care, prior to mating, in such species may further attest to the robustness of the mechanism, such that full activation of the system (i.e., mate presence) is not required for some aspects of the behavior to be shown. In contrast, species with optional or facultative paternal care should retain a degree of system flexibility, such that the neural machinery can be more responsive to environmental inputs, such as seasonal changes that impact litter survival (e.g., Wynne-Edwards, 1995) or amount of paternal care received (Roberts, Williams, Wang, & Carter, 1998; see Cushing & Kramer, 2005).

In other biparental rodents, such as *Peromyscus* mice, alternate neurohormonal pathways to paternal behavior may have evolved. In such species, the pathways may be more similar to those described for maternal behavior in the rat (e.g., involving the MPOA), such that hormonal activation in the presence of appropriate social cues (pups) is required to establish parental responsiveness.

The extent to which paternal and nonpaternal rodents and other mammals share neural machinery for the expression of paternal behavior is, as yet, unknown. While it is possible that paternal species have unique neuroendocrine pathways to parental behavior (Wynne-Edwards & Timonin, 2007), it is likely that some common evolutionarily conserved mechanisms will be discovered, which have been modified in particular species to cope with the ecological demands under which each species evolved social and parental behavior.

Glucocorticoids and Paternal Responsiveness

The next theme we develop from the Mileva and Fleming chapter is the relationship between parental behavior and so-called glucocorticoid "stress hormones," such as cortisol and corticosterone, which are associated with both positive and negative aspects of parenting. For example, Fleming and her colleagues have shown that women with traumatic early life experiences had higher early morning cortisol levels than women without traumatic events (Gonzales, Jenkins, Steiner, & Fleming, 2009). They also noted that elevated cortisol is often associated with depression. These are the kinds of observations that support the general view of cortisol (and other gluco- corticoids) as "stress" hormones. But on the positive response side, Fleming has also found that mothers with higher levels of cortisol were more responsive to their new- borns than women with lower cortisol (Fleming, Steiner, & Corter, 1997; Fleming, Ruble, Krieger, & Wong, 1997). These results, which initially surprised people but have been repeatedly confirmed, suggest that elevated cortisol helps new mothers focus on this new environmental challenge of responding to a new baby.

We have also found that cortisol is involved in both positive and negative aspects of parental functioning. Cortisol levels increase from early to late pregnancy in both mothers and fathers and then decline in the postpartum period (Storey, Walsh, Quinton, & Wynne-Edwards, 2000). Just prior to becoming fathers, we asked men to report on their emotional responses to the infant stimuli we presented (cries and birth video). When tested later holding their own babies, men who reported concern (C) or "wanting to comfort the baby" (WCB) at the prenatal tests had a different pattern of cortisol change compared to men not reporting those feelings (non-C/ WCB). Non-C/WCB men showed the typical drop in cortisol seen at the end of a brief stressful stimulus (experimenters arriving and taking the first blood sample). In contrast, C/WCB men showed no decrease when cortisol levels were compared before and after they held their babies (Storey, Delahunty, & McKay, 2007). These findings are consistent with Fleming's results that cortisol is positively related to heightened sensitivity and attentiveness to infant cues.

Paternal contributions may indirectly benefit offspring by assisting the mother with tasks that free her time to engage in direct parental care. A positive aspect of elevated stress hormones is that they are associated with an increase in activity (Astheimer, Buttemer, and Wingfield, 1992; Belthoff & Dufty, 1998) that can benefit the offspring. When their babies were 2 months old, we asked fathers whether their domestic workload had changed. Men who reported an increase in meal preparation, confirmed by the mother, had higher cortisol than men reporting no change in their domestic work (Storey, Delahunty, & McKay, 2007). This associa- tion between increased workload and elevated cortisol levels is consistent with some of the animal literature to be discussed later.

New mothers with postpartum depression are reported to have cortisol levels that are either higher (e.g., Ehlert, Patalla, Kirschbaum, Piedmont, & Hellhammer, 1990) or lower (e.g., Groer & Morgan, 2007; Taylor, Glover, Marks, & Kammerer, 2009) than levels in nondepressed new mothers. Variable time of testing and the use of different stress tests and depression measures may account for some of these differences across studies. About half of the new mothers in our study reported that they found parenting more difficult than expected, a rating than was independent of how difficult mothers judged their own babies to be relative to other babies. Mothers with greater parenting difficulties had higher cortisol levels than mothers without unexpected difficulties, as did their partners (Storey, Delahunty, & McKay, 2007). These results suggest that the mother's stress may be communicated to her partner. We noted significant cortisol correlations within pregnant and new parent couples; these correlations were largely absent in nonpregnant controls.

Together, these results for cortisol highlight some of the complexities in the relationship between cortisol and parental behavior. Elevations in cortisol can be used to mobilize the organism to deal with the challenge of being an effective parent. Elevations in cortisol with no effective action component, however, may contribute to less effective parental responses, accompanied by distress.

Animal Model of Parental Behavior: Common Murres

The other major theme we develop from the Mileva and Fleming chapter is the use of animal models to help us understand the evolution of parental behavior. Alison Fleming chose the rat, a species with many physiological similarities to humans. Mileva and Fleming do, however, point out several differences from humans, namely, that rats are nocturnal, bear large litters, and are short-lived. Another important difference from our perspective is that adult male rats are not naturally involved in paternal care. Our animal model is the common murre (*U. aalge*), a long-lived north temperate seabird that maintains long-term pair-bonds and raises only a single chick per year. Unlike mammals, paternal care is very common in birds, occurring in more than 90% of species. Given external gestation of the young in the egg and no specialized maternal physiology for feeding young, there are more opportunities for male birds to increase their reproductive success by caring for young than is typically the case in mammals.

Common murres are colony-nesting diving seabirds. Males and females share all phases of parental care equally except that the male alone takes the chick to sea once it leaves the colony. One parent is always with the egg or chick to defend against predators while the other is foraging, so biparental care is obligatory. Parents bring a single fish per trip to the colony to feed their chicks. Both parents lose body mass during chick rearing, and they must balance the cost of rearing their single chick against their own and their partner's deteriorating body condition (Jones, Ruxton, & Monaghan, 2002). Chick rearing is particularly difficult in years when the inshore arrival of spawning capelin (*Mallotus villosus*) is delayed until after chicks hatch. We found that the same birds (with the same partners and nest sites) had higher corticosterone in the year of late capelin arrival compared to levels in 2 normal years (Doody, Wilhelm, McKay, & Storey, 2008). Birds with higher than average corticosterone levels for the late capelin year brought back more fish to their chicks than birds with lower corticosterone, in keeping with the idea that higher hormone levels can mobilize individuals to meet this extraordinary challenge of feeding a chick under conditions of sparse food availability. In the normal year, however, the birds with lower than average corticosterone levels brought back more fish than murres with higher corticosterone. If we had only looked at this relationship in any one year, we would have concluded very different things about the relationship between corticosterone and parental work.

Recent models suggest that organisms may have different physiological responses to life events that are either predictable (e.g., any breeding season) or unpredictable and/or extraordinary (e.g., a particularly difficult breeding season; McEwen & Wingfield, 2003; Romero, Dickens, & Cyr, 2009). These models may help explain the opposite relationships we found between corticosterone levels and parental provisioning rates in murres for different years. Most organisms should be able to cope with predictable changes (normal breeding season), so lower corticosterone should be associated with more effective parental responses (higher feeding rates, hence a negative relationship between feeding and corticosterone). According to the models, an organism's responses to unpredictable changes should depend on its reactive scope, defined as its ability to increase mediators such as corticosterone, without exceeding a threshold that causes this once-adaptive response to now become pathological. This threshold could be different for animals in better or worse body condition; in an extremely bad year, those organisms that can mount the greatest physiological response (higher corticosterone) will be the more effective parents (i.e., have the higher chick-feeding rates).

How do these bird–mammal comparisons contribute to our understanding of the evolution of effective fathering? In seabirds such as the murre, obligatory biparental care allowed successful dispersal into, and exploitation of, prey-rich foraging areas in northern climates. In mammals, maintaining pair-bonds after fertilization may have been a behavioral solution to environmental difficulties (e.g., keeping helpless young warm in colder climates in rodents, or group hunting in social carnivores). In rodents, those males taking advantage of the extra warmth from being allowed to stay in the burrow, but without harming the pups, would have had a fitness advantage in some seasons over more aggressive males. Being with the pups more may have activated neuroendocrine responses, and the ease with which this activation occurred may have had a heritable component. Thus, in most paternal species of mammals, care is generally activated by experience-induced changes in hormonal response, and flexibility is important. For humans, we see that paternal behavior has evolved in much the same way as in most other paternal mammals, being variable and primarily expressed after considerable social experience.

References

Alvergne, A., Faurie, C., & Raymond, M. (2009). Father–offspring resemblance predicts paternal investment in humans. *Animal Behavior*, 78, 61–69.
Astheimer, L. B., Buttemer, W. A., & Wingfield, J. C. (1992). Interactions of corticosterone with feeding, activity and metabolism in passerine birds. *Ornis Scandinavica*, 23, 355–365.

Barry, H., & Paxson, L. M. (1971). Infancy and early childhood: cross cultural codes 2. *Ethnology, 10*, 466–508.

Belsky, J., Steinberg, L., & Draper, P. (1991). Childhood experience, interpersonal development, and reproductive strategy: an evolutionary theory of socialization. *Child Development, 62*, 647–670.

Belthoff, J. R., & Dufty, A. M. (1998). Corticosterone, body condition and locomotor activity: a model for dispersal in screech-owls. *Animal Behavior, 55*, 405–415.

Berg, S. J., & Wynne–Edwards, K. E. (2001). Changes in testosterone, cortisol, and estradiol levels in men becoming fathers. *Mayo Clinic Proceedings, 76*, 582–592.

Brooks, P. L., Vella, E. T., & Wynne–Edwards, K. E. (2005). Dopamine agonist treatment before and after the birth reduces prolactin concentration but does not impair paternal responsiveness in Djungarian hamsters, *Phodopus campbelli*. *Hormones and Behavior, 47*, 358–366.

Brown, R. E., Murdoch, T., Murphy, P. R., & Moger, W. H. (1995). Hormonal responses of male gerbils to stimuli from their mate and pups. *Hormones and Behavior, 29*, 474–491.

Buchan, J.C., Alberts, S.C., Silk, J.B., & Altmann, J. (2003). True paternal care in a multi–male primate society. *Nature, 425*, 179–181.

Carpentier, M. J. E., Van Horn, R. C., Altmann, J., & Alberts, S. C. (2008). Paternal effects of offspring fitness in a multimale primate society. *Proceedings of the Royal Society of London, Series B, Biological Science, 105*, 1988–1992.

Clark, M. M., & Galef, B. G. (1999). A testosterone mediated trade–off between parental and sexual effort in male Mongolian gerbils, *Meriones unguiculatus*. *Journal of Comparative Psychology, 113*, 388–395.

Cushing, B. S., & Kramer, K. M. (2005). Mechanisms underlying epigenetic effects of early social experience: The role of neuropeptides and steroids. *Neuroscience and Biobehavioral Reviews, 29*, 1089–1105.

Cushing, B. S., Perry, A., Musatov, S., Ogawa, S., & Papademetriou, E. (2008). Estrogen receptors in the medial amydala inhibit the expression of male prosocial behavior. *Journal of Neuroscience, 28*, 10399–10403.

Cushing, B. S., Razzoli, M., Murphy, A. Z., Epperson, P. M., Le, W–W., & Hoffman, G. E. (2004). Intraspecific variation in estrogen receptor alpha and the expression of male sociosexual behavior in two populations of prairie voles. *Brain Research, 1016*, 247–254.

Cushing, B. S., & Wynne–Edwards, K. E. (2006). Estrogen receptor-α distribution in male rodents is associated with social organization. *Journal of Comparative Neurology, 494*, 595–605.

de Jong, T. R., Chauke, M., Harris, B. N., & Saltzman, W. (2009). From here to paternity: Neural correlates of the onset of paternal behavior in California mice (*Peromyscus californicus*). *Hormones and Behavior, 56*, 220–231.

Delahunty, K. M, McKay, D. W., Noseworthy, D. E., & Storey, A. E. (2007). Prolactin responses to infant cues in men and women: effects of parental experience and recent infant contact. *Hormones and Behavior, 51*, 213–220.

Doody, L. M., Wilhelm, S. I., McKay, D. W., & Storey, A. E. (2008). The effects of variable foraging conditions on common murre (*Uria aalge*) parental behavior and corticosterone concentrations. *Hormones and Behavior, 53*, 140–148.

Ehlert, U., Patalla, U., Kirschbaum, C., Piedmont, E., & Hellhammer, D. H. (1990). Postpartum blues: salivary cortisol and psychological factors. *Journal of Psychosomatic Medicine, 34*, 319–325.

Fleming, A. S., Corter, C., Stallings, J., & Steiner, M. (2002). Testosterone and prolactin are associated with emotional responses to infant cries in new fathers. *Hormones and Behavior, 42*, 399–413.

Fleming, A. S., Ruble, D., Krieger, H., & Wong, P. Y. (1997). Hormonal and experiential correlates of maternal responsiveness during pregnancy and the puerperium in human mothers. *Hormones and Behavior, 31*, 145–158.

Fleming, A. S., Steiner, M., & Corter, C. (1997). Cortisol, hedonics, and maternal responsiveness in human mothers. *Hormones and Behavior, 32*, 85–98.

Gonzales, A., Jenkins, J. M, Steiner, M., & Fleming, A. S. (2009). The relation between early life adversity, cortisol awakening response and diurnal salivary cortisol levels in postpartum women. *Psychoneuroendocrinology, 34*, 76–86.

Gray, P. B., Kathlenberg, S. M., Barrett E. S., Lipson S. F., & Ellison P. T. (2002). Marriage and fatherhood are associated with lower testosterone in males. *Evolution and Human Behavior, 23,* 193–201.

Groer, M. W., & Morgan, K. (2007). Immune, health and endocrine characteristics of depressed postpartum mothers. *Psychoneuroendocrinology, 32,* 133–139.

Gubernick, D. J., Schneider, K. A., & Jeannotte, L. A. (1994). Individual differences in the mechanisms underlying the onset and maintenance of paternal behavior and the inhibition of infanticide in the monogamous biparental California mouse, *Peromyscus californicus. Behavioral Ecology and Sociobiology, 34,* 225–231.

Gubernick, D. J., Wright, S. L., & Brown, R. E. (1993). The significance of father's Presence for offspring survival in the monogamous California mouse, *Peromyscus californicus. Animal Behavior, 46,* 539–546.

Han, T. M., & De Vries, G. J. (2003). Organizational effects of testosterone, estradiol, and dihydrotestosterone on vasopressin mRNA expression in the bed nucleus of the stria terminalis. *Journal of Neurobiology, 54,* 502–510.

Hewlett, B. S. (1992). Husband–wife reciprocity and the father–infant relationship among Aka Pygmies. In B. S. Hewlett (Ed.), *Father–child Relations: Cultural and biosocial contexts* (pp. 31–55). New York: Aldine de Gruyter.

Huber, S., Millesi, E., & Dittami, J. P. (2002). Paternal effort and its relation to mating success in the European ground squirrel. *Animal Behavior, 63,* 157–164.

Hurtado, A. M., & Hill, K. R. (1992). Paternal effects of offspring survivorship among Ache and Hiwi hunter–gatherers: implications for modeling pair–bond stability. In B. S. Hewlett (Ed.), *Father–child relations: Cultural and biosocial contexts* (pp. 153–176). New York: Aldine de Gruyter.

Iwaniuk, A. N. (2005). Evolution. In I. Q. Whishaw & B. Kolb (Eds.), *The behavior of the laboratory rat: A handbook with tests* (pp. 3–14). New York: Oxford University Press.

Jia, R., Tai, F., An, S., Zhang, X., & Broders, H. (2009). Effects of neonatal paternal deprivation or early deprivation on anxiety and social behaviors of the adults in maderin voles. *Behavioral Processes, 82,* 271–278.

Jones, J. S., & Wynne–Edwards, K. E. (2001). Paternal behavior in biparental hamsters, *Phodopus campbelli,* does not require contact with the pregnant female. *Animal Behavior, 62,* 453–464.

Jones, K.M., Ruxton, G.D., & Monaghan, P. (2002). Model parents: is full compensation for reduced partner nest attendance compatible with stable biparental care? *Behavioral Ecology, 13,* 838–843.

Kleiman, D. G., & Malcolm, J. R. (1981). The evolution of male parental investment in mammals. *Quarterly Review of Biology, 52,* 39–68.

Kramer, K. K., Perry, A. N., Golbin, D., & Cushing, B. S. (2009). Sex steroids are necessary in the second postnatal week for the expression of male alloparental behavior in prairie voles (*Microtus ochragaster*). *Behavioral Neuroscience, 123,* 958–963.

Luis, J., Ramirez, L., Carmona, A., Ortiz, G., Delgado, J., & Cárdenas, R. (2009). Paternal behavior and testosterone plasma levels in the Volcano Mouse *Neotomodon alstoni* (Rodentia: Muridae). *International Journal of Tropical Biology, 57,* 433–439.

Madison, D. M., Fitzgerald, R. W., & McShea, W. J. (1984). Dynamics of social nesting in overwintering meadow voles, *Microtus pennsylvanicus*: possible consequences for population cycling. *Behavioral Ecology and Sociobiology, 15,* 9–17.

McEwen, B.S., & Wingfield, J.C. (2003). The concept of allostasis in biology and biomedicine. *Hormones and Behavior, 43,* 2–15.

McGuire, B. (1988). Effects of cross–fostering on parental behavior in the meadow vole (*Microtus pennsylvanicus*). *Journal of Mammalogy, 69,* 332–341.

Oliveras, D., & Novak, M. (1986). A comparison of paternal behavior in the meadow vole (*Microtus pennsylvanicus*), the pine vole (*M. pinetorum*) and the prairie vole (*M. ochrogaster*). *Animal Behavior, 34,* 519–526.

Parker, K. J., & Lee, T. M. (2001). Central vasopressin administration regulates the onset of paternal behavior in *Microtus pennsylvanicus. Hormones and Behavior, 39,* 285–294.

Reburn, C.J., & Wynne–Edwards, K.E. (1999). Hormonal changes in males of a naturally biparental and a uniparental mammal. *Hormones and Behavior, 35*, 163–176.

Roberts, R. L., Jenkins, K. T., Lawler, T., Jr., Wegner, F. H., & Newman, J. D. (2001). Bromocriptine administration lowers serum prolactin and disrupts parental responsiveness in common marmosets (*Callithrix j. jacchus*). *Hormones and Behavior, 39*, 106–112.

Roberts, R. L., Williams, J. R., Wang, A. K., & Carter, C. S. (1998). Cooperative breeding and monogamy in prairie voles: influence of the sire and geographic variation. *Animal Behavior, 55*, 1131–1140.

Romero, M., Dickens, M. J., & Cyr, N. E. (2009). The reactive scope model – A new model integrating homeostasis, allostasis, and stress. *Hormones and Behavior, 55*, 375–389.

Schradin, C., & Pillay, N. (2004). The influence of the father on offspring development in the striped mouse. *Behavioral Ecology, 16*, 450–455.

Seifritz, E., Esposito, F., Neuhoff, J. G., Luthi, A., Mustovic, H., Dammann G., et al. (2003). Differential sex–independent amygdala response to infant crying and laughing in parents versus nonparents. *Biological Psychiatry, 54*, 1367–1375.

Storey, A. E., Bradbury, C. G., & Joyce, T. L. (1994). Nest attendance in male meadow voles: the role of the female in regulating male interactions with pups. *Animal Behavior, 47*, 1037–1046.

Storey, A. E., Delahunty, K. M., McKay, D. M., Walsh, C. J., & Wilhelm, S. I. (2006). Social and hormonal bases for individual differences in the parental behavior of bird and mammals. *Canadian Journal of Experimental Psychology, 60*, 237–245.

Storey, A. E., Delahunty, K. M., & McKay, D. W. (2007). Are elevated cortisol levels associated with enhanced or reduced parental responsiveness? Poster presented at the Parental Brain Conference, Boston.

Storey, A. E., & Joyce, T. L. (1995). Pup contact promotes paternal responsiveness in male meadow voles. *Animal Behavior, 49*, 1–10.

Storey, A. E., & Snow, D. T. (1987). Male identity and enclosure size affect paternal attendance of meadow voles, *Microtus pennsylvanicus*. *Animal Behavior, 35*, 411–419.

Storey, A. E. & Walsh, C. J. (1994). The role of physical contact from females and pups in the development of paternal responsiveness in meadow voles. *Behavior, 131*, 139–151.

Storey, A. E., Walsh, C. J., Quinton, R., & Wynne–Edwards, K. E. (2000). Hormonal correlates of paternal responsiveness in new and expectant fathers. *Evolution and Human Behavior, 21*, 79–95.

Taylor, A., Glover, V., Marks, M., & Kammerer, M. (2009). Diurnal pattern of cortisol output in postnatal depression. *Psychoneuronedocrinology, 34*, 1184–1188.

Timonin, M. E., & Wynne–Edwards, K. E. (2008). Aromatase inhibition during adolescence reduces adult sexual and paternal behavior in the biparental dwarf hamster *Phodopus campbelli*. *Hormones and Behavior, 54*, 748–757.

Tinbergen, N. (1963). On aims and methods of ethology. *Zeitschrift für Tierpsychology, 20*, 410–433.

Trainor, B. C., & Marler, C. A. (2002). Testosterone promotes paternal behavior in a monogamous mammal via conversion to oestrogen. *Proceedings of the Royal Society of London, Series B, 269*, 823–829.

Woodroffe, R., & Vincent, A. (1994). Mother's little helpers: patterns of male care in mammals. *Trends in Ecology and Evolution, 9*, 294–297.

Wright, H. W. Y. (2006). Paternal den attendance is the best predictor of offspring survival in the socially monogamous bat–eared fox. *Animal Behavior, 71*, 503–510.

Wynne–Edwards, K. (1995). Biparental care in Djungarian but not Siberian dwarf hamsters (*Phodopus*). *Animal Behavior, 50*, 1571–1585.

Wynne–Edwards, K. E., & Lisk, R. D. (1989). Differential effects of paternal presence on pup survival in two species of dwarf hamster (*Phodopus sungorus and Phodopus campbelli*). *Physiology and Behavior, 45*, 465–469.

Wynne–Edwards, K. E., & Timonin, M. E. (2007). Parental care in rodents: weakening support for hormonal regulation of transition to behavioral fatherhood in rodent animal models of biparental care. *Hormones and Behavior, 52*, 114–121.

Yamamoto, Y., Carter, C. S., & Cushing, B. S. (2006). Neonatal manipulation of oxytocin affects expression of estrogen receptor alpha. *Neuroscience, 137*, 157–164.

Young, K. A., Liu, Y., & Wang Z. (2008). The neurobiology of social attachment: A comparative approach to behavioral, neuroanatomical, and neurochemical studies. *Comparative Biochemistry and Physiology C, 148*, 401–410.

Chapter 3
Caregiving as Coregulation: Psychobiological Processes and Child Functioning

Susan D. Calkins

Abstract Although considerable research has sought to understand the relations between parental behavior and a range of child developmental outcomes, much of this work has been conducted at a very broad level of analysis. Psychobiological theory and research point to the need for models of caregiving that offer greater specificity regarding processes that may be implicated in the effects of these relationships. Recent work on animals and some work on humans have focused more on the proximal mechanisms through which caregivers and infants affect one another. This chapter presents a model of the caregiver–child relationship that focuses on proximal processes operating within both caregiver and child. This model uses a self-regulatory framework to capture the levels of influence of the caregiver's behavior on the child's functioning. Next, I present an overview of physiological regulation and findings that support its role as foundational to more sophisticated emotional and behavioral regulation. Then, I provide evidence for the effects of caregiver behavior on physiological regulation. Finally, I offer general recommendations for future research that could illuminate how specific types of caregiver behavior influence multiple levels of child behavior.

Introduction

Psychobiological approaches to the study of early behavioral development remind us that a range of biological mechanisms is implicated in functioning at all levels of analysis. And, as our understanding of the role of these genetic and biological processes has grown, a shift in focus has occurred in our attempt to understand *how* specific behavioral developments emerge and influence children's outcomes. Researchers have come to view development as a dynamic process involving transactions between the child and his or her environment that affect children's development,

S.D. Calkins (✉)
Department of Psychology, The University of North Carolina, Greensboro, NC, USA
e-mail: sdcalkin@uncg.edu

A. Booth et al. (eds.), *Biosocial Foundations of Family Processes*,
National Symposium on Family Issues, DOI 10.1007/978-1-4419-7361-0_3,
© Springer Science+Business Media, LLC 2011

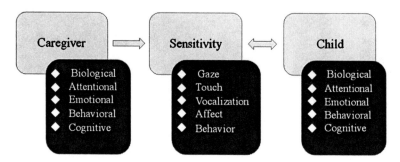

Fig. 3.1 Proximal regulatory mechanisms in caregiver–child relationships

and caregiver behavior, at multiple biological and behavioral levels (e.g., Blair, 2002; Wachs, 1999; Chap. 1). And, as Mileva and Fleming demonstrate quite convincingly, analysis across levels of caregiver functioning provides us with insight into the more proximal processes that affect both caregiver behavior and child functioning. Here, I use a self-regulatory framework to explore in some depth the way in which caregiver behavior supports the emergence and elaboration of a set of skills necessary for child functioning. Specifically, Fig. 3.1 extends Mileva and Fleming's analysis and provides a framework for understanding caregiver behavior as both regulated (i.e., within the caregiver) and regulatory (i.e., between caregiver and child).

Very broadly, self-regulation can be defined as one's *own* ability to control emotions and behaviors in order to cope effectively with environmental demands. Although the term self-regulation has been used as a rubric for a wide range of behaviors, we use the term to refer to a *specific* set of processes: control mechanisms that function at the biological and behavioral level that enable an individual to manage arousal, attention, emotion, behavior, and cognition in an adaptive way (Baumeister & Vohs, 2004). Mileva and Fleming (Chap. 1) describe how many of these skills operate in the adult caregiver. The development of self-regulation in children is marked by the acquisition of an integrated set of domain-specific (biological, attentional, emotional, behavioral, cognitive) self-regulatory mechanisms that are hierarchical in nature and that build upon each other over the course of development. The rationale for hypothesizing the differentiation, development, and integration of these regulatory processes over the course of childhood emanates from recent work in the area of developmental neuroscience that has identified specific brain regions that may play a functional role in the deployment of attention and in the processing and regulation of emotion, cognition, and behavior (Posner & Rothbart, 1992, 1998). This work suggests that because of its dependence on the maturation of prefrontal–limbic connections, the development of self-regulatory processes is relatively protracted (Beauregard, Levesque, & Paquette, 2004), from the development of basic and automatic regulation of physiology in infancy and toddlerhood to the more self-conscious and intentional regulation of cognition emerging in middle childhood (Ochsner & Gross, 2004). From a developmental perspective, understanding how these skills emerge is critical to facilitating their development and deployment in a range of contexts throughout development.

One important assumption of much of the research on the acquisition of self-regulation skills is that parental caregiving practices may support or undermine such development and thus contribute to observed individual differences among young children's emotional, cognitive, and behavioral skills (Morris, Silk, Steinberg, Myers, & Robinson, 2007; Thompson, 1994). In infancy, there is an almost exclusive reliance on parents for the regulation of arousal, attention, and emotion. Over time, interactions with parents in a variety of contexts teach children that the use of particular strategies may be more useful for the reduction of emotional arousal, for example, than other strategies (Sroufe, 1996). Although caregiving practices are often attributed a role in the development of self-regulation, the specific processes by which these practices affect children's development are often discussed at a mostly global level (Fox & Calkins, 2003). Greater specificity in *how* caregiving affects children requires a consideration of the multiple levels of child self-regulation that are emerging during early development. Clearly, biological regulation is one candidate process that may allow greater specificity in understanding how caregiving affects child behavior. Theories of self-regulation that focus on underlying biological components assume that maturation of different biological support systems lays the foundation for increasingly sophisticated emotional, cognitive, and behavioral regulation that is observed across childhood.

Recent psychophysiological research highlights the role of one such system, the autonomic nervous system, in regulating many biobehavioral processes. The autonomic nervous system functions as a complex system of afferent and efferent feedback pathways that are integrated with other neurophysiological and neuroanatomical processes, reciprocally linking cardiac activity with central nervous system processes (Chambers & Allen, 2007). Pathways of the parasympathetic nervous system, in particular, are implicated in these processes and, consequently, they play a key role in the regulation of state, motor activity, emotion, and cognition (Porges, 2003). Specifically, the myelinated vagus nerve, originating in the brainstem nucleus ambiguus, provides input to the sinoatrial node of the heart, producing dynamic changes in cardiac activity that allow the organism to transition between sustaining metabolic processes and generating more complex responses to environmental events (Porges, 2007). This central–peripheral neural feedback loop is functional relatively early in development (Porges, 2007), though there is good evidence that individual differences in the integrity of these processes are a consequence of both organic characteristics and postnatal experiences (Calkins & Hill, 2007).

Parasympathetic influences on heart rate can be easily quantified in young humans by measuring heart rate variability. Variability in heart rate that occurs at the frequency of spontaneous respiration [respiratory sinus arrhythmia (RSA)] can be measured noninvasively and is considered a good estimate of the parasympathetic influence on heart rate variability via the vagus nerve. Porges and colleagues developed a method that measures the amplitude and period of the oscillations associated with inhalation and exhalation, referred to as vagal tone (Vna; Porges, 1985, 1991, 1996; Porges & Byrne, 1992). Of particular interest to researchers studying self-regulation, though, has been measurement of vagal *regulation* of the heart when the organism is challenged. Such regulation is indexed by a decrease in

RSA or vagal tone (vagal withdrawal) during situations where coping or emotional and behavioral regulation is required (Porges, 2003, 2007). Vagal regulation in the form of decreases in RSA is often described as the functioning of "the vagal brake" because a decrease, or *withdrawal*, of vagal input to the heart has the effect of stimulating increases in heart rate. During demanding tasks, such a response reflects physiological processes that allow the child to shift focus from internal homeostatic demands to demands that require internal processing or the generation of coping strategies to control affective or behavioral arousal. Thus, vagal withdrawal is thought to be a physiological strategy that results in greater cardiac output in the form of HR acceleration, and that supports behaviors indicative of active coping (Calkins, Graziano, & Keane, 2007; El-Sheikh, Harger, & Whitson, 2006; Porges, 1991, 1996; Propper & Moore, 2006; Wilson & Gottman, 1996).

What, specifically, can studies of physiological regulation in children tell us about the effects of caregiver behavior? A number of fundamental predictions and hypotheses regarding development, contextual effects, and links to behavioral functioning may be usefully examined with RSA measures, and these findings may shed light on the role of physiological regulation in emerging adaptive behavioral functioning and behavioral problems and, importantly, how caregivers may affect these relations. Considerable research suggests that cardiac vagal withdrawal is linked to a range of behavioral processes that are regulatory in nature and that are observable quite early in development, and that caregiver–child relationships affect and are affected by these processes. In the next sections, I examine some of these findings with data from a series of cross-sectional and longitudinal studies my colleagues and I have conducted in which both physiological and behavioral measures of self-regulation were collected.

Cardiac vagal regulation and child functioning across early development. One question that we have investigated concerns how early in development we can observe the ability to suppress cardiac vagal tone in support of an adaptive behavioral response. In one study, we observed mothers and 3-month-old infants interacting in a series of tasks, including the Still Face Paradigm, which involves both positive and negative interactions with the caregiver (Moore & Calkins, 2004). We observed that infants display significant cardiac vagal withdrawal, or suppression, to the negative tasks and increases to the positive tasks. These data demonstrate that the physiological response to challenge is present quite early in life. We continue to see a similar pattern of responding among toddlers (Calkins & Dedmon, 2000), preschoolers (Calkins & Keane, 2004), and school-age children (Calkins, Graziano, Berdan, Keane, & Degnan, 2008).

A second question that has been less well explored concerns the specific demands of the challenge and whether these differential demands elicit a differential RSA response. That is, is RSA suppression a sensitive measure of the degree of challenge faced by the individual? We have explored this question in several samples of infants and children (Calkins, 1997; Calkins & Dedmon, 2000; Calkins, Dedmon, Gill, Lomax, & Johnson, 2002; Calkins et al., 2008; Calkins & Keane, 2004; Calkins, Smith, & Gill, 1998). Across these studies, our results have been remarkably consistent. First, tasks that elicit negative affect typically yield a greater

RSA suppression response than do tasks that elicit positive affect. Second, tasks that elicit negative affect elicit a greater RSA response than those that have attentional, but not affective domains. Thus, the RSA suppression measures do seem to be an indicator of both the degree of challenge the task imposes on the child's regulatory ability and the extent to which the child can generate a coping response. Third, the pattern of physiological regulation parallels the pattern of behavioral regulation we observe; children with greater physiological regulation use more emotion regulation strategies and display more on-task behaviors (Calkins & Dedmon, 2000).

The extension of our research findings is that while the ability to suppress RSA may be related to complex responses involving the regulation of attention and behavior, a deficiency in this ability may be related to early behavior problems, particularly problems characterized by a lack of behavioral and emotional control (Calkins & Dedmon; Porges, 1996; Wilson & Gottman, 1996). In the next section, I discuss data more directly relevant to the question of whether deficits in the regulation of physiological arousal underlie the behavioral characteristics of children with early disruptive behavior problems.

Vagal regulation and disruptive behavior problems. Lack of behavioral and emotional control is considered a core deficit for children with disruptive behavior problems (Gilliom & Shaw, 2004; Keenan & Shaw, 2003). Moreover, children with externalizing problems display patterns of aggressive, destructive, and undercontrolled behavior that remains stable from preschool to middle childhood (Gilliom & Shaw, 2004) and that often results in more severe conduct problems in adolescence and young adulthood (Olweus, 1979). Given that such problems are believed to have both biological and socialization origins (Moffitt, 1993), one question that may be asked is whether these children display a pattern of physiological dysregulation that impairs their ability to generate and engage appropriate regulatory strategies in situations that are emotionally or behaviorally challenging.

In one study, we identified children at high risk for the development of aggressive behavior problems at age 2 and assessed them in a number of challenging emotion and cognitive tasks (Calkins & Dedmon, 2000). These children displayed significantly lower RSA suppression across these tasks than did children at low risk for behavior problems. In a follow-up of these same children, continued behavioral difficulties, including social problems and difficulties with emotion regulation, were characteristic of the children who displayed, across the preschool period, a stable pattern of physiological dysregulation, in the form of lower RSA suppression to challenge (Calkins & Keane, 2004). Interestingly, children who displayed a pattern of lower suppression at age 2 but who were observed to suppress RSA at age 4 showed continued difficulties, suggesting that the early pattern of cardiac vagal regulation may have constrained the acquisition of regulatory skill that affected behavior later in the preschool period.

These findings suggest that there may be a physiological profile of poorer vagal regulation of HR activity that may be characteristic of children with early externalizing problems. However, one challenge to the study of physiological regulation among children with behavior problems characterized by aggression is that these problems often present with co-occurring internalizing symptoms (anxiety, withdrawal) (Achenbach, Howell, Quay, & Connors, 1991; Gilliom & Shaw, 2004). These co-occurring problems are often ignored, either because they are thought to be a consequence of single-reporter bias or because the sample sizes in most studies of children's behavior problems are too small to allow for separate consideration of pure vs. co-occurring problems (Calkins & Dedmon, 2000).

We explored this issue in a large sample of 5-year-old children, some of whom were at high risk for externalizing problems, others of whom displayed early externalizing problems with co-occurring internalizing problems, and a third group of children with no behavioral problems (Calkins et al., 2007). The children were assessed in a battery of tasks that were emotionally and behaviorally challenging. We found that children displaying a mixed profile of externalizing and internalizing behavior problems displayed the greatest cardiac vagal regulation, whereas children with a pure externalizing profile displayed the least cardiac vagal regulation. These data suggest that either the pattern of greater vagal regulation leads to anxiety symptoms or that children with emergent anxiety become more regulated physiologically. Alternatively, these children may in fact be overregulated physiologically, which may explain the high level of internalizing symptoms. Recent research in the study of emotion regulation suggests that both underregulation and overregulation of emotion may be characteristic of children with very different patterns of behavioral difficulties (Eisenberg, Smith, Sadovsky, & Spinrad, 2004). Studies of physiological regulation have yet to address the question of whether greater vagal regulation may, in some instances, be an indicator of overregulation.

The effects of caregiver behavior on cardiac vagal regulation. In every study we have conducted using physiological measures of regulation, we have observed that infants and children engaged in a challenging task with a caregiver typically display a greater magnitude of RSA suppression than when they are engaged in a task alone (cf. Calkins & Dedmon, 2000; Calkins et al., 2008). Thus, the RSA suppression measures do seem to be an indicator of both the degree of challenge the task imposes on the child's regulatory ability and the extent to which the child can generate a coping response independently vs. with environmental support. However, an important issue not addressed by this kind of analysis is whether caregivers contribute to the *development* of physiological regulation and how that regulation might influence subsequent dyadic interactions.

Much recent conceptual work and empirical research supports the view that caregiver behavior affects the development of behavioral self-regulation skills (Calkins, 2004; Crockenberg & Leerkes, 2004), as well as the functioning of numerous biological regulatory and stress systems (Calkins & Hill, 2007; Gunnar, 2006; Propper & Moore, 2006). Importantly, evidence from animal models suggests that caregiving affects infants' biological and behavioral systems of regulation through the environment the caregiver provides rather than through shared inherited traits. For example, Meeney and colleagues have shown that high levels of maternal licking/grooming and arched backed nursing in rats affects the neurological systems associated with the stress response, a process that has a long-term influence on stress-related illness, certain cognitive functions, and physiological functions

(Caldji et al., 1998; Champagne & Meaney, 2001; Francis, Caldji, Champagne, Plotsky, & Meaney, 1999). Furthermore, cross-fostering studies demonstrate convincingly that these maternal behaviors are transmitted behaviorally through the nursing mother and not through the biological mother, indicating that early caregiving is a crucial factor in early development and may affect the organism's level of emotional reactivity even when they reach adulthood (Calatayud, Coubard, & Belzung, 2004; Champagne & Meaney, 2001).

This psychobiological influence on self-regulation is important because, as we have shown, children who have characteristically low thresholds for arousal, or who have difficulty managing that physiological arousal, are at a disadvantage because emergent behavioral self-regulation strategies are dependent on the basic control of physiological processes (Porges, 2003). To the extent that caregivers can provide the support for such physiological control early in development, children should be more successful at using attentional and behavioral strategies to control emotion, behavior, and cognitive processes. They should also be better prepared to engage in interactions with caregivers, facilitating the transactional relationship that reinforces sensitive and responsive caregiving. We have explored these issues in several cross-sectional and longitudinal studies.

In one of our studies (Moore & Calkins, 2004), we found that infants who displayed a pattern of vagal regulation to challenge engaged in more positive interactions with caregivers. These infants also showed a "recovery" from disruption in their interactions with the caregiver, by displaying less negative affect toward the caregiver after the disruption. These findings confirm our hypothesis that good physiological regulation may facilitate social interactions with others, which, in the case of caregiver–child interactions, may support the ongoing relationship that is needed for children to acquire more sophisticated regulatory skills.

Longitudinal studies that we have conducted have been more informative about the relations over time between caregiving and physiological regulation in infants. In one recent study (Propper et al., 2008), we identified children who might be at genetic risk for problems with regulation because they carried the "risk" allele of the dopamine transmitter gene *DRD2*. We assessed vagal regulation and caregiver sensitivity across the first year of life. We observed that infants without the risk allele displayed appropriate vagal regulation in a laboratory paradigm that was challenging to the infants, and that this pattern held across the first year. Infants with the risk allele, however, displayed a different pattern of results, depending on the level of caregiver sensitivity to which they were exposed. For infants with the risk allele and mothers who were not sensitive, poor physiological regulation was observed across the first year. Infants with the risk allele and mothers who were sensitive displayed poor physiological regulation during assessments at 3 and 6 months of age, but by the end of the first year, their pattern of physiological responding to challenge was no different from that of the infants without the risk allele. This G × E interaction demonstrates convincingly that infants and caregivers each bring something to the developmental process of acquiring regulatory skills very early in development.

One final question that we have addressed concerns the effects of caregiving behavior on physiological regulation beyond infancy. The challenge to studying this question, though, is that the relations between physiological and behavioral functioning emerge quite early in development (Moore & Calkins, 2004), so disentangling the direction of effects between caregiver behavior and child biological vs. behavioral functioning is difficult. We examined these effects longitudinally from the toddler period, as this is a period of rapid growth in self-regulatory abilities (Kopp, 1982), to the early childhood period, when physiological regulation has been demonstrated to support more sophisticated emotional and cognitive self-regulation skills (Calkins & Keane, 2004). Prior research indicates that there are concurrent relations between externalizing spectrum behavior problems and physiological regulation across childhood (Calkins, 1997; Calkins et al., 2007; El-Sheikh, et al., 2006) and between maternal positive and negative behavior and vagal regulation (Calkins et al., 1998). In this study, we examined whether the quality of the maternal–child relationship during toddlerhood (indexed by maternal behavior characterized by low hostility, high positive affect and responsiveness, and low stress attributed to the maternal–child relationship) would affect physiological regulation at age 5, *beyond the effects of prior and current levels of behavioral functioning*. We also controlled for *earlier physiological regulation* to ensure that the effects of the maternal–child relationship on the development of physiological regulation would be above and beyond the effects of prior regulation skills. The findings from this study were clear: across each of the six self-regulation tasks, whether the child was working independently or in collaboration with the caregiver, children who had harmonious relationships with their mothers in toddlerhood showed greater physiological regulation than children with less harmonious relationships, and this effect was over and above the effect of prior level of physiological regulation and prior and current behavioral problems. Earlier caregiving behavior predicted growth in physiological regulation across the toddler to preschool period of development.

An important question unaddressed in this study is whether maternal–child relationship problems during toddlerhood are a function of child or maternal problems. That is, it is possible that the relationship effects observed in this study were a function of manifestations of child behavioral difficulties that are observable earlier, in infancy perhaps and that affect parents' experiences and behaviors with their offspring. Recent work suggests that toddler behavior that is aversive, problematic, and normative affects caregiver's experience of stress in both the short (Calkins, 2002) and the long term (Williford, Calkins, & Keane, 2007). It is possible that fundamental problems in physiological regulation lead to patterns of unpredictable, unmanageable, and difficult behavior that stresses the emerging parent–child relationship. Under conditions that exacerbate such stress, such as those that accompany social and economic challenge, normative child behavioral difficulties may lead to negative, hostile, and nonsupportive parenting that undermines the acquisition of basic regulatory skills of the sort that are integral to adaptive functioning during early childhood.

Although our data clearly support a model of transactions, or coregulation, between caregivers and children, it is obvious that many more questions remain, the answers to which would provide greater specificity such as that proposed by the model in Fig. 3.1. First, the modes of caregiving behavior depicted in the model have not been adequately measured in our research, nor in most research examining caregiver behavior and physiological regulation (but see Feldman, 2006). Second, the model as depicted is insufficiently developmental, and given what we know about how regulatory processes come "on line" and how parenting varies with child developmental level (Calkins & Hill, 2007), it will be important to examine these child and caregiver behaviors across time. Third, and as Mileva and Fleming (Chap. 1) clearly demonstrate, we need to better understand the factors that predict caregiver regulation in order to understand the meditational effects of parenting on child self-regulation. Each of these issues can be best addressed in multilevel longitudinal studies that assess both biological and behavioral indices of self-regulation.

Acknowledgment The writing of this manuscript was supported in part by a National Institute of Health Research Scientist Career Development Award (K02) to Susan D. Calkins (MH 74077).

References

Achenbach, T. M., Howell, C. T., Quay, H. C., & Connors, C. K. (1991). National survey of problems and competencies among four- to sixteen-year-olds: Parents' reports for normative and clinical samples. *Monogr Soc Res Child Dev, 56*, (Serial No. 225, Whole No. 3).

Baumeister, R. F., & Vohs, K. D. (2004). *Handbook of self-regulation: Research, theory, and application.* New York: Guilford.

Beauregard, M., Levesque, J., & Paquette, V. (2004). Neural basis of conscious and voluntary self-regulation of emotion. In M. Beauregard (Ed.), *Consciousness, emotional self-regulation and the brain* (pp. 163–194). Philadelphia, PA: John Benjamins.

Blair, C. (2002). School readiness: Integrating cognition and emotion in a neurobiological conceptualization of children's functioning at school entry. *American Psychologist, 57*, 111–127.

Calatayud, F., Coubard, S., & Belzung, C. (2004). Emotional reactivity may not be inherited but influenced by parents. *Physiological Behavior, 80*, 465–474.

Caldji, C., Tannenbaum, B., Sharma, S., Francis, D., Plotsky, P. M., & Meaney, M. J. (1998). Maternal care during infancy regulates the development of neural systems mediating the expression of fearfulness in the rat. *Neurobiology, 9*, 5335–5340.

Calkins, S. D. (1997). Cardiac vagal tone indices of temperamental reactivity and behavioral regulation in young children. *Developmental Psychobiology, 31*, 125–135.

Calkins, S. D. (2002). Does aversive behavior during toddlerhood matter? The effects of difficult temperament on maternal perceptions and behavior. *Infant Mental Health Journal, 23*, 381–402.

Calkins, S. D. (2004). Early attachment processes and the development of emotional self-regulation. In R. Baumeister & K. Vohs (Eds.), *Handbook of self-regulation: Research, theory, and applications* (pp. 324–339). New York: Guilford.

Calkins, S. D., & Dedmon, S. E. (2000). Physiological and behavioral regulation in two-year-old children with aggressive/destructive behavior problems. *Journal of Abnormal Child Psychology, 28*, 103–118.

Calkins, S. D., Dedmon, S., Gill, K., Lomax, L., & Johnson, L. (2002). Frustration in infancy: Implications for emotion regulation, physiological processes, and temperament. *Infancy, 3*, 175–198.

Calkins, S. D., Graziano, P. A., & Keane, S. P. (2007). Cardiac vagal regulation differentiates among children at risk for behavior problems. *Biological Psychology, 74*, 144–153.

Calkins, S. D., Graziano, P., Berdan, L., Keane, S. P., & Degnan, K. (2008). Predicting cardiac vagal regulation in early childhood from maternal–child relationship quality during toddlerhood. *Developmental Psychobiology, 50*, 751–766.

Calkins, S. D., & Hill, A. L. (2007). Caregiver influences on emerging emotion regulation: Biological and environmental transactions in early development. In J. Gross (Ed.), *Handbook of emotion regulation* (pp. 229–248). New York: Guilford.

Calkins, S. D., & Keane, S. P. (2004). Cardiac vagal regulation across the preschool period: Stability, continuity, and implications for childhood adjustment. *Developmental Psychobiology, 45,* 101–112.

Calkins, S. D., Smith, C. L, & Gill, K. L. (1998). Maternal interactive style across contexts: Relations to emotional, behavioral, and physiological regulation during toddlerhood. *Social Development, 7,* 350–369.

Chambers, A., & Allen, J. (2007). Cardiac vagal control, emotion, psychopathology, and health. *Biological Psychology, 74,* 113–115.

Champagne, F., & Meaney, M. J. (2001). Like mother, like daughter: Evidence for non-genetic transmission of parental behavior and stress responsivity. *Progressive Brain Research, 133,* 287–302.

Crockenberg, S., & Leerkes, E. (2004). Infant and maternal behaviors regulate infant reactivity to novelty at 6 months. *Developmental Psychology, 40,* 1123–1132.

Eisenberg, N., Smith, C., Sadovsky, A., & Spinrad, T. (2004). Effortful control: Relations with emotion regulation, adjustment, and socialization in childhood. In R. Baumeister & K. Vohs (Eds.), *Handbook of self-regulation: Research, theory, and applications* (pp. 259–282). New York: Guilford.

El-Sheik, M., Harger, T., & Whitson, S. (2006). Longitudinal relations between marital conflict and child adjustment: Vagal regulation as a protective factor. *Journal of Family Psychology, 20,* 30–39.

Feldman, R. (2006). From biological rhythms to social rhythms: Physiological precursors of mother–infant synchrony. *Developmental Psychology, 42,* 175–188.

Fox, N., & Calkins, S. D. (2003). The development of self-control of emotion: Intrinsic and extrinsic influences. *Motivation and Emotion, 23,* 7–26.

Francis, D. D., Caldji, C., Champagne, F., Plotsky, P. M., & Meaney, M. J. (1999). The role of cortcotropin-releasing factor – norepinephrine systems in mediating the effects of early experience on the development of behavioral and endocrine responses to stress. *Biological Psychiatry, 46,* 1153–1166.

Gilliom, M., & Shaw, D. S. (2004). Codevelopment of externalizing and internalizing problems in early childhood. *Development and Psychopathology, 16,* 313–333.

Gunnar, M. R. (2006). Social regulation of stress in early child development. In K. McCartney & D. Phillips (Eds.), *Blackwell handbook of early childhood development* (pp. 106–125). Malden, MA: Blackwell Publishing.

Keenan, K., & Shaw, D. S. (2003). Exploring the etiology of antisocial behavior in the first years of life. In B. B. Lahey, T. E. Moffitt, & A. Caspi (Eds.), *Causes of conduct disorder and juvenile delinquency* (pp. 153–181). New York: Guilford.

Kopp, C. (1982). Antecedents of self–regulation: A developmental perspective. *Developmental Psychology, 18,* 199–214.

Moffitt, T. E. (1993). Adolescence-limited and life-course-persistent antisocial behavior: A developmental taxonomy. *Psychological Review, 100*(4), 674–701.

Moore, G., & Calkins, S. D. (2004). Infants' vagal regulation in the still-face paradigm is related to dyadic coordination of mother-infant interaction. *Developmental Psychology, 40,* 1068–1080.

Morris, A., Silk, J., Steinberg, L., Myers, S., & Robinson, L. (2007). The role of the family context in the development of emotion regulation. *Social Development, 16,* 361–388.

Ochsner, K. N., & Gross, J. J. (2004). Thinking makes it so: A social cognitive neuroscience approach to emotion regulation. In R. F. Baumeister & K. D. Vohs (Eds.), *Handbook of self-regulation: Research, theory, and applications* (pp. 229–255). New York: Guilford.

Olweus, D. (1979). Stability of aggressive reactive patterns in males: A review. *Psychological Bulletin, 86,* 852–875.

Porges, S. W. (1985). Method and apparatus for evaluating rhythmic oscillations in aperiodic physiological response systems. US Patent No. 4520944.

Porges, S. W. (1991). Vagal tone: An autonomic mediator of affect. In J. Garber & K. A. Dodge (Eds.), *The development of emotional regulation and dysregulation* (pp. 111–128). Cambridge: Cambridge University Press.

Porges, S. W. (1996). Physiological regulation in high-risk infants: A model for assessment and potential intervention. *Development and Psychopathology, 8,* 43–58.

Porges, S. W. (2003). The polyvagal theory: Phylogenetic contributions to social behavior. *Physiology and Behavior, 79,* 503–513.

Porges, S. W. (2007). The polyvagal perspective. *Biological Psychology, 74,* 116–143.

Porges, S. W., & Byrne, E. A. (1992). Research methods for measurement of heart rate and respiration. *Biological Psychology, 34,* 93–130.

Posner, M. I., & Rothbart, M. K. (1992). Attentional mechanisms and conscious experience. In D. A. Milner & M. D. Rugg (Eds.), *The neuropsychology of consciousness* (pp. 91–111). San Diego, CA: Academic Press.

Posner, M. I., & Rothbart, M. K. (1998). Summary and commentary: Developing attentional skills. In J. E. Richards (Ed.), *Cognitive neuroscience of attention: A developmental perspective* (pp. 317–323). Mahwah, NJ: Lawrence Erlbaum Associates.

Propper, C., & Moore, G. (2006). The influence of parenting on infant emotionality: A multi-level psychobiological perspective. *Developmental Review, 26,* 427–460.

Propper, C., Moore, G., Mills-Koonce, R., Halpern, C., Hill, A., Calkins, S., et al. (2008). Gene–environment contributions to the development of vagal tone. *Child Development, 79,* 1378–1395.

Sroufe, A. L. (1996). *Emotional development: The organization of emotional life in the early years.* New York: Cambridge University Press.

Thompson, R. A. (1994). Emotion regulation: A theme in search of definition. In N. A. Fox (Ed.), *The development of emotion regulation: Biological and behavioral considerations.* Monographs of the Society for Research in Child Development, *59,* 25–52.

Wachs, T. D. (1999). The what, why, and how of temperament: A piece of the action. In L. Balter & C. S. Tamis-LeMonda (Eds.), *Child psychology: A handbook of contemporary issues* (pp. 23–44). Philadelphia, PA: Taylor & Francis.

Williford, A. P., Calkins, S. D., & Keane, S. P. (2007). Predicting change in parenting stress across early childhood: Child and maternal factors. *Journal of Abnormal Child Psychology, 35,* 251–263.

Wilson, B., & Gottman, J. (1996). Attention – the shuttle between emotion and cognition: Risk, resiliency, and physiological bases. In E. Hetherington & E. Blechman (Eds.), *Stress, coping and resiliency in children and families.* Mahwah, NJ: Lawrence Erlbaum Associates.

Chapter 4
The Determinants of Parenting in GxE Perspective: A Case of Differential Susceptibility?

Jay Belsky

Abstract Much research on how the environment affects development, especially that pertaining to the conditions under which environmental influence operates, is informed by the diathesis-stress model of environmental action. This stipulates that certain individuals are particularly vulnerable to the negative effects of contextual adversity due to personal characteristics, whereas others lacking these attributes are resilient. Mileva and Fleming interpret some of their own and others' research on the determinants of parenting from this perspective. I offer an alternative framework for thinking about the issue. The differential susceptibility perspective stipulates that some are more and others are less susceptible to both adverse and supportive environments (i.e., not just "vulnerable" to adversity). Evidence consistent with this claim is highlighted.

Introduction

Even though concerted study of the *determinants* of parenting emerged well after extensive work had been initiated on the *effects* of parenting on child development (Belsky, 1984), it is indisputable that much progress has been made over the past 25 years in answering the question "why do parents parent the way they do?" (Belsky & Jaffee, 2006). Whereas early work with humans focused principally on parent's social class, developmental history (i.e., maltreated or not) and, eventually, psychological well-being (i.e., depression), an ecological and developmental focus called attention as well to not just child factors, such as difficult temperament, but intrafamilial and extrafamilial ones, too, including marital relations (Belsky, 1981), social support, and occupational experience (Belsky, 1984). More recently, those studying human parenting have turned their attention to biological sources of

J. Belsky (✉)
Institute for the Study of Children, Families and Social Issues, Birkbeck College,
University of London, London, UK
e-mail: j.belsky@bbk.ac.uk

A. Booth et al. (eds.), *Biosocial Foundations of Family Processes*,
National Symposium on Family Issues, DOI 10.1007/978-1-4419-7361-0_4,
© Springer Science+Business Media, LLC 2011

influeence, including hormones and genes. And much of the latter work has followed in the footsteps of nonhuman research programs, including that of Fleming and collaborators who, using elegant experimental methods, have done so much to illuminate the complex and fascinating nature of biological pathways of causation, often themselves shaped by social experience. It comes as no surprise, then, to see this research team even further extending their work on rats and humans, insightfully illuminating multiple factors and processes that shape early mothering, as well as the many physiological mechanisms and neural pathways involved.

Of special interest to this reader were the findings pertaining to effects of experience on parenting, particularly in the case of human mothers. Also of particular interest were the data pertaining to Gene-x-Environment (GxE) interaction. In this commentary, I briefly call attention to the evidence cited on the first subject, eventually raising a core question about it upon turning attention to the issue of GxE interaction while also offering an alternative reading of what such evidence may actually reflect. Of importance is that this alternative viewpoint will challenge the prevailing focus in so much GxE work on the negative effects of adversity, including on parenting, and thus the diathesis-stress thinking that underlies so much of it.

The Role of Experience in Shaping Parenting

Repeatedly, Mileva and Fleming (Chap. 1) highlight evidence that variation in parental behavior (or physiological functioning) is related to experience. One might think of such evidence in terms of how nurture experienced shapes nurture provided (or its mediating physiological mechanisms). Consider in this regard the following observations made by Mileva and Fleming: experiences interacting with the young enhances maternal responsiveness to the very infant olfactory, auditory, and visual cues that orient, arouse, and direct mother's attention (Fleming et al., 1993; Fleming, Steiner, & Corter, 1997; Schaal & Porter, 1991), perhaps because early postpartum contact and interactional experience enhance maternal *attraction* to the general body odors of infants (Fleming et al., 1993); being a mother is related to elevated levels of sympathy and alertness in response to infant cries (Stallings, Fleming, Corter, Worthman, & Steiner, 2001); a history of neglect or adversity in a mother's family of origin predicts, as a result of mediating (and experimentally evaluated) attentional mechanisms, less sensitive care of 6-month olds (Gonzalez, Jenkins, Steiner & Fleming, 2009, this Chapter 1); multiparous animals reinduced to be maternal through sensitization or continuous exposure to pups show greater dopamine response to pups than multiparous animals lacking such exposure (Afonso, Grella, Chatterjee, & Fleming, 2008); the expression of genes likely to influence parenting are themselves affected by being a parent, as revealed via comparisons of virgin ad postpartum animals (Akbari et al., in prep).

Also of note are findings reported that do not *directly* illuminate effects of experience on parenting but which, nevertheless, raise this issue, at least implicitly. Consider in this regard evidence that increases in the ratio of estradiol to progesterone during pregnancy predicts greater attachment of mother to her newborn, with some of this effect being mediated by effects on mother's psychological well-being (Fleming, Ruble, Krieger & Wong, 1997). The question that arises, of course, is why some mothers experienced an increase in this influential hormonal ratio and thus its apparent positive effects, while others experienced a decrease? A similar question arises following the observation that postpartum hormone cortisol influences responses to newborn baby odors (Fleming et al., 1997). Are such influential cortisol levels themselves shaped by experience, either during the postpartum period or during pregnancy or even earlier in the mother's developmental history, as some of Boyce and Ellis' (2005) theorizing about biological sensitivity to context might suggest? Then, there are the findings showing that mothers with higher circulating levels of cortisol and higher baseline heartrates tend to respond more sympathetically when experimentally exposed to infant cries (Stallings et al., 2001), raising the question of whether concurrent or prior experience – of what kind? – affects these physiological features.

GxE and Parenting

Recent research on GxE interaction, most of which is focused on explaining psychological disorder rather than variation in parenting, makes it clear that not all individuals – and in this case parents – are likely to be affected in the same manner even by the very same experience. Indeed, perhaps one reason that questions regarding effects of early postpartum contact on maternal attachment and behavior remain unresolved, as Mileva and Fleming (Chap. 1) note, is because the possibility of GxE interaction has not been considered. That is, perhaps some mothers, for genetic reasons, are more responsive than others to the putative beneficial effects of early postpartum contact (Bystrova et al., 2009). This seems quite possible because it was, at least in part, due to inconsistencies in research linking child maltreatment with antisocial behavior and negative life events with depression that led Caspi et al. (2002, 2003) to consider – and document – GxE interactions reflective of the fact that the presumed across-the-board effects of such adverse experiences proved more pronounced in some and rather limited – or entirely absent – in others.

Like the groundbreaking work by Caspi, Moffitt, and their collaborators (2002, 2003), most GxE research to date is guided by diathesis-stress thinking, which stipulates that some individuals are more susceptible to the negative effects of adversity as a result of their genetic makeup; that is, some individuals carry "vulnerability genes" or "risk alleles." Of note is that Mileva and Fleming (Chap. 1) in discussing GxE research, including their own, appear to interpret relevant evidence from the same vantage point – though not entirely, as we see here. Notable for the time being is their discussion of the just mentioned GxE work by Caspi et al. (2003) and related work on life events, the serotonin-transporter gene (*5-HTTLPR*), and ADHD severity (Muller et al., 2008). Even more important, though, is their apparent misrepresentation of Dutch research purporting to show, in line with the traditional diathesis-stress view, that DRD4 alleles associated with less efficient transmission of dopamine "predict decreased sensitivity in mothers with high levels of self-reported daily hassles (van IJzendoorn, Bakermans-Kranenburg, & Mesman, 2008)" (Chap. 1).

Beyond Diathesis Stress

What the cited Dutch work reveals, consistent with Belsky's (1997a, 1997b; 2005) differential susceptibility hypothesis, which the research was designed explicitly to test, was that it was not just the case, as diathesis-stress thinking presumes, that those mothers experiencing many daily hassles proved less sensitive interacting with their infants if – and only if – they carried the 7-repeat version of the DRD4 gene. Critically – and in addition – mothers carrying this same putative "risk allele" manifested the highest level of sensitivity when daily hassles were very limited (or not present at all). In other words, although mothers not carrying this allele were unaffected by daily hassles, at least insofar as their observed parenting was concerned, those carrying it were affected in a "for-better-*and*-for-worse" manner (Belsky, Bakermans-Kranenburg, & van IJzendoorn, 2007). Although their parenting was undermined by high levels of hassles relative to those not carrying DRD4 – 7R, it also was enhanced, also relative to those without this allele, if they were not hassled.

Such findings are in line with the view that there exist individual differences in developmental plasticity, with some individuals being more and some less affected by experience and with the nature of the effect determined by the quality of the experience (Belsky et al., 2009; Belsky & Pluess, 2009a,b). Thus, it may not be the case, as diathesis-stress thinking and research has long presumed, that some are simply more susceptible to the negative effects of adversity but that the very same individuals also benefit disproportionately from supportive contextual conditions, including ones defined sometimes by just the absence of adversity (e.g., limited hassles). Of interest in this regard is that multiple GxE findings from studies of psychological disturbance designed to test diathesis-stress propositions actually provide evidence of differential susceptibility, though this is often not noticed or at least commented on, even by investigators generating such findings (Belsky et al., 2009; Belsky & Pluess, 2009a,b).

Therefore, of special interest is at least one set of findings cited by Mileva and Fleming (Chap. 1) that actually chronicles evidence seemingly consistent with differential susceptibility rather than diathesis stress: "Animals with one of the DRD2 genotypes, if raised in a deprived environment, show lower dopamine receptor density than those raised in a normal environment. Environment has no impact on receptor density in the NAC in animals carrying the alternative genotype (Lovic et al., 2010)."

Inspection of Figs. 1.4 and 1.5 provided by Mileva and Fleming (Chap. 1) and based on preliminary data from the MAVAN project involving some 250 women, followed from pregnancy, and their infants does not, it must be noted, seem to provide any additional evidence consistent with differential susceptibility in the case of parents and parenting. It is difficult to know why this is the case. On the one hand, it could be that the MAVAN findings could change as more cases are added or as parenting is studied at older ages or via other means. On the other, it could very well prove to be the case that the for-better-*and*-for-worse pattern of environmental effects for some, but not other individuals, may simply not apply, or at least not often, to parents and parenting. In fact, with the exception of the two studies already cited, one focused on parental sensitivity (van IJzendoorn et al., 2008) and the other on dopamine receptor density (Lovic et al., 2010), virtually all GxE findings consistent with differential susceptibility pertain to nonparenting phenotypes (e.g., depression, aggression, physiological reactivity) (Belsky & Pluess, 2009a,b).

But there is another, perhaps less obvious, explanation for the absence of evidence from the MALVAN project consistent with differential susceptibility, one that applies to – in fact, *plagues* – much of the existent GxE literature involving the prediction of psychological and behavioral phenotypes. And, that is that a full range of environments is not measured when it comes to examining environmental influences and thus GxE interaction. Note in this regard that all the data presented by Mileva and Fleming (Chap. 1) – see Figs. 1.4 and 1.5 – concern putative effects of early adversity. As a result, the positive side of the environmental continuum does not reflect a positive or high quality rearing environment necessarily, but simply the *absence* of adversity. In many cases, as Belsky and Pluess' (2009b) review of evidence consistent with differential susceptibility reveals, such "truncated" measurement of the environment or of developmental experience may be sufficient. But, in other cases, there is reason to wonder whether the absence of a differential-susceptibility-like GxE interaction – in which a cross-over interaction reveals one set of genotypes to be apparently unaffected at all by the experience in question and another set to be affected both positively and negatively, depending on the experience – could simply be an artifact of limitations of measurement.

Beyond Single Genes

With a very few exceptions (see below), virtually all GxE research on human psychological and behavioral functioning has, in addition to being guided by diathesis-stress thinking, examined one gene at a time, just as Mileva and Fleming (Chap. 1) report doing in their MAVAN project. The fact, though, that (a) it is now widely acknowledged that most phenotypes are influenced by many genes (that have small effects) (Plomin, DeFries, McClearn, & McGuffin, 2008) and (b) that multiple so-called vulnerability genes have been found to operate in a differential-susceptibility-like manner (Belsky et al., 2009; Belsky & Pluess, 2009a,b), the question arises as to what would be discerned if GxE studies evaluating the moderating role of genetic makeup vis-à-vis environmental effects used indices of *cumulative* genetic risk or plasticity rather than just single genes? The answer to this question comes from three recent studies.

Working from a "vulnerability" perspective, informed as it was by diathesis-stress thinking, Beaver Ratchford and Ferguson (2009) and Beaver, Sak, Vaske, & Nilsson (2009) scored adolescents participating in the Add Health Study (Harris et al., 2003, Harris, Halpern, Smolen, & Haberstick, 2006) in terms of the number of "risk alleles" they carried (out of a total of five polymorphisms), to determine if *degree* of genetic risk moderated the effect of negative parenting on antisocial behavior. Results clearly showed that the more risk alleles an adolescent carried, the more likely it was that problematic parent–child relations predicted high levels of antisocial behavior.

Working from a plasticity perspective and thus guided by differential-susceptibility thinking, Belsky and Beaver (in press) scored adolescents in terms of whether they carried 0, 1, 2, or 3 putative plasticity alleles, with each of five genes measured being able to contribute one such plasticity point to an individual's cumulative-genetic plasticity score. When it came to predicting relationship instability in adolescents from divorce exposure in childhood, results showed that this anticipated relation emerged but revealing a veritable plasticity gradient: The more plasticity alleles an adolescent carried, the stronger the relation between parenting experienced and self-control in the case of males (only).

Conclusion

Great strides have been made since 1984 when this scholar pulled together the limited evidence then available to answer the question "why do parents parent the way they do?" (Belsky, 1984). The conclusion reached 25 years ago – that parenting is "multiply determined" – remains as true today as it did then. What has changed dramatically, though, are the potential sources of influence shaping human parenting that students of human (and animal) development consider worthy of investigation. As Mileva and Fleming (Chap. 1) make clear, this set of factors now not only includes ecological and developmental-history factors but biological ones as well. And, perhaps most notably, their work and that of others show that we can move beyond the empirical observation that parenting, too, is heritable (Neiderhiser, Reiss, Lichtenstein, Spotts, & Ganiban, 2007) reveal some of the neurological and hormonal factors and processes shaping it.

But, what their work also makes clear is that experience continues to matter, whether experiences in childhood or the experience of becoming a parent in adulthood, to cite but two contextual sources of influence. What this commentary has highlighted, much as GxE research has done more generally, is to remind us that there are likely individual differences in responsiveness to experiences, be they had in the past or the present, and that this should be true with respect to parents and parenting. But it may not just be the case as so much diathesis-stress research, including GxE work, has led us to expect, namely, that there exist "vulnerability genes" making some people especially susceptible to the negative effects of adversity. Rather, it may be that many of those most vulnerable for genetic (and other organismic) reasons are simultaneously most likely to benefit from supportive experiences, including sometimes just the absence of adversity.

Whether this proves true when it comes to predicting and explaining variation in parenting remains, for the most part, to be determined, as so little GxE research has been carried out predicting parenting. Before the null or especially diathesis-stress conclusions are embraced, two questions will need to be considered: Has the investigation assessed a full (positive–negative) range of environments, not just adversity and its absence; have the effects of multiple genes and thus "cumulative genetic plasticity" been considered?

References

Afonso, V. M., Grella, S. L., Chatterjee, D., & Fleming, A. S. (2008). Previous maternal experience affects accumbal dopaminergic responses to pup stimuli. *Brain Research, 1198*, 115–123.

Akbari, E., Shams, S., Westwood, T., Kent, C., Sokolowski, M., & Fleming, A. S. (2010). Effects of pup stimulation on gene expression in the MPOA and amygdala of postpartum and virgin females: A microarray study. Manuscript in preparation.

Beaver, K. M., Ratchford, M., & Ferguson, C. J. (2009). Evidence of genetic and environmental effects on the development of low self-control. *Criminal Justice and Behavior*. Forthcoming.

Beaver, K. M., Sak, A., Vaske, J., & Nilsson, J. (2009). Genetic risk, parent–child relations, and antisocial phenotypes in a sample of African-American males. *Psychiatry Research*.

Belsky, J. (1981). Early human experience: A family perspective. *Developmental Psychology, 17*, 3–23.

Belsky, J. (1984). The determinants of parenting: A process model. *Child Development, 55*, 83–96.

Belsky, J. (1997a). Theory testing, effect–size evaluation, and differential susceptibility to rearing influence: the case of mothering and attachment. *Child Development, 68*(4), 598–600.

Belsky, J. (1997b). Variation in susceptibility to rearing influences: An evolutionary argument. *Psychological Inquiry, 8*, 182–186.

Belsky, J. (2005). Differential susceptibility to rearing influences: An evolutionary hypothesis and some evidence. In B. Ellis & D. Bjorklund (Eds.), *Origins of the social mind: Evolutionary Psychology and Child Development* (pp. 139–163). New York: Guildford.

Belsky, J., Bakermans-Kranenburg, M. J., & van Ijzendoorn, M. H. (2007). For better and for worse: Differential Susceptibility to environmental influences. *Current Directions in Psychological Science, 16*(6), 300–304.

Belsky, J., & Beaver, K.M. (in press). Cumulative-genetic plasticity, parenting and adolescent self-control/*Journal of child Psychology & Psychiatry*.

Belsky, J., & Jaffee, S. (2006). The multiple determinants of parenting. In D. Cicchetti & D. Cohen (Eds.), *Developmental psychopathology*, 2nd ed., *Risk, disorder and adaptation* (2nd ed., Vol. 3, pp. 38–85). New York: Wiley.

Belsky, J., Jonassaint, C., Pluess, M., Stanton, M., Brummett, B., & Williams, R. (2009). Vulnerability genes or plasticity genes? *Molecular Psychiatry, 14*, 746–754.

Belsky, J., & Pluess, M. (2009a). The nature (and nurture?) of plasticity in early human development. *Perspectives on Psychological Science, 4*(4), 345–351.

Belsky, J., & Pluess, M. (2009b). Beyond diathesis-stress: Differential susceptibility to environmental influence. *Psychological Bulletin, 135*, 885–908.

Boyce, W. T., & Ellis, B. J. (2005). Biological sensitivity to context: I. An evolutionary-developmental theory of the origins and functions of stress reactivity. *Development and Psychopathology, 17*(2), 271–301.

Bystrova, K., Ivanova, V., Edhborg, M., Matthiesen, A. S., Ransjö-Arvidson, A. B., Mukhamedrakhimov, R., et al. (2009). Early contact versus separation: Effects on mother–infant interaction one year later. *Birth, 36*, 97–109.

Caspi, A., McClay, J., Moffitt, T. E., Mill, J., Martin, J., Craig, I. W., et al. (2002). Role of genotype in the cycle of violence in maltreated children. *Science, 297*(5582), 851–854.

Caspi, A., Sugden, K., Moffitt, T. E., Taylor, A., Craig, I. W., Harrington, H., et al. (2003). Influence of life stress on depression: moderation by a polymorphism in the 5-HTT gene. *Science, 301*(5631), 386–389.

Fleming, A. S., Corter, C., Franks, P., Surbey, M., Schneider, B., & Steiner, M. (1993). Postpartum factors related to mother's attraction to newborn infant odors. *Developmental Psychobiology, 26*, 115–132.

Fleming, A. S., Ruble, D., Krieger, H., & Wong, P. Y. (1997). Hormonal and experiential correlates of maternal responsiveness during pregnancy and the puerperium in human mothers. *Hormones and Behavior, 31*, 145–158.

Fleming, A. S., Steiner, M., & Corter, C. (1997). Cortisol, hedonics, and maternal responsiveness in human mothers. *Hormones and Behavior, 32*, 85–98.

Gonzalez, A., Jenkins, J., Steiner, M., & Fleming, A. S. (submitted, under review). Neuropsychology and physiology: intervening variables between maternal early adversity and parenting.

Harris, K. M., Florey, F., Tabor, J., Bearman, P. S., Jones, J., & Udry, J. R. (2003). *The national longitudinal study of adolescent health: Research design.* Retrieved June 29, 2009, from http://www.cpc.unc.edu/projects/addhealth/design

Harris, K. M., Halpern, C. T., Smolen, A., & Haberstick, B. C. (2006). The National Longitudinal Study of Adolescent Health (Add Health) twin data. *Twin Research and Human Genetics, 9*, 988–997.

Lovic, V., Keer, D., Fletcher, P. J., & Fleming, A. S. (2010). Dissociative effects of early-life maternal separation and social isolation through artificial rearing on different forms of impulsivity. Manuscript submitted for publication.

Mileva, V. M., & Fleming, A. S. (2010). How mothers are born: A psychobiological analysis of mothering. In A. Booth, S. McHale, & N. S. Lansdale (Eds.), *Biosocial foundations of family processes* (pp. 3–34). New York: Springer.

Müller, D. J., Mandelli, L., Serretti, A., DeYoung, C. G., De Luca, V., Sicard, T., et al. (2008). Serotonin transporter gene and adverse life events in adult ADHD. *American Journal of Medical Genetics Part B (Neuropsychiatric Genetics), 147B*, 1461–1469.

Neiderhiser J. M., Reiss, D., Lichtenstein, P., Spotts, E. L., & Ganiban, J. (2007). Father-adolescent relationships and the role of genotype-environment correlation. *Journal of Family Psychology, 21*, 560–571.

Plomin, R., DeFries, J.C., McClearn, G.E., & McGuffin, P. (2008). *Behavioral genetics* (5th ed.). New York: Worth.

Schaal, B., & Porter, R. H., (1991). Microsmatic humans revisited: The generation and perception of chemical signals. *Advances in the Study of Behavior, 20*, 135–199.

Stallings, J., Fleming, A. S., Corter, C., Worthman, C., & Steiner, M. (2001). The effects of infant cries on affective, hormonal, and autonomic responses in new mothers and non-parturient women. *Parenting: Science & Practice, 1*, 71–100.

van IJzendoorn, M. H., Bakermans-Kranenburg, M. J., & Mesman J. (2008). Dopamine system genes associated with parenting in the context of daily hassles. *Genes, Brain and Behavavior, 7*, 403–410.

Part II
Development and Adjustment
in Adolescence

Chapter 5
Gene–Environment Interplay Helps to Explain Influences of Family Relationships on Adolescent Adjustment and Development

Jenae M. Neiderhiser

Abstract It is clear that the family relationships have important and lasting influences on adolescent adjustment and development. Genetically informed studies have provided additional information suggesting that these influences are due, at least in part, to the interplay of genetic and environmental factors via genotype–environment correlation and interaction. Understanding the relative contributions of genes and environment and how they operate together through family relationships to influence development and adjustment is critical for advancing our understanding of the mechanisms involved. With the rapid advances being made in molecular genetics and in brain function, the added value of the use of quantitative genetic strategies has become less clear. This chapter describes different aspects of gene–environment interplay as related to family relationships, discusses relevant findings that help to elucidate mechanisms, and proposes a strategy that combines advances across fields to better understand how family relationships influence adolescent adjustment and development.

Introduction

An extensive and established literature reports that family relationships have important and lasting influences on adolescent adjustment and development (e.g., Baumrind, 1991; Dishion & Bullock, 2002; Patterson, Dishion, & Yoerger, 2000). Most studies examining the impact of family relationships on child and adolescent development have not considered how genetic and environmental factors may operate in these associations. Until fairly recently, associations between family factors and the adjustment of children and adolescents have been assumed to reflect environmental influences of the family on development. Now that many studies have shown evidence for genetic influences on measures of family relationships (see Towers, Spotts, & Neiderhiser, 2002; Ulbricht & Neiderhiser, 2009 for reviews), including the effects of

J.M. Neiderhiser (✉)
Department of Psychology, The Pennsylvania State University, University Park, PA, USA
e-mail: jenaemn@psu.edu

A. Booth et al. (eds.), *Biosocial Foundations of Family Processes*,
National Symposium on Family Issues, DOI 10.1007/978-1-4419-7361-0_5,
© Springer Science+Business Media, LLC 2011

specific genes (e.g., Bakermans-Kranenburg & Van Ijzendoorn, 2008; Walum et al., 2008), it has become clear that the mechanisms of associations between family relationships and child and adolescent development are more complex.

In this chapter, I review work that has examined genetic influences on family relationships with a focus on studies of adolescents. Emphasis is given to studies that have considered how best to characterize and capture gene–environment interplay (genotype–environment correlation and genotype × environment interaction). A discussion of work that has attempted to translate findings from animal research into human designs is included to underscore the importance of gene–environment interplay across disciplines. Finally, I underscore the continued importance of quantitative genetic research as a tool for advancing our understanding of how genes and environments operate together.

Family Relationships and Adolescent Development

One of the most studied relationships within the family is that between parents and children. In general, such research has shown that high levels of parent–adolescent conflict and low levels of parental monitoring increase the likelihood that adolescents will develop conduct problems and participate in delinquent activities (Dishion & Kavanaugh, 2002; Fletcher, Steinberg, & Williams-Wheeler, 2004). As noted above, this association was often considered unidirectional – from the parents to the child. There were calls to consider the role of the child in parent–child relationships as early as the 1960s1968 (Bell, 1979) and, later, the role of parent characteristics and contextual factors (Belsky, 1984; Woodworth, Belsky, & Crnic, 1996). While researchers focused on parenting were beginning to recognize the role of the individual – both child and parent – in the parent–child relationship, researchers using genetically informed designs (studies of family members who vary in genetic relatedness) were beginning to examine individual differences in parent–child relationships in regard to genetic and environmental influences (Rowe, 1981, 1983). In both cases, the findings converged on the importance of the individual in influencing parent–child relationships and, subsequently, child and adolescent development.

Although parenting has been one of the most thoroughly studied family influences on child functioning, other aspects of family relationships have also been examined. Sibling relationships have been found to have an important influence on the development of adolescent behavior problems with more controlling and conflictual sibling behaviors increasing the risk of problems (e.g., Conger, Conger, & Scaramella, 1997; Kim, McHale, Crouter, & Osgood, 2007). The ways in which sibling relationships influence the adjustment of the children is somewhat less clear. It has been proposed that older siblings "train" their younger siblings to deviant behavior (Patterson, Dishion, & Bank, 1984), although at least one report suggests that the direction of effects for training is not always from the older to younger child (Natsuaki, Ge, Reiss, & Neiderhiser, 2009).

Marital relationship also has an impact on children and adolescents, both in regard to their healthy development (e.g., Cummings & Davies, 2002) and in their development of subsequent relationships with others (e.g., Amato & Booth, 2001). Recognizing that each dyad within the family does not operate in a vacuum, a number of studies have also examined how these family relationships operate together and/or have examined the family as a system in influencing child and adolescent development. Taken as a whole, it is clear that understanding how family relationships influence adolescent adjustment is crucial for understanding the development of problems.

As noted above, relatively few studies have examined associations among family relationships and adolescent adjustment using genetically informed designs. This is generally due to the fact that studies focused on measuring relationships of family members typically do not include family members who vary in the degree of genetic relatedness, while studies using genetically informed approaches typically do not include detailed measures of the family. The exceptions to this (e.g., Boivin et al., 2005; Leve, Neiderhiser, Scaramella, & Reiss, 2008; Neiderhiser & Lichtenstein, 2008; Neiderhiser, Reiss, & Hetherington, 2007) provide powerful evidence of the importance of genetic influences on the family factors (genotype–environment correlation: rGE) and of the role of family factors in moderating the genetic (and environmental) effects (genotype × environment interaction: G × E). Molecular genetic studies have examined both rGE and G × E, although such research tends to focus on cross-sectional data and/ or a single point in time with a single gene. Quantitative genetic designs – twin, sibling, adoption, and combination studies – on the other hand, have examined these questions within the framework of longitudinal studies and using complex assessments of the family relationships (e.g., Reiss, Neiderhiser, Hetherington, & Plomin, 2000).

The rapid advances being made in molecular genetics and in brain function raise the question of whether there is still a continued use for quantitative genetic research. The advances in molecular genetics and brain function are providing much more specific information on the biological mechanisms involved in influencing adjustment, and in some cases on environmental mechanisms. However, much remains to be gained from quantitative genetic studies, especially longitudinal approaches that carefully measure family relationships and other aspects of the social environment. These studies provide another tool that can continue to contribute to advancing our understanding of adjustment and to the complex interplay of genes and environment. Others have recently argued that such research is important for helping to understand causal influences, and particularly to better identify environmental influences on behavioral outcomes (Johnson, Turkheimer, Gottesman, & Bouchard, 2009). In order to better specify environmental influences on behavior it is essential to consider how genes and environments work together – gene–environment interplay.

Gene–Environment Interplay

Genotype–environment correlation (rGE). Correlations between genotype and environment have been recognized for several decades (Plomin, DeFries, & Loehlin, 1977; Scarr, 1992; Scarr & McCartney, 1983). Typically, three types of rGE are described: passive, evocative, and active. Passive rGE is the result of sharing both genes and environment simply because of the family you are reared in. Passive rGE is one explanation of correlations between children and their parents and other family members when the children are reared in a household with their biological relatives. When an individual's genes evoke a change or response in the environment evocative rGE is operating. For example, a temperamentally exuberant child may receive more supervision than a child who is more subdued in temperament. Finally, active rGE refers to an individual seeking out environments correlated with his/her genotype. A musically gifted adolescent (presuming musical ability is genetically influenced) may be more likely to seek the company of other musicians, thus providing himself/herself with a more musical environment. Understanding which type of rGE is operating helps to clarify the types of mechanisms that may be involved in influencing adjustment as well as informing us how the social environment may be operating.

Only fairly recently, however, have efforts been made to identify both when rGE is present and to understand the type of rGE operating. There has been a great deal of study of rGE, especially in relation to parenting and adolescent adjustment. A number of studies have examined genetic influences on parenting using studies of children who are twins (e.g., Boivin et al., 2005; McGue, Elkins, Walden, & Iacono, 2005) as well as of parents who are twins (e.g., Kendler, 1996; Losoya, Callor, Rowe, & Goldsmith, 1997). Generally, such studies have provided evidence for genetic influences on parental warmth and conflict and occasionally control, but less or no genetic influences on monitoring. Shared environmental influences, or those nongenetic factors that increase the similarity of family members, are important for studies of child twins, but less so for studies of parent twins. Nonshared environmental influences (nongenetic factors that account for differences in family members including measurement error) are more important for studies of parent twins, although they are also present in studies of child twins. These findings can be interpreted as indicating that the within-family environment has an important influence on parent–adolescent relationships. In studies of child twins, this is illustrated by shared environmental influences on parent–adolescent relationships. The same within-family environmental factors will result in *nonshared environmental* effects in a study of twin parents as they are parents of different children in different households. This set of findings provides strong evidence for the importance of the within-family environment *as well as* genetic influences of parents and children on parent–child relationships. In other words, these findings suggest that both passive and evocative rGE and nongenetic environmental factors are influencing the relationships of parents and children.

In an effort to specify the type(s) of rGE for parent–adolescent relationships, one set of studies used a comparison of two studies of the parenting of adolescents. Specifically, a study of twin parents of an adolescent child and of adolescent twins and their parents using identical measures of parenting estimated genetic and environmental influences on mother–adolescent and father–adolescent relationships (Neiderhiser, Reiss, Lichtenstein, Spotts, & Ganiban, 2007; Neiderhiser et al., 2004). Four broad constructs of parent–adolescent relationships were examined: positivity (closeness, warmth, and support), negativity (conflict, harsh discipline), monitoring (knowledge of child's behavior and whereabouts), and control (both attempts and success in controlling your child's behavior). Although there was some variation based on reporters, this set of studies found evidence for both passive and evocative *r*GE for parent–adolescent relationships with some evidence that evocative *r*GE is more important for father's positivity, while mother's positivity was best explained by passive *r*GE. There was also clear evidence of nongenetic contributions to parent–adolescent relationships, with sizable shared and nonshared environmental influences in the adolescent twin sample and primarily nonshared environmental influences in the twin parent sample.

The focus of research on parenting is how it influences child and adolescent development and functioning. There are a number of studies that have examined genetic and environmental influences on associations between parent–adolescent relationships and adolescent adjustment (e.g., Pike, McGuire, Hetherington, & Reiss, 1996). Because these studies are decomposing covariation between parenting and adolescent adjustment, they all focus on children who vary in the degree of genetic relatedness. Thus, it is implied that genetic influences on these associations are best described as evocative *r*GE correlations. Some studies have attempted to understand how child characteristics may mediate these associations – in other words, what is the process through which children evoke responses from their parents that then influence their later behavior (e.g., Narusyte, Andershed, Neiderhiser, & Lichtenstein, 2007). Other studies have taken advantage of longitudinal designs to specify the order of influences – from parenting to adolescent behavior or vice versa – thus allowing evocative *r*GE to be identified (Burt, McGue, Krueger, & Iacono, 2005; Neiderhiser, Reiss, Hetherington, & Plomin, 1999). Although all of these efforts have contributed to our understanding of *r*GE and helped to clarify how these processes operate for adolescents, none have been able to clearly distinguish, within the same model, passive from evocative *r*GE.

A combination design that includes parents who are twins and their children (Children of Twins (COT)) was first proposed as a solution to understanding the contributions of genes and environment within the full family context (Silberg & Eaves, 2004). Specifically, a COT design helps to disentangle passive *r*GE from purely environmental influences of parents on children. However, if one is equally interested in identifying both evocative and passive *r*GE, an additional step of including children who are twins must be taken, thus resulting in an Extended COT (ECOT) design (Narusyte et al., 2008). In this design, parenting and child adjustment are examined simultaneously using a causal model in an effort to tease apart passive and evocative *r*GE and direct environmental effects. One such report examined maternal emotional overinvolvement and adolescent internalizing problems and found that evocative *r*GE provided the best explanation for this association (Narusyte et al.). In other words, adolescents who had higher levels of internalizing behavior elicited more emotional overinvolvement from their mothers.

These findings provide clear evidence that genotype–environment correlation is operating in the parent–child relationship. Some of these findings are also beginning to provide clues about how this is operating. For example, finding evidence of child aggressive temperament explains half of the genetic covariation between parental criticism and adolescent delinquency (Narusyte et al., 2007). This not only indicates that evocative *r*GE is operating but provides an opening for potentially changing the outcome. Understanding how *r*GE operates and what type of *r*GE is important for which family relationships can help us to change behaviors in order to improve outcomes and reduce the likelihood of problematic outcomes. For example, parents who do not respond to the adolescent's aggression with criticism may be able to decrease the likelihood of adolescent delinquency, thus improving the likely outcome of the adolescent while also eliminating the genotype–environment correlation.

The above example provides one explanation for why understanding *r*GE is important – to help provide additional information about likely targets for intervention. A second reason that *r*GE is important is that it is likely to be ubiquitous, especially within the family. A handful of studies have found genetic influences on marital relationships (Reiss et al., 2000; Spotts, Neiderhiser, Towers, et al., 2004; Spotts, Prescott, & Kendler, 2006), divorce (McGue & Lykken, 1992), and associations between marital relationships and the adjustment of adult twins (Spotts, Neiderhiser, Ganiban, et al., 2004; Spotts, Pederson, et al., 2005). The findings from these studies also suggest a role for *r*GE, with additional analyses indicating that the personality of the adult twins accounts for some or all of the genetic influences on marital quality (Spotts, Lichtenstein, et al., 2005) and divorce (Jocklin, McGue, & Lykken, 1996). It is less clear in the context of marital relationships and adult adjustment how to conceptualize the types of *r*GE, however. Of particular relevance to the current chapter are the findings that the covariation between marital conflict about the adolescent and adolescent antisocial behavior is due in large part to the genetic influences of the child (Reiss et al., 2000). In other words, adolescents who are getting into more trouble are eliciting more conflict between their parents for reasons to do with the adolescent's genes, an evocative *r*GE.

In sum, a now sizable literature has examined genetic influences on family relationships. Not all of these studies have considered the role of *r*GE, although inferences about how *r*GE is operating can still be drawn. The clear conclusion of this body of work is that *r*GE is important for parenting, marital relationships, and adolescent adjustment. The type of *r*GE operating appears to be both passive and evocative *r*GE, with genetically influenced characteristics of the adolescents influencing both the way they are parented or parent–adolescent relationships as well as conflict within the marriage. Although some of this work has relied on "traditional" twin or sibling studies, the use of novel and combination designs is allowing us to better understand the processes involved in *r*GE and permit us to have more confidence in our findings.

Genotype × environment interaction (G × E). It is now possible to examine G × E within quantitative genetic designs using normative samples (Purcell, 2002; Purcell & Koenen, 2005). Specifically, differences in genetic, shared environmental and nonshared environmental influences on a particular construct (i.e., adolescent conduct problems) can be examined as a function of a variation in a specific environment. The specific environment may be dichotomous (i.e., presence or absence of child abuse) or continuous (i.e., parent–child conflict). These methodological advances have provided the field with the tools necessary to begin to disentangle how specific constructs may moderate the genetic and latent environmental factors typically estimated in quantitative genetic studies. Prior to these methodological advances it was only possible to consider G × E when dramatic differences in the environment were available (e.g., Heath et al., 1985) or by using adoption designs (e.g., Cadoret, Cain, & Crowe, 1983). Although both strategies were powerful, these constraints severely limited the work that was able to be done in this area.

A plethora of quantitative genetic studies now are examining G × E, with most finding evidence of the moderation of genetic influences as a function of some measured environmental factor (e.g., Button, Scourfield, Martin, Purcell, & McGuffin, 2005; Dick, Rose, Viken, Kaprio, & Koskenvuo, 2001; Lau, Gregory, Goldwin, Pine, & Eley, 2007). For example, in a sample of Swedish adolescent twins, genetic influences on antisocial behavior were greater when social economic status (SES) was high, while shared environmental influences were greater when SES was low (Tuvblad, Grann, & Lichtenstein, 2006). A similar pattern of findings was found for SES and IQ in young children (Turkheimer, Haley, Waldron, D'Onofrio, & Gottesman, 2003). In general, studies examining moderation of genetic and environmental influences have found that genetic, shared environmental, and nonshared environmental influences may vary as a function of the environment.

Many of the published studies of G × E have typically used moderators that are general, like SES, and/or constructs that may comprise social environmental risk factors and other commonly measured variables like negative life events (e.g., Hicks, South, DiRago, Iacono, & McGue, 2009; Lau et al., 2007). However, a number of studies have examined family environment constructs as potential moderators (e.g., Button, Lau, Maughan, & Eley, 2008; Dick et al., 2007; Feinberg, Button, Neiderhiser, Reiss, & Hetherington, 2007; Leve et al., 2010). One study focused on adolescent smoking behavior found that when parental monitoring was high genetic influences on adolescent smoking were low and shared environmental influences were high, while the reverse was true when parental monitoring was low (Dick et al., 2007). In other words, if parents closely monitor their adolescents any genetic propensity toward smoking becomes less important, only coming into play when parental monitoring is low. A different report examining antisocial behavior in adolescent twins and siblings found that when levels of parental negativity were high or parental warmth was low that genetic influences were greater (Feinberg et al., 2007). Taken together, these two sets of findings suggest that when overall parenting is poor – low monitoring, high conflict, and low warmth – an adolescent's genetic propensities toward problematic behaviors are higher. In other words, adolescents at risk for genetic reasons are at increased risk when the environment is also problematic. What is still unclear in this work is why this is the case. Some have proposed that "genetic risk" or "genetic vulnerability" would be better characterized as genetically influenced sensitivity to the environment (e.g., Belsky & Pluess, 2009; Caspi & Moffitt, 2006; Kim-Cohen & Gold, 2009; Reiss & Leve, 2007). Additional work, especially work combining neuroscience with genetics, is needed to better specify how G × E is operating.

Finally, studies have now begun to consider how constructs other than "environment" may moderate genetic and environmental influences on behavior. These studies are worth mentioning here as they are advancing our understanding of how genetic and environmental influences on behavior may operate. For example, a recent report found that the patterns of genetic and environmental influences on aggressive and nonaggressive delinquent antisocial behavior in adolescents varied as a function of the age of the adolescents (Burt & Neiderhiser, 2009). Specifically, the relative levels of genetic and environmental influences on aggressive antisocial behavior remained stable across adolescence, while genetic influences on nonaggressive delinquency increased with age and shared environmental influences decreased. A similar strategy of using age as a moderator of genetic and environmental influences has been used to examine daily diary reports of emotional distress in an adult sample (Neiss & Almeida, 2004). Both of the above reports represent a novel approach to better understanding how genes and environments influence development and help to advance our understanding of the underlying processes that may be involved.

Considering both rGE and G × E. We are now beginning to examine how measures of social environment may operate and interact together to influence child and adolescent adjustment. Specifically, we have found evidence for the moderation of parent–adolescent negativity by marital conflict, with higher levels of marital conflict increasing evocative rGE for mother's negativity and increasing the influence of nonshared environmental influences for father's negativity (Ulbricht, 2009). In other words, there is now evidence of an rGE × E interaction. Evidence for rGE × E interaction has also been found using data from a sample of adopted infants, their adopted parents, and their birth parent(s) (Hajal et al., 2008). Specifically, evocative rGE effects were found for father's overreactive parenting only in families with high levels of marital warmth, and no evidence of rGE was found for mother's parenting. A different study found that adolescent personality moderated genetic and environmental influences on parent–adolescent relationships in a large sample of 17-year-old twins (South, Krueger, Johnson, & Iacono, 2008). In other words, adolescents' personality may have an impact on the relevance of rGE in their relationship with their parents.

The importance of considering rGE when examining G × E is underscored by the studies described above. If rGE changes as a function of variation in other aspects of the family environment and/or as a function of the child's personality, a more nuanced approach is needed for considering both rGE and G × E. One such approach is suggested by Price and Jaffee (2008), although their focus is on passive rGE. Most studies of G × E that include a measure of family environment or relationships use a strategy that first accounts for the main effects of the moderator on the behavior under study (Purcell & Koenen, 2005), although, as noted by Price and Jaffee (2008), this does not control for the effects of passive rGE. What is clear from the work to date is that the field is rapidly moving from a focus on relative proportions of genetic and environmental influences on behavior to one that considers how genetic and environmental factors may operate together. By combining approaches, samples, and methods we are likely to get a more complete understanding of the interplay between genes and environments.

Crossing the Divide

One strategy for moving beyond a focus on genetic and environmental influences on behaviors is to integrate across multiple disciplines to better understand the mechanisms of behavior and of gene–environment interplay. In this section, an example of how a particular set of genetic findings in animal research on relational behaviors were extended into human molecular genetic research is described, with the objective of helping to underscore how findings from different areas can help to inform one another. Finally, the chapter concludes with a discussion of how quantitative genetic research can continue to inform the field, especially in regard to family relationships.

Voles and humans. In a series of studies Young and colleagues were able to establish that differences in social pair bonding behaviors in two species of voles could be explained by variation in a particular gene in males (Hammock & Young, 2005; Lim et al., 2004). The *vasopressin 1a receptor (avpr1a)* gene regulates vasopressin 1a receptor expression in the brain of voles, and variation in the *avpr1a* gene in males, but not females, explains species differences in social pair bonding for prairie voles vs. montane voles. Additional work in this area suggests that oxytocin receptors operate similarly in female voles, although the genetic factors contributing to this difference are not yet known (Donaldson & Young, 2008; Young & Wang, 2004). In order to extend this work to human behavior, a recent report examined associations between variation in the human *AVPR1A* gene and a measure of partner-bonding in male and female couples (Walum et al., 2008). Findings from this study indicated that men who had a particular allele (334) of polymorphism RS3 on the *AVPR1A* gene had significantly lower levels of partner bonding than men who did not carry this allele. This effect was not found for women. Another natural extension of this work with voles is to examine the role of oxytocin receptor genes (*OXTR*) in explaining differences in parenting behaviors as caretaking of offspring is characteristic of the social bonding behavior in voles. In one such study, associations of *OXTR* and maternal sensitivity were found with some evidence of a gene–gene interaction between the serotonin transporter gene and *OXTR* (Bakermans-Kranenburg & Van Ijzendoorn, 2008).

The work with *avpr1a* in voles is groundbreaking in that it was one of the earliest efforts to establish a clear link between a specific gene and a pattern of social behaviors. The human extensions of this work have focused on family relationships in areas similar to the behaviors observable in voles and have found findings that support the cross-species comparisons. Other studies have examined other aspects of social pair bonding behavior and the *AVPR1A* gene in humans (e.g., Wassink et al., 2004; Yirmiya et al., 2006), although a review of this work is beyond the scope of the current report. The findings from the literature on humans extend the work in voles in that subtle variations in social behavior within the family are associated with the same gene variations that result in gross differences in species of voles. This emphasizes the value of carefully considering all of the literature – regardless of discipline – when attempting to understand how genes and environments may operate together to influence behavior.

Conclusion

This chapter has attempted to provide a brief overview of work focused on understanding how genes and environments work together to influence adolescent adjustment – particularly externalizing behaviors. The role of family relationships has been a guiding theme throughout, both because of the importance of family relationships in helping to shape adolescent adjustment and because there is now evidence that genetic factors may influence behavior *through* family relationships. Understanding the types of genotype–environment correlations can help us to understand more about the processes through which genetic factors shape the environment, and considering both genotype–environment correlation and interaction in influencing developmental outcomes is critical.

Although the traditional twin study focused on estimating genetic and environmental influences on various behaviors is not likely to contribute much to our understanding of gene–environment interplay, there is still an important role for quantitative genetics. A number of strategies can continue to inform us about how genes and environment work together and may also be able to provide information about the direction of effects or causation (Johnson et al., 2009; Vitaro, Brendgen, & Arseneault, 2009). Specifically, combining studies of child twins and twin parents can help us to disentangle passive and evocative rGE from direct environmental influences. Examining identical twin differences clarifies direct effects of nonshared environment, and adoption designs eliminate the confounder of passive rGE and facilitate the identification of both evocative rGE and G × E interactions. These designs will only help to advance the field, however, if they also include careful and precise measurement of the environment including family relationships over time. It is unlikely that any one study can meet all of these requirements. By combining our efforts, across disciplines, samples, and designs, we will be able to better specify the mechanisms involved in development and thus be able to design more targeted interventions that may be more likely to have a positive impact.

References

Amato, P. R., & Booth, A. (2001). The legacy of parents' marital discord: Consequences for children's marital quality. *Journal of Personality and Social Psychology, 81*(4), 627–638.

Bakermans-Kranenburg, M. J., & Van Ijzendoorn, M. H. (2008). Oxytocin receptor (OXTR) and serotonin transporter (5-HTT) genes associated with observed parenting. *Social Cognitive and Affective Neuroscience, 3*, 138–134.

Baumrind, D. (1991). The influence of parenting style on adolescent competence and substance use. *Journal of Early Adolescence, 11*(1), 56–95.

Bell, R. Q. (1968). A reinterpretation of the direction of effects in studies of socialization. *Psychological Review, 75*, 81–95.

Bell, R. Q. (1979). Parent, child and reciprocal influences. *American Psychologist, 34*, 821–826.

Belsky, J. (1984). The determinants of parenting: A process model. *Child Development, 55*(1), 83–96.

Belsky, J., & Pluess, M. (2009). The nature (and nurture?) of plasticity in early human development. *Perspectives on Psychological Science, 4*(4), 345–351.

Boivin, M., Perusse, D., Dionne, G., Saysset, V., Zoccolillo, M., Tarabulsy, G. M., et al. (2005). The genetic–environmental etiology of parents' perceptions and self-assessed behaviours toward their 5-month-old infants in a large twin and singleton sample. *Journal of Child Psychology and Psychiatry, 46*(6), 612–630.

Burt, S. A., McGue, M., Krueger, R. F., & Iacono, W. G. (2005). How are parent-child conflict and childhood externalizing symptoms related over time? Results from a genetically informative cross-lagged study. *Development and Psychopathology, 17*, 145–165.

Burt, S. A., & Neiderhiser, J. M. (2009). Aggressive versus nonaggressive antisocial behavior: Distinctive etiological moderation by age. *Developmental Psychology, 45*(4), 11.

Button, T. M. M., Lau, J. Y. F., Maughan, B., & Eley, T. C. (2008). Parental punitive discipline, negative life events and gene–environment interplay in the development of externalizing behavior. *Psychological Medicine, 38*(1), 29–39.

Button, T. M. M., Scourfield, J., Martin, N., Purcell, S., & McGuffin, P. (2005). Family dysfunction interacts with genes in the causation of antisocial symptoms. *Behavior Genetics, 35*(2), 115–120.

Cadoret, R., Cain, C. A., & Crowe, R. R. (1983). Evidence for gene-environment interaction in the development of adolescent antisocial behavior. *Behavior Genetics, 13*(3), 301–310.

Caspi, A., & Moffitt, T. E. (2006). Gene-environment interactions in psychiatry: Joining forces with neuroscience. *Nature Reviews. Neuroscience, 7*, 583–590.

Conger, K. J., Conger, R. D., & Scaramella, L. V. (1997). Parents, siblings, psychological control, and adolescent adjustment. *Journal of Adolescent Research, 12*(1), 113–138.

Cummings, E., & Davies, P. T. (2002). Effects of marital conflict on children: Recent advances and emerging themes in process-oriented research. *Journal of Child Psychology and Psychiatry, 43*(1), 31–63.

Dick, D. M., Rose, R. J., Viken, R. J., Kaprio, J., & Koskenvuo, M. (2001). Exploring gene-environment interactions: Socioregional moderation of alcohol use. *Journal of Abnormal Psychology, 110*(4), 625–632.

Dick, D. M., Viken, R., Purcell, S., Kaprio, J., Pulkkinen, L., & Rose, R. J. (2007). Parental monitoring moderates the importance of genetic and environmental influences on adolescent smoking. *Journal of Abnormal Psychology, 116*(1), 213–218.

Dishion, T. J., & Bullock. (2002). Parenting and adolescent problem behavior: An ecological analysis of the nurturance hypothesis. In J. G. Borkowski, S. L. Ramey, & M. Bristol-Power (Eds.), *Parenting and the child's world: Influences on academic, intellectual, and social-emotional development*. Mahwah, NJ: Lawrence Erlbaum Associates.

Dishion, T. J., Kavanaugh, K, J.B. Reid, G.R. Patterson & J.J. Snyde B. M. (2002). The Adolescent Transitions Program: A family-centered prevention strategy for schools. In J. B. Reid, G. R. Patterson, et al. (Eds.), *Antisocial behavior in children and adolescents: A developmental analysis and model for intervention* (pp. 257–272). Washington, DC: American Psychological Association.

Donaldson, Z. R., & Young, L. J. (2008). Oxytocin, vasopressin, and the neurogenetics of sociality. *Science, 322*(5903), 900–904.

Feinberg, M. E., Button, T. M. M., Neiderhiser, J. M., Reiss, D., & Hetherington, E. M. (2007). Parenting and adolescent antisocial behavior and depression: Evidence of genotype x parenting environment interaction. *Archives of General Psychiatry, 64*(4), 457–465.

Fletcher, A. C., Steinberg, L., & Williams-Wheeler, M. (2004). Parental influences on adolescent problem behavior: Revisiting Stattin and Kerr. *Child Development, 75*(3), 781–796.

Hajal, N. J., Moore, G. A., Shaw, D. S., Leve, L. D., Neiderhiser, J. M., & Reiss, D. (2008). Infant Temperament, Marital Relationship, and Parenting in Adoptive Families. (abstract). *Behavior Genetics, 38*, 629.

Hammock, E. A. D., & Young, L. J. (2005). Microsatellite instability generates diversity in brain and sociobehavioral traits. *Science, 308*, 1630–1634.

Heath, A. C., Berg, K., Eaves, L. J., Sclaas, M. H., Corey, L. A., Sunder, J., et al. (1985). Education policy and the heritability of educational attainment. *Nature, 314*(6013), 734–736.

Hicks, B. M., South, S. C., DiRago, A. C., Iacono, W. G., & McGue, M. (2009). Environmental adversity and increasing genetic risk for externalizing disorders. *Archives of General Psychiatry, 66*(6), 3.

Jocklin, V., McGue, M., & Lykken, D. T. (1996). Personality and divorce: A genetic analysis. *Journal of Personality and Social Psychology, 71*(2), 288–299.

Johnson, W., Turkheimer, E., Gottesman, I. I., & Bouchard, T. J., Jr. (2009). Beyond heritability: Twin studies in behavioral research. *Current Directions in Psychological Science, 18*(4), 217–220.

Kendler, K. S. (1996). Parenting: A genetic-epidemiologic perspective. *American Journal of Psychiatry, 153*(1), 11–20.

Kim-Cohen, J., & Gold, A. L. (2009). Measured gene-environment interactions and mechanisms promoting resilient development. *Current Directions in Psychological Science, 18*(3), 138–142.

Kim, J. Y., McHale, S. M., Crouter, A. C., & Osgood, D. W. (2007). Longitudinal linkages between sibling relationships and adjustment from middle childhood through adolescence. *Developmental Psychology, 43*, 960–973.

Lau, J. Y. F., Gregory, A. M., Goldwin, M. A., Pine, D. S., & Eley, T. C. (2007). Assessing gene–environment interactions on anxiety symptom subtypes across childhood and adolescence. *Development and Psychopathology. Special Issue: Gene-Environment Interaction, 19*(4), 1129–1146.

Leve, L. D., Kerr, D. C., Shaw, D., Ge, X., Neiderhiser, J. M., Scaramella, L. V., et al. (2010). Infant pathways to externalizing behavior: Evidence of genotype x environment interaction. *Child Development, 81*(1), 340–356.

Leve, L. D., Neiderhiser, J. M., Scaramella, L. V., & Reiss, D. (2008). The Early Growth and Development Study: Using the prospective adoption design to examine genotype-environment interplay. *Acta Psychologica Sinica, 40*(10), 1106–1115.

Lim, M. M., Wang, Z., Olazabal, D. E., Ren, X., Terwilliger, E. F., & Young, L. J. (2004). Enhanced partner preference in a promiscuous species by manipulating the expression of a single gene. *Nature, 429*, 754–757.

Losoya, S. H., Callor, S., Rowe, D. C., & Goldsmith, H. H. (1997). Origins of familial similarity in parenting: A study of twins and adoptive siblings. *Developmental Psychology, 33*(6), 1012–1023.

McGue, M., Elkins, I., Walden, B., & Iacono, W. G. (2005). Perceptions of the parent–adolescent relationship: A longitudinal investigation. *Developmental Psychology, 41*(6), 971–984.

McGue, M., & Lykken, D. T. (1992). Genetic influence on risk of divorce. *Psychological Science, 3*(6), 368–373.

Narusyte, J., Andershed, A.-K., Neiderhiser, J. M., & Lichtenstein, P. (2007). Aggression as a mediator of genetic contributions to the association between negative parent-child relationships and adolescent antisocial behavior. *European Child & Adolescent Psychiatry, 16*(2), 128–137.

Narusyte, J., Neiderhiser, J. M., D'Onofrio, B., Reiss, D., Spotts, E. L., Ganiban, J., et al. (2008). Testing different types of genotype–environment correlation: An extended children-of-twins model. *Developmental Psychology, 44*(6), 1591–1603.

Natsuaki, M. N., Ge, X., Reiss, D., & Neiderhiser, J. M. (2009). Aggressive behavior between siblings and the development of externalizing problems: Evidence from a genetically sensitive study. *Developmental Psychology, 45*(4), 11.

Neiderhiser, J. M., & Lichtenstein, P. (2008). The Twin and Offspring Study in Sweden: Advancing our understanding of genotype–environment interplay by studying twins and their families. *Acta Psychologica Sinica, 40*(10), 1116–1123.

Neiderhiser, J. M., Reiss, D., Hetherington, E., & Plomin, R. (1999). Relationships between parenting and adolescent adjustment over time: Genetic and environmental contributions. *Developmental Psychology, 35*(3), 680–692.

Neiderhiser, J. M., Reiss, D., & Hetherington, E. M. (2007). The Nonshared Environment in Adolescent Development (NEAD) Project: A longitudinal family study of twins and siblings from adolescence to young adulthood. *Twin Research and Human Genetics, 10*(1), 74–83.

Neiderhiser, J. M., Reiss, D., Lichtenstein, P., Spotts, E. L., & Ganiban, J. (2007). Father–adolescent relationships and the role of genotype-environment correlation. *Journal of Family Psychology, 21*(4), 560–571.

Neiderhiser, J. M., Reiss, D., Pedersen, N. L., Lichtenstein, P., Spotts, E. L., Hansson, K., et al. (2004). Genetic and environmental influences on mothering of adolescents: A comparison of two samples. *Developmental Psychology, 40*(3), 335–351.

Neiss, M., & Almeida, D. M. (2004). Age differences in the heritability of mean and intraindividual variation of psychological distress. *Gerontology, 50*, 22–27.

Patterson, G. R., Dishion, T., & Bank, L. (1984). Family interaction: A process model of deviancy training. *Aggressive Behavior, 10*(3), 253–267.

Patterson, G. R., Dishion, T. J., & Yoerger, K. (2000). Adolescent growth in new forms of problem behavior: Macro- and micro-peer dynamics. *Prevention Science, 1*(1), 3–13.

Pike, A., McGuire, S., Hetherington, E., & Reiss, D. (1996). Family environment and adolescent depressive symptoms and antisocial behavior: A multivariate genetic analysis. *Developmental Psychology, 32*(4), 590–604.

Plomin, R., DeFries, J. C., & Loehlin, J. C. (1977). Genotype-environment interaction and correlation in the analysis of human behavior. *Psychological Bulletin, 84*, 309–322.

Price, T. S., & Jaffee, S. (2008). Effects of the family environment: Gene-environment interaction and passive gene-environment correlation. *Developmental Psychology, 44*(2), 305–315.

Purcell, S. (2002). Variance components models for gene-environment interaction in twin analysis. *Twin Research, 5*(6), 554–571.

Purcell, S., & Koenen, K. C. (2005). Environmental mediation and the twin design. *Behavior Genetics, 35*(4), 491–498.

Reiss, D., & Leve, L. D. (2007). Genetic expression outside the skin: Clues to mechanisms of genotype x environment interaction. *Development and Psychopathology, 19*, 1005–1027.

Reiss, D., Neiderhiser, J. M., Hetherington, E. M., & Plomin, R. (2000). *The relationship code: Deciphering genetic and social influences on adolescent development.* Cambridge, MA: Harvard University Press.

Rowe, D. C. (1981). Environmental and genetic influences on dimensions of perceived parenting: A twin study. *Developmental Psychology, 17*, 203–208.

Rowe, D. C. (1983). A biometrical analysis of perceptions of family environment: A study of twins and singleton sibling kinships. *Child Development, 54*, 416–423.

Scarr, S. (1992). Developmental theories for the 1990's: Development and individual differences. *Child Development, 63*(1), 1–19.

Scarr, S., & McCartney, K. (1983). How people make their own environments: A theory of genotype –> environment effects. *Child Development, 54*, 424–435.

Silberg, J., & Eaves, L. (2004). Analysing the contributions of genes and parent–child interaction to childhood behavioural and emotional problems: A model for the children of twins. *Psychological Medicine, 34*(2), 347–356.

South, S. C., Krueger, R. F., Johnson, W., & Iacono, W. G. (2008). Adolescent personality moderates genetic and environmental influences on relationships with parents. *Journal of Personality and Social Psychology, 94*(5), 899–912.

Spotts, E. L., Lichtenstein, P., Pedersen, N., Neiderhiser, J. M., Hansson, K., Cederblad, M., et al. (2005). Personality and marital satisfaction: A behavioural genetic analysis. *European Journal of Personality, 19*(3), 205–227.

Spotts, E. L., Neiderhiser, J. M., Ganiban, J., Reiss, D., Lichtenstein, P., Hansson, K., et al. (2004). Accounting for depressive symptoms in women: A twin study of associations with interpersonal relationships. *Journal of Affective Disorders, 82*(1), 101–111.

Spotts, E. L., Neiderhiser, J. M., Towers, H., Hansson, K., Lichtenstein, P., Cederblad, M., et al. (2004). Genetic and environmental influences on marital relationships. *Journal of Family Psychology, 18*(1), 107–119.

Spotts, E. L., Pederson, N. L., Neiderhiser, J. M., Reiss, D., Lichtenstein, P., Hansson, K., et al. (2005). Genetic effects on women's positive mental health: Do marital relationships and social support matter? *Journal of Family Psychology, 19*(3), 339–349.

Spotts, E. L., Prescott, C., & Kendler, K. (2006). Examining the origins of gender differences in marital quality: A behavior genetic analysis. *Journal of Family Psychology, 20*(4), 605–613.

Towers, H., Spotts, E. L., & Neiderhiser, J. M. (2002). Genetic and environmental influences on parenting and marital relationships: Current findings and future directions. *Marriage & Family Review, 33*(1), 11–29.

Turkheimer, E., Haley, A., Waldron, M., D'Onofrio, B., & Gottesman, I. I. (2003). Socioeconomic status modifies heritability of IQ in young children. *Psychological Science, 14*(6), 623–628.

Tuvblad, C., Grann, M., & Lichtenstein, P. (2006). Heritability for adolescent antisocial behavior differs with socioeconomic status: Gene-environment interaction. *Journal of Child Psychology and Psychiatry, 47*(7), 734–743.

Ulbricht, J. (2009). *The role of gene and environment interplay in the interaction of family subsystems.* Washington, DC: George Washington University.

Ulbricht, J. A., & Neiderhiser, J. M. (2009). Genotype-environment correlation and family relationships. New York: Springer Science+Business Media.

Vitaro, F., Brendgen, M., & Arseneault, L. (2009). The discordant MZ-twin method: One step closer to the holy grail of causality. *International Journal of Behavioral Development, 33*(4), 376–382.

Walum, H., Westberg, L., Henningsson, S., Neiderhiser, J. M., Reiss, D., Igl, W., et al. (2008). Genetic variation in the vasopressin receptor 1a gene (AVPR1A) associates with pair-bonding behavior in humans. *Proceedings of the National Academy of Sciences of the United States of America, 105*(37), 20.

Wassink, T. H., Priven, J., Vieland, V. J., Pietila, J., Goedken, R. J., Folstein, S. E., et al. (2004). Examination of *AVPR1a* as an autism susceptibility gene. *Molecular Psychiatry, 9*, 968–972.

Woodworth, S., Belsky, J., & Crnic, K. (1996). The determinants of fathering during the child's second and third years of life: A developmental analysis. *Journal of Marriage and the Family, 58*(3), 679–692.

Yirmiya, N., Rosenberg, C., Levi, S., Salomon, S., Shulman, C., Nemanov, L., et al. (2006). Association between the arginine vasopressin 1a receptor (*AVPR1a*) gene and autism in a family-based study: Mediation by socialization skills. *Molecular Psychiatry, 11*(5), 488–494.

Young, L. J., & Wang, Z. (2004). The neurobiology of pair bonding. *Nature Neuroscience, 7*(10), 1048–1054.

Chapter 6
The Importance of the Phenotype
in Explorations of Gene–Environment Interplay

S. Alexandra Burt

Abstract Prior research has ably highlighted the likely role of gene–environment interplay in adolescent development, with a specific focus on gene–environment transactions involving the family of origin. One issue that researchers should attend to closely when exploring gene–environment interplay, however, is that of the phenotype (or observed behavior) under study. Namely, given the different demographic patterns, behavioral expressions, and developmental trajectories that characterize various adolescent outcomes (e.g., depression vs. substance abuse), one would a priori expect the role of gene–environment interplay to also vary across these outcomes. In this chapter, I argue that gene–environment interplay is not a "one-size-fits-all phenomenon" via the use of a specific example. In particular, I illustrate the differential role of gene–environment interplay across two related forms of antisocial behavior (i.e., physical aggression and nonaggressive rule breaking).

Introduction

Neiderhiser (Chap. 5) ably discussed the role of gene–environment interplay in adolescent adjustment and development, with a specific focus on gene–environment transactions involving the family of origin. It is hoped that these sorts of incisive reviews will stimulate researchers to substantively consider the probable role of gene–environment interplay in both normative and atypical development. One issue that researchers should attend to closely when exploring gene–environment interplay, however, is that of the phenotype (or observed behavior) under study. Namely, given the different demographic patterns, behavioral expressions, and developmental trajectories that characterize various adolescent outcomes (e.g., antisocial behavior as compared to depression), one would not necessarily expect the role of gene–environment interplay to be invariant across these outcomes.

S.A. Burt (✉)
Department of Psychology, Michigan State University, East Lansing, MI, USA
e-mail: burts@msu.edu

A. Booth et al. (eds.), *Biosocial Foundations of Family Processes*,
National Symposium on Family Issues, DOI 10.1007/978-1-4419-7361-0_6,
© Springer Science+Business Media, LLC 2011

Even so, a quick review of the relevant literature clearly suggests that phenotype in question is only rarely considered. Instead, it appears that researchers are considering possible gene–environment interactions across virtually all phenotypes, regardless of their their developmental patterns or phenotypic expression.

Below, I argue that gene–environment interplay is not a "one-size-fits-all phenomenon" via the use a specific example. I specifically illustrate the differential role of gene–environment interplay across two related forms of antisocial behavior (a particularly trenchant example given that both subtypes are subsumed within the broader construct of antisocial behavior). In doing so, I first present evidence of meaningful demographic, developmental, and etiologic differences between physically aggressive (AGG) and nonaggressive, rule-breaking (RB) forms of antisocial behavior. I then discuss differences in the timing of genetic expression across these behavioral subtypes and the implications these results have for the respective role of gene–environment interplay in AGG as compared to RB. I close by offering hypotheses as to the origin of these differences.

Meaningful Differences Between AGG and RB

Antisocial behavior describes a wide variety of actions and attitudes that violate societal norms and the personal or property rights of others (e.g., running away, vandalism, hurting animals, setting fires, theft, and bullying/assault). Though generally conceptualized as a single construct, extant research has begun to illuminate meaningful distinctions within the broader construct of antisocial behavior. For example, the factor analytic literature has consistently indicated that there are at least two oblique factors within antisocial behavior, an "overt" or aggressive/oppositional factor and a "covert" or nonaggressive/delinquent factor (DeMarte, 2008; Frick et al., 1993; Loeber & Schmaling, 1985; Tackett, Krueger, Sawyer, & Graetz, 2003; Tackett, Krueger, Iacono, & McGue, 2005). Of note, this AGG/RB distinction appears to roughly map onto the other primary approach to subtyping the heterogeneity of antisocial behavior, that regarding age-of-onset (Moffitt, 1993, 2003). Research has indicated that those with childhood-onset antisocial behavior exhibited higher rates of aggressive behaviors than those with adolescent-onset antisocial behavior, but roughly the same prevalence of nonaggressive, rule-breaking behaviors (Lahey et al., 1998). These results extended previous findings indicating that the median age of onset of aggressive behaviors is earlier than that of nonaggressive but delinquent behaviors (Lahey, Loeber, Quay, Frick, & Grimm, 1992). Such findings collectively indicate that the age of onset of antisocial behavior may be intimately tied to the presence or absence of physical aggression.

Developmental trajectories also vary across AGG and RB. Physical aggression appears to be a relatively stable interpersonal trait such that those who are most aggressive in early childhood (roughly 5% of children, mostly boys) continue to be so later in life (Stanger, Achenbach, & Verhulst, 1997; Tremblay, 2003). Even so, overall levels of aggression decrease precipitously from early childhood to adulthood, with only a slight (and temporary) increase again during mid-adolescence (Stanger et al., 1997; Tremblay, 2003). By contrast, nonaggressive delinquency shows a steep increase over the course of adolescence, less rank-order stability, and although this subtype is also more common in males, the gender difference is less pronounced (Moffitt, 2003; Stanger et al., 1997).

There is also mounting evidence of etiologically driven distinctions between AGG and RB. Recent evidence points to emotional dysfunction as one source of such variability. AGG appears to be more closely linked to indices of autonomic and neuroendocrine functioning than is nonaggressive but rule-breaking behavior (Lahey, Hart, Pliszka, Applegate, & McBurnett, 1993). As low autonomic arousal and lack of autonomic responsiveness represent a form of affective deficit (Raine, 2002), such findings suggest that affective dysfunction may be particularly characteristic of AGG. Similarly, activity in the hypothalamic–pituitary–adrenal axis, a core component of the stress response, is restricted only in those high in AGG (McBurnett, Lahey, Rathouz, & Loeber, 2000; Ramirez, 2003) and does not extend to either nonaggressive antisocial behavior or impulsivity in general (Krueger, Schedlowski, & Meyer, 2005; McBurnett et al., 2000). Lack of empathy also appears to be largely exclusive to AGG (Cohen & Strayer, 1996; Pardini, Lochman, & Frick, 2003), again highlighting the role of affective dysfunction in aggression. Lastly, a recent study has found that the potentiation of negative affect following the completion of an aversive task appears to be specific to those high in AGG and does not persist to those high in RB (Burt & Larson, 2007), a pattern of results that was subsequently extended to trait levels of negative emotionality (Burt & Donnellan, 2008; DeMarte, 2008). Together, such findings suggest that affective dysfunction may represent a core deficit specifically in those with aggressive antisocial behavior.

By contrast, several studies have indicated that the well-replicated association between diminished central serotonin functioning and impulsive-aggressive behavior in animals (Mehlman et al., 1994) and humans (Manuck et al., 1998; Siever et al., 1999; Virkkunen, Goldman, Nielson, & Linnoila, 1995) extends to impulsive but nonaggressive behaviors (LeMarquand, Benkelfat, Pihl, Palmour, & Young, 1999; Pihl & Peterson, 1995), but not to premeditated, nonimpulsive aggression (Davidson, Putnam, & Larson, 2000; Linnoila et al., 1983). Indeed, recent studies have indicated that the personality trait of impulsivity is far more strongly associated with rule-breaking delinquency than with aggression (Burt & Donnellan, 2008; DeMarte, 2008). Such findings collectively disambiguate impulsivity and physical aggression per se while also suggesting that impulsivity may be specifically associated with RB.

Finally, and most importantly, a handful of twin and adoption studies have compared aggressive and nonaggressive antisocial behavior (see meta-analysis by Burt, 2009). Results collectively reveal that aggressive behaviors are more heritable than rule-breaking behaviors, whereas rule-breaking behaviors are more highly influenced by shared environmental factors (i.e., those environmental factors that create similarities between siblings). In particular, additive genetic influences were significantly larger for AGG as compared to RB (65 vs. 48%, respectively), whereas shared environmental influences were larger for RB than for AGG (18 vs. 5%, respectively). Nonshared environmental influences were also slightly, albeit significantly, larger for RB than for AGG (34 vs. 30%, respectively). Importantly, these results generally persisted across sex, age, and various informants. Such findings collectively highlight etiological differences between AGG and RB and thus offer yet another strong source of support for meaningful distinctions between these subtypes.

Different Roles for Gene–Environment Interplay across AGG and RB?

Considerations of the Timing of Genetic Expression

Given these developmental and etiologic differences in the phenotypic expression of AGG and RB, a recent study asked whether the developmental timing of genetic expression also varied across the two subtypes (Burt & Neiderhiser, 2009). Burt & Neiderhiser (2009) examined age-related etiological change in aggressive versus rule-breaking antisocial behavior (as assessed using the Behavior Problems Index) in a sample of 720 adolescent sibling pairs with varying degrees of genetic related-ness. Cross-sectional analyses revealed that the magnitude of genetic and environ-mental influences on aggression remained stable across adolescence, whereas genetic influences on rule-breaking nearly tripled in magnitude from age 10 to age 15, after which they slowly decreased (see Fig. 6.1). Additional longitudinal analy-ses in these data fully supported these findings. When combined with prior research indicating that genetic influences on aggression increase from age 3 to age 7 and then stabilize (van Beijsterveldt, Bartels, Hudziak, & Boomsma, 2003), such find-ings imply that genetic influences on aggression and rule breaking are expressed during childhood and adolescence, respectively.

Subsequent analyses provided a constructive replication of these results, examin-ing different measures of AGG and RB in a different type of sample (a twin sample, as compared to the twin-sibling sample analyzed above). More specifically, Burt and Klump (2009) examined AGG and RB scales from the well-known Child Behavior Checklist in an independent sample of early adolescent twins. Results again revealed that AGG remained etiologically stable across adolescence, whereas genetic influ-ences on RB increased substantially (more than doubling in magnitude) from age 10 to age 15. Such findings offer key support for prior findings of distinctive patterns of etiological moderation by age across aggressive and rule-breaking forms of anti-social behavior and indicate that these results are largely robust to sampling variation and persist across multiple measures of these constructs.

As discussed by Neiderhiser (Chap. 5), one prominent theoretical concept that may explain at least some of these developmental shifts in genetic expression is that of the active gene–environment correlation (i.e., active rGE), in which individuals select environmental experiences consistent with their genotype (Plomin, DeFries,

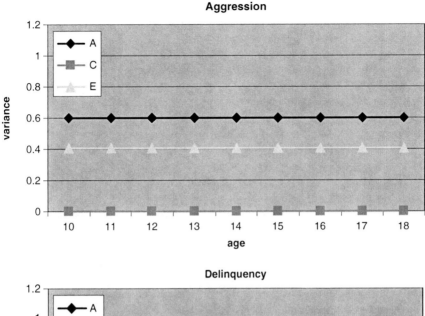

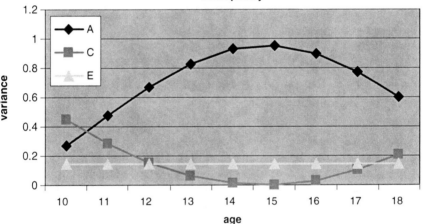

Fig. 6.1 Unstandardized variance components in AGG and RB across Adolescence. *Note*: *A, C,* and *E* represent genetic, shared, and nonshared environmental variance components, respectively. These estimates index the absolute changes in genetic and environmental variance from ages 10 to 18. As presented in Burt and Neiderhiser (2009). Reprinted with permission from *Developmental Psychology*

& Loehlin, 1977; Scarr & McCartney, 1983). Scarr and McCartney (1983) postulated that as children age, they exert increasingly greater control over the environments they experience, progressively shaping their environments to be consistent with their genetic predispositions. The relative importance of active rGE is thus thought to change across development such that it has less impact in childhood and becomes progressively more important as children transition into adolescence and adulthood. This increasing influence of active rGE should manifest as increasing genetic influences from childhood to adulthood. Put differently, as individuals exert an increasingly greater impact on the environments they experience, their genetic predispositions should be more fully expressed.

Given this, the results of Burt and Neiderhiser (2009) imply that AGG and RB may be differentially susceptible to active rGE. In particular, because active rGE seems likely to induce increasing heritability during adolescence in particular (the developmental period most characterized by increasing independence from parental decision making), it may be that RB is particularly responsive to active rGE. By contrast, if the genes contributing to AGG are first expressed during early- to mid-childhood (as suggested by van Beijsterveldt et al., 2003), a more limited role for active rGE processes in aggression may be implied.

That said, the very high and stable levels of genetic influence observed for AGG (as reviewed previously) may imply that gene–environment interactions (G × E) are particularly important for this phenotype. Indeed, because gene–environment interactions typically load on the genetic proportion of variance in standard twin modeling, the finding of higher genetic influences on AGG than on RB is circumstantially consistent with this possibility. Moreover, given that the timing of genetic expression for AGG appears to be early to mid-childhood, such findings are collectively consistent with the possibility that G × E during early childhood are particularly important for the development of AGG.

Theoretical Rationale for Differential Gene–Environment Interplay in AGG and RB

It is worthwhile to spend a moment speculating on the origins of differential gene–environment interplay between AGG and RB. Such conjecture is warranted not only because it offers a more compelling framework for the above interpretations but also because any discussion of genetic influences invites reflection on the possible role of evolution. As background for this discussion, it should be noted that the average level of a trait is presumed to be "ideal" in evolutionary terms. The developmental period in which a given trait is most prevalent (or the most "average") would, therefore, be critical to establish its evolutionary basis. I discuss AGG and RB using this framework.

The high prevalence of physical aggression during the toddler years (more than 50% of toddlers bite, kick, and hit; as discussed in Tremblay, 2003) is consistent with the notion that aggression may have been highly selected for at some time in our evolutionary past. Indeed, although it is very costly to individuals and society in general, physical aggression does have advantages in certain contexts. In times of scarcity, for instance, physical aggression could provide access to additional resources (i.e., simply taking food or shelter from others). It can also provide protection against outsiders for yourself, your kin, and your social group. How does one rectify the advantages of aggression in these contexts with its clear disadvantages to the social group overall? One possibility is that although humans have a capacity for aggression, our penchant for living in social groups requires that this be expressed only in times of necessity (e.g., war) and not within our social group. Indeed, the rather profound reduction in mean levels of physical aggression over the course of childhood suggests an active attempt to reduce and/or divert aggressive impulses in children. In other words, rather than learning to be aggressive, it appears that children learn *not* to be aggressive (Tremblay, 2003). As nicely discussed by Tremblay (2003), it may be that the real difficulty faced by those who engage in unusually high levels aggression is an inability to be socialized (i.e., "learning to regulate one's pleasure seeking to that of others"; Tremblay, 2003, p. 205) and/or a lack of exposure to socialization. This sort of process would be particularly amenable to G × E, as it would suggest that inadequate socialization (or inadequate response to socialization) may result in a failure to "turn off" genes related to human aggression.

Rule breaking, by contrast, is notably less frequent than AGG during childhood, but becomes nearly ubiquitous during adolescence (especially among boys); indeed, only 7% of 18-year-old boys deny all forms of RB (as discussed in Moffitt, 1993). In her seminal theory on the development of antisocial behavior, Moffitt (1993) made sense of this normalization of otherwise pathological behavior. Essentially, she argued that adolescent-onset RB served an adaptive purpose from the perspective of contemporary teens: access to some of the freedoms and privileges of adult life. As an example, one study found that, among high school students, 61% of marijuana users were sexually experienced (a highly valued outcome by many adolescent males) as compared to only 18% of nonusers (Jessor, 1991). Adolescent RB can, thus, be reframed as an adaptive and circumscribed response to the particular developmental challenges of adolescence.

Given the above, active rGE in RB could be a function of peer selection or deviant peer affiliation, particularly as there is evidence to suggest that affiliation with deviant peers exacerbates antisocial behaviors (Deater-Deckard, 2001) and moreover that rule-breaking is more frequently committed in the company of peers (Gardner & Steinberg, 2005). Alternately, it could be a function of familial influences, in which adolescents are aiming to become independent from their family of origin and assume an adult role. Consistent with the latter possibility, Burt et al. (2005) evaluated the longitudinal relationship between parenting and adolescent externalizing behaviors using a novel cross-lagged twin design. Results suggested that environmental triggers, provoked by the adolescent's externalizing behaviors, were in turn responsible for maintaining and even exacerbating the adolescent's behavior, findings that neatly capture rGE.

Conclusion

The above review of AGG and RB provides a concrete example of the need to consider the phenotype in question when examining contributions of gene–environment interplay. In the case presented above, for example, there are both empirical and theoretical reasons to suspect that pattern and influence of gene–environment interplay is phenotype-specific. Such findings are particularly noteworthy given that AGG and RB, while clearly distinguishable from one another, are empirically (r ~0.5) and conceptually related. In short, the above review strongly suggests that rather than assuming that G × E and or rGE will be applicable across all disorders and outcomes, *scientists must meaningfully consider the developmental and etiologic influences on a given phenotype when exploring the possible role of gene–environment interplay.*

References

Burt, S. A. (2009). Are there meaningful etiological differences within antisocial behavior? Results of a meta-analysis. *Clinical Psychology Review, 29*, 163–178.

Burt, S. A., & Donnellan, M. B. (2008). Personality correlates of aggressive and non-aggressive antisocial behavior. *Personality and Individual Differences, 44*, 53–63.

Burt, S. A., & Larson, C. L. (2007). Differential affective responses in those with aggressive versus non-aggressive antisocial behaviors. *Personality and Individual Differences, 43*, 1481–1492.

Burt, S. A., & Neiderhiser, J. M. (2009). Aggressive versus non-aggressive antisocial behavior: Distinctive etiological moderation by age. *Developmental Psychology, 45*, 1164–1176.

Burt, S.A. & Klump, K.L. (2009). The etiological moderation of aggressive and nonaggressive antisocial behavior by age. *Twin Research & Human Genetics, 12*, 343–350.

Burt, S. A., McGue, M., Krueger, R.F., & Iacono, W.G. (2005). How are parent-child conflict and childhood externalizing symptoms related over time? Results from a genetically-informative cross-lagged study. *Development and Psychopathology, 17*, 145–165.

Cohen, D., & Strayer, J. (1996). Empathy in conduct-disordered and comparison youth. *Developmental Psychology, 32*, 988–998.

Davidson, R. J., Putnam, K. M., & Larson, C. L. (2000). Dysfunction in the neural circuitry of emotion regulation – A possible prelude to violence. *Science, 289*, 591–594.

Deater-Deckard, K. (2001). Annotation: Recent research examining the role of peer relationships in the development of psychopathology. *Journal of Child Psychology and Psychiatry, 42*, 565–579.

DeMarte, J. A. (2008). *The heterogeneity of antisocial behavior: Evidence for distinct dimensions of physical aggression, rule-breaking, and social aggression.* Unpublished doctoral dissertation, Michigan State University, East Lansing, MI.

Frick, P. J., Lahey, B. B., Loeber, R., Tannenbaum, L., Van Horn, Y., Christ, M. A. G., et al. (1993). Oppositional defiant disorder and conduct disorder: A meta-analytic review of factor analyses and cross–validation in a clinic sample. *Clinical Psychology Review, 13*, 319–340.

Gardner, M., & Steinberg, L. (2005). Peer influence on risk taking, risk preference, and risky decision making in adolescence and adulthood: An experimental study. *Developmental Psychology, 41*, 625–635.

Jessor, R. (1991). Risk behavior in adolescence: A psychosocial framework for understanding and action. *Journal of Adolescent Health, 12*, 597–605.

Krueger, T. H. C., Schedlowski, M., & Meyer, G. (2005). Cortisol and heart rate measures during casino gambling in relation to impulsivity. *Neuropsychobiology, 52*, 206–211.

Lahey, B. B., Hart, E. L., Pliszka, S., Applegate, B., & McBurnett, K. (1993). Neurophysiological correlates of conduct disorder: A rationale and a review of research. *Journal of Clinical Child Psychology, 22*, 141–153.

Lahey, B. B., Loeber, R., Quay, H. C., Applegate, B., Shaffer, D., Waldman, I., et al. (1998). Validity of DSM-IV subtypes of conduct disorder based on age of onset. *Journal of the American Academy of Child and Adolescent Psychiatry, 37*, 435–442.

Lahey, B. B., Loeber, R., Quay, H. C., Frick, P. J., & Grimm, J. (1992). Oppositional defiant and conduct disorders: Issues to be resolved for DSM-IV. *Journal of the American Academy of Child and Adolescent Psychiatry, 31*, 539–546.

LeMarquand, D. G., Benkelfat, C., Pihl, R. O., Palmour, R. M., & Young, S. N. (1999). Behavioral disinhibition induced by tryptophan depletion in nonalcoholic young men with multigenerational family histories of paternal alcoholism. *American Journal of Psychiatry, 156*, 1771–1779.

Linnoila, M., Virkkunen, M., Scheinin, M., Nuutla, A., Rimon, R., & Goodwin, F. K. (1983). Low cerebrospinal fliud 5-hydroxyindoleacetic acid concentration differentiates impulsive from non-impulsive violent behavior. *Life Sciences, 33*, 2609–2614.

Loeber, R., & Schmaling, K. B. (1985). Empirical evidence for overt and covert patterns of antisocial conduct problems: A meta-analysis. *Journal of Abnormal Child Psychology, 13*, 337–352.

Manuck, S. B., Flory, J. D., McCaffery, J. M., Matthews, K. A., Mann, J. J., Muldoon, M. F. (1998). Aggression, impulsivity, and central nervous system serotonergic responsivity in a non-patient sample. *Neuropsychopharmocology, 19*, 287–299.

McBurnett, K., Lahey, B., Rathouz, P. J., & Loeber, R. (2000). Low salivary cortisol and persistent aggression in boys referred for disruptive behavior. *Archives of General Psychiatry, 57*, 38–43.

Mehlman, P. T., Higley, J. D., Faucher, L., Lilly, A. A., Taub, D. N., Suomi, S. J., Linnoila, M. (1994). Low CSF 5-HIAA concentrations and sever aggression and impaired impulse control in non-human primates. *American Journal of Psychiatry, 151*, 1485–1491.

Moffitt, T. E. (1993). Adolescence-limited and life-course-persistent antisocial behavior: A developmental taxonomy. *Psychological Review, 100*, 674–701.

Moffitt, T. E. (2003). Life-course persistent and adolescence-limited antisocial behavior: A research review and a research agenda. In B. Lahey, T. E. Moffitt, & A. Caspi (Eds.), *The causes of conduct disorder and serious juvenile delinquency*. New York: Guilford Press.

Pardini, D. A., Lochman, J. E., & Frick, P. J. (2003). Callous/unemotional traits and social cognitive processes in adjudicated youth. *Journal of the American Academy of Child and Adolescent Psychiatry, 42*, 364–371.

Pihl, R. O., & Peterson, J. (1995). Drugs and aggression: Correlations, crime and human manipulative studies and some proposed mechanisms. *Journal of Psychiatry and Neuroscience, 20*, 141–149.

Plomin, R., DeFries, J. C., & Loehlin, J. C. (1977). Genotype-environment interaction and correlation in the analysis of human behavior. *Psychological Bulletin, 84*, 309–322.

Raine, A. (2002). Annotation: The role of prefrontal deficits, low autonomic arousal, and early health factors in the development of antisocial and aggressive behavior in children. *Journal of Child Psychology and Psychiatry, 43*, 417–434.

Ramirez, J. M. (2003). Hormones and aggression in childhood and adolescence. *Aggression and Violent Behavior, 8*, 621–644.

Scarr, S., & McCartney, K. (1983). How people make their own environments: A theory of genotype-environment effects. *Child Development, 54*, 424–435.

Siever, L. J., Buchsbaum, M. S., New, A. S., Spiegel-Cohen, J., Wei, T., Hazlett, E. A., et al. (1999). d,l-fenfluramine response to impulsive personality disorder assessed with [^{18}F] fluorodeoxyglucose positron emission tomography. *Neuropsychopharmocology, 20*, 413–423.

Stanger, C., Achenbach, T. A., & Verhulst, F. C. (1997). Accelerated longitudinal comparisons of aggressive versus delinquent syndromes. *Development and Psychopathology, 9*, 43–58.

Tackett, J. L., Krueger, R. F., Iacono, W. G., & McGue, M. (2005). Symptom-based subfactors of DSM-defined conduct disorder: Evidence for etiologic distinctions. *Journal of Abnormal Psychology, 114*, 483–487.

Tackett, J. L., Krueger, R., Sawyer, M. G., & Graetz, B. W. (2003). Subfactors of DSM-IV conduct disorder: Evidence and connections with syndromes from the child behavior checklist. *Journal of Abnormal Child Psychology, 31*(6), 647–654.

Tremblay, R. E. (2003). Why socialization fails: The case of chronic physical aggression. In B. Lahey, T. E. Moffitt & A. Caspi (Eds.), *The causes of conduct disorder and serious juvenile delinquency*. New York: Guilford Press.

van Beijsterveldt, C. E. M., Bartels, M., Hudziak, J. J., & Boomsma, D. I. (2003). Causes of stabil-
    ity of aggression from early childhood to adolescence: A longitudinal genetic analysis in
    Dutch twins. *Behavioral Genetics, 33*, 591–605.
Virkkunen, M., Goldman, D., Nielson, D. A., & Linnoila, M. (1995). Low brain serotonin turnover
    rate (low CSF 5-HIAAA) and impulsive violence. *Journal of Psychiatry and Neuroscience, 20*,
    271–275.

Chapter 7
The Importance of Puberty in Adolescent Development

Sheri A. Berenbaum

Abstract Adolescence is a good time to study the influences of physiology and social environmental factors within the family because it is a time of major biological change with substantial implications for psychological change. Puberty represents a key transition in psychological function, and many studies of adolescent development consider the effects of puberty. Key questions concern mechanisms by which puberty affects psychological function and the psychological consequences and antecedents of variations in pubertal timing. Examples of these questions are considered in this chapter, with consideration of the ways in which they can be integrated with behavior genetics studies.

Introduction

Neiderhiser (Chap. 5) has highlighted the extent to which genes and the environment operate individually and jointly to shape family influences (especially parenting) on adolescent adjustment and development. Behavior genetic studies have been valuable for pointing to the importance of different forms of behavioral transmission, that is, in telling us how much of the variance in a particular characteristic or covariance among characteristics is due to genes, shared environment, nonshared environment, gene–environment correlation, gene–environment interaction, or other complex joint effects.

Behavior genetic studies can do more than that, however. The power of behavior genetics studies comes from the ability to control genetic factors and selection biases to examine environmental influences on the characteristics of interest; they enable causal inferences not possible with traditional studies (Johnson, Turkheimer, Gottesman, & Bouchard, 2009; Rutter, 2007). Thus, behavior genetics studies can help us understand the mechanisms that underlie variation in a characteristic or covariation among characteristics.

S.A. Berenbaum (✉)
Department of Psychology, The Pennsylvania State University,
University Park, PA, USA
e-mail: sberenbaun@psu.edu

A. Booth et al. (eds.), *Biosocial Foundations of Family Processes*,
National Symposium on Family Issues, DOI 10.1007/978-1-4419-7361-0_7,

How might this be exploited in studying development in adolescence? Adolescence is a particularly good time to study the influences of physiology and social environmental factors within the family because it is a time of major biological change with substantial implications for psychological change. Puberty represents a key transition in psychological function and many studies of adolescent development consider the effects of puberty. Some of the key questions are: How does puberty affect psychological function directly through changes in the brain induced by sex hormones or by other factors related to age? How does puberty affect psychological function indirectly through alterations of social responses to a youth's changing body, including the responses of teens themselves and of others in the social environment, such as peers and relatives? What is the significance for psychological adjustment of variations in developmental timing (maturing early or late)? Examples of these questions are considered in this chapter, with consideration of the ways in which they can be integrated with behavior genetics studies.

Puberty as a Transition

Adolescence is a time of major physical change brought on by the activation of the hypothalamic–pituitary–gonadal axis and consequent increases in sex hormones leading to mature reproductive capacity. The brain develops throughout adolescence, with increased connections and synaptic pruning (resulting in reduced volume), and sex differences in trajectories (e.g., girls have an earlier peak of gray matter volume) (Lenroot et al., 2007; Lenroot & Giedd, 2006).

Many psychological characteristics increase in frequency or become more salient in adolescence compared to childhood, and many psychological sex differences emerge or increase at this time; the type and nature of social relationships also change (e.g., Lerner & Steinberg, 2004). There appear to be different developmental trajectories of and influences on cognition versus affect: Improvements in cognition and their underlying neural substrates are linked more closely with age and experience than with pubertal maturation; changes in affect and their neural substrates appear to be associated with pubertal changes and thus tied to changes in sex hormones. Changes in risk-taking are suggested to be associated with multiple processes tied to brain development (Steinberg, 2008): increased risk-taking from childhood to adolescence is associated with increased reward seeking, whereas decreased risk-taking from adolescence to adulthood is associated with increased cognitive control and self-regulation. The different timetables for the development of intellectual ability and psychosocial maturity may account for adolescents' increased risk for behavior problems (Steinberg, 2008).

Pubertal changes in both physical and psychological characteristics are likely due to changes in gene expression: genes become activated ("turned on") by factors that change at puberty. This has been seen in studies showing that genetic influences on behavior problems increase at puberty (e.g., Culbert, Burt, McGue, Iacono, & Klump, 2009; Klump, Burt, McGue, & Iacono, 2007; Van Hulle et al., 2009).

For example, in a longitudinal twin study of disordered eating, genetic factors were shown to account for a small proportion of the variation at age 11, but almost half the variation at ages 14 and 18; the authors suggested that "the transition from early to mid-adolescence (is) a critical time for the emergence of a genetic diathesis for disordered eating" (Klump, Burt, McGue, & Iacono, 2007). In general, the triggers for gene expression are both intrinsic (e.g., hormones) and extrinsic (e.g., diet and maternal care), so gene regulation can help us understand both biological and social influences on adolescent development.

Puberty also changes a child's social world, including relationships with family members. Although it is not easy to separate effects of chronological age from specific aspects of pubertal development, evidence suggests that some changes in social relationships are tied to puberty per se. But it is unclear whether these puberty-associated changes occur directly via brain maturation or indirectly via social responses to physical changes. Most of what we know concerns relationships with parents. When children go through puberty, they spend less time with their parents (especially with opposite-sex parents) and have more conflict with their parents (especially between mothers and daughters). These conflicts are characterized as having more intense negative affect than earlier conflicts (Whiteman, McHale, & Crouter, 2007).

Most work has focused on effects of pubertal changes on the child him or herself. But some work has focused on the ways in which changed parent–child relationships at puberty affect other aspects of the family system, especially the relationship between parents (Whiteman et al., 2007). In general, marital quality was seen to decline when offspring experienced puberty, but the decline varied across indicators of marital quality and was moderated by sex of parent and child birth order. For example, marital conflict was associated with pubertal development of same-sex firstborn offspring; there was some evidence that pubertal development in second borns had different effects on mothers and fathers (increasing conflict in mothers and decreasing it in fathers). This work emphasizes the need to consider the ways in which the entire family system may be changed by a child's pubertal development, and how this effect may further change the child's development. It is also important to note that these effects may change across the development of the family (from first born to second born).

Consequences of Variations in Pubertal Timing

Children vary considerably in the timing of their pubertal development, and there is good evidence that these variations have psychological consequences. Most work has documented adverse psychological outcomes associated with early puberty in girls. For example, early-maturing girls have more emotional distress and problem behavior (e.g., delinquency, substance use, early sexuality) than on-time peers (e.g., Ge, Conger, & Elder, 1996) and at least some of these problems persist into adulthood (Weichold, Silbereisen, & Schmitt-Rodermund, 2003). There is good evidence that these effects are mediated and moderated by socialization. Mediators include peers and parents: Girls who mature early associate with older and male peers who expose them to risky substances and activities (Weichold et al., 2003); early maturers' higher rate of externalizing behavior has been linked to parents' use of harsh inconsistent discipline (Ge, Brody, Conger, Simons, & Murry, 2002). Moderators include social context: Early-maturing children living in disadvantaged neighborhoods were significantly more likely to affiliate with deviant peers (Ge et al., 2002); problem behaviors were higher in early-maturing girls who attended coeducational schools than in their counterparts in all-girls' schools (Caspi, Lynam, Moffitt, & Silva, 1993).

There is now also reason to think that some of these effects may reflect direct effects of hormones on brain organization. Hormonal influences on adolescent behavior have traditionally been considered to be "activational," affecting brain function only when the hormone is present; thus, increased hormones at puberty facilitate the function of structures that were "organized" early in life. However, recent hypotheses and evidence from rodents suggest that hormones may also have "organizational" effects at puberty, producing permanent changes to the brain (e.g., Schulz, Molenda–Figueira, & Sisk, 2009; Sisk & Zehr, 2005). Thus, animals exposed to high levels of sex hormones at a time when the brain is relatively immature are behaviorally different than animals exposed to those high levels of hormones at the typical age (e.g., Schulz et al., 2009; Sisk & Zehr, 2005). If this mechanism is found to operate in people – and it is likely that it will, given all the other ways in which animal models of hormone–behavior links have been confirmed in human beings – then brain organization would vary with the timing of hormone increase and with corresponding permanent behavioral changes. For example, early-maturing children might engage in more risk-taking and thus be more vulnerable to behavior problems because they experience an extended time of mismatch between the maturation of the reward and cognitive control systems (Steinberg, 2008). Thus, it is important to consider how behavioral risks associated with early puberty are mediated by permanent changes in the brain.

Most work on the consequences of variations in pubertal timing concern early maturation in girls; less is known about effects of early puberty in boys, probably because of issues in measuring puberty. Girls' pubertal development is generally measured by menarche, but boys lack such a clearly demarcated event that can easily be reported. Measurement issues will be discussed in detail below. There is also little known about the consequences of late development in either boys or girls, and such work is important for helping us to understand mechanisms underlying the consequences of pubertal timing. That is, studying children who are later maturers will help us to know whether observed effects of early timing reflect special risks associated with early development or a type of nonnormative development, in which late maturers should also be at risk for problems compared to children who mature on-time. Late development might be expected to affect psychological development through social factors (being different than peers) or through hormonal effects on the brain (being exposed to hormones at a later time than is typical).

Our understanding of the significance of pubertal timing for adjustment could be substantially enhanced by using within-family designs. Within-family designs enable causal inferences about mechanisms underlying associations and are the only way to identify mechanisms that operate within families (traditional studies confound between- and within-family effects). This potential is illustrated in a twin study of links between pubertal timing and substance use (Dick, Rose, Viken, & Kaprio, 2000). Pubertal timing is heritable, but not completely so, and dissimilarity in timing among pairs of identical twins was exploited. Monozygotic twins who were discordant for pubertal timing also were found to be discordant for substance use, with the early-maturing twin drinking more than the late-maturing twin. Neither peers nor personality were found to mediate the effect (perhaps because twins have peers in common), but residence moderated it: the effect was found only in families living in urban areas, not in rural areas. Although this study primarily serves to confirm results from between-family studies, it shows the power of behavior genetics designs for determining causative mechanism because discordances in monozygotic twins must be due to something in the environment that they do not share.

Within-family designs should be extended to identify the ways in which puberty affects the family system to influence adolescent development (e.g., McHale et al., 2003). Because children's puberty changes the family system (Whiteman et al., 2007), it is reasonable to hypothesize that the outcome of pubertal timing might reflect, at least in part, a change in the family system. This effect might depend on the child's birth order. It seems likely that the family disruption created by an early-maturer will depend on whether she is a first- or later born, and how her development compares to that of her siblings. Thus, pubertal timing effects on psychological outcome would be expected to be larger for first-born girls than for later-born girls, and, within families, a first-born's pubertal timing should have consequences for her siblings as well as for herself.

Antecedents of Variations in Pubertal Timing

Family relationships are important not just as a reaction to a child's pubertal development, and thus as a potential influence on psychological development, but as a potential *cause* of those variations. Data from nonhuman animals clearly show that pubertal development is affected by the environment, both physical and social. For example, puberty in female mice is accelerated by exposure to a pheromone in adult male urine (termed the "Vandenbergh effect"). In people, it is well known that physical factors can affect pubertal development. Most discussed factors act to delay puberty, such as poor nutrition or excessive exercise. But there are factors known to accelerate puberty, including international adoption: girls who are born in developing countries and adopted into families in western countries experience earlier menarche than girls who remain in the country of origin and girls born in the adopted country (e.g., Mason & Narad, 2005). The exact reasons for the accelerated puberty are not clear, but have been suggested to include catch-up growth due to improved diet and nutrition in the adoptive country and from exposure to environmental toxins that act as endocrine disrupters.

Social experiences may also affect pubertal timing in human beings. This work is generally driven by hypotheses proposed by Belsky, Steinberg, and Draper (1991), who considered the ways in which childhood experiences (especially the father–daughter relationship) provide information that serves to guide future reproductive strategies. In essence, these experiences are hypothesized to induce an understanding about resources, others' trustworthiness, and enduringness of close relationships, which, in turn, affect reproductive effort. Belsky et al. (1991) focused on effects of father absence, which was hypothesized to accelerate puberty, leading to "quantity" (vs. "quality") mating, and an emphasis on mating more than parenting. The evidence linking family function to girls' pubertal timing is not entirely consistent, and the relevant aspects of the family environment vary across studies, but the topic is worthy of further consideration.

A key question is whether the association is truly environmental or is mediated by genes. For example, a woman with early puberty is likely to have had sexual activity at an earlier age than one with a later puberty; the other correlates of early puberty (e.g., delinquency, substance use) may have also led her to choose a partner whose characteristics increase the likelihood of relationship instability so her daughter is likely to grow up in a "father absent" home. Thus, the mother with early puberty transmits to her daughter genes for early puberty, and, through those genes, also provides her daughter with an unstable early childhood family environment.

An opportunity to disentangle genetic from environmental effects is provided by within-family studies, comparing pubertal timing in siblings with differential exposure to the putative environmental risk factor. For example, a study of pubertal timing in sisters with different early family experiences showed that age at menarche was related to joint effects of birth order, family disruption, and father dysfunction (Tither & Ellis, 2008): Younger sisters from disrupted families who were exposed to serious paternal dysfunction in early childhood attained menarche 11 months earlier than either their older sisters or other younger sisters from disrupted families who were not exposed to such dysfunction.

These results are intriguing, but it is important to have additional data to confirm that pubertal timing is environmentally linked to early family factors related specifically to father absence or poor fathering. For example, interventions designed to improve family function (especially related to the father) should also delay puberty in girls. If the association is, in fact, a true environmental effect, is the mechanism as Belsky et al. (1991) suggested or through some other social mechanism that is linked to father absence? And what is the physiological pathway through which the social effect operates?

Findings linking early childhood family factors to pubertal timing have other implications. Some apparent consequences of pubertal timing might actually reflect family antecedents. For example, the link between early puberty and delinquency might reflect initial effects of family dysfunction, so that family problems could lead to both early puberty and delinquency through separate paths. Further, genes could play a mediating role: Genes predisposing to antisocial behavior might lead to poor family function and separately to child antisocial behavior (and thus delinquency); women with early puberty might be especially likely to marry men with antisociality, giving their daughters genes for early puberty and antisocial fathers (and perhaps their own genes for antisociality). It is likely that multiple pathways operate, with both genes and family environment important for adolescent development.

Measurement of Puberty

Given the importance of pubertal development in adolescent development, there is increasing interest in including measures of puberty in developmental studies. Most studies involve some version of adolescent self-report of puberty: assessing the age at which a girl reached menarche and asking children of both sexes to rate their current physical status using a standard scale based on the pubertal stages described by Tanner (e.g., Tanner, 1978). But, it is considerably more complicated to measure puberty (e.g., Dorn, Dahl, & Biro, 2006). Puberty is a process (or a series of processes), not a single event, and different features and different stages might have different significance, both for brain development and as social signals. For example, brain changes might accompany initial increases in hormones, whereas social responses are likely to be most pronounced during mid-puberty when physical maturation becomes apparent to others; different aspects of appearance mature at different ages with different signaling value. Further, children vary not just in the age at which they reach a particular pubertal milestone, but in how long it takes them to go through all stages (tempo).

Pubertal measures should correspond to hypotheses about the mechanisms underlying links between puberty and behavior, but most studies rely on measures of convenience. Most studies measure age at menarche, which is late in puberty and not obvious to others, whereas most hypothesized mechanisms of puberty–behavior links concern changes that occur early in puberty (e.g., genes activated by sex hormones) or mid-puberty (social responses to youth's changing appearance). This issue is nicely illustrated in work on eating disorders: genetic influences are seen to emerge at puberty when puberty is measured with an early indicator but not when it is measured by menarche (Culbert et al., 2009).

A child's pubertal development is best measured through a physical exam by a trained health professional; the development of each of several indicators, such as pubic hair, underarm hair, and genitalia (breasts in girls and penis in boys) is described in terms of Tanner stages. But this method is rarely used because it is costly to implement and invasive (requiring that the child be undressed). Instead, most investigators use children's self-reports of their pubertal status, with children asked to rate themselves on the basis of verbal or pictorial descriptions of different features at different pubertal stages (e.g., Brooks-Gunn, 1987; Petersen, Crockett, Richards, & Boxer, 1988). Although different features of pubertal change (e.g., genital development and pubic hair development) are usually assessed, the data are generally aggregated in order to increase reliability. Thus, an overall score is derived from the different indicators, making it difficult to capture the complexity of puberty. Self-report measures have limited validity because they reflect children's perceptions of their pubertal development rather than their objective physical status (Dorn et al., 2006). Some investigators also obtain parent reports, but parents are not good respondents because they do not often see the bodies of their developing teens. Surprisingly, hormones themselves may not be very good indicators, because they vary within the day and across days in pubertal children, so multiple measures of hormones are needed for reliable and valid indicators of pubertal status. Estradiol is especially difficult to measure at low levels, so an ultrasensitive assay is needed. Concordance among the different indicators of pubertal status is not as high as might be expected (Shirtcliff, Dahl, & Pollak, 2009).

Retrospective measures of pubertal timing are even more problematic. Such studies generally rely on a single indicator in a single sex, menarcheal age in females. Because there is not a parallel, easily recalled discrete event in boys, there are few retrospective studies in males. Reporting may be improved if people are asked to compare their development to their peers, and to report if they were early, on-time, or late relative to same-age others.

Conclusion

It is useful to return to the question addressed in this section "How do physiological and social environmental factors within the family influence development and adjustment in adolescence?" and emphasize the need to consider the physiological *mechanisms* through which genetic and environmental factors affect development in adolescence. Puberty is a key mechanism because it is associated with major psychological changes, including cognition, affect, and social relationships. These changes occur as a result of brain changes with maturation, some of which are linked to the activation of the hypothalamic–pituitary–gonadal axis. Behavioral risk may occur because reward seeking develops earlier than cognitive control. A child's puberty (whenever it occurs) affects the family system. There are also variations that need to be considered: variations in the timing of puberty may derive from early experiences with the father and have consequences for behavioral problems in the youth; youth's pubertal development has varying effects on the family system (depending, for example, on interactions among the child's sex, the parent's sex, and the child's birth order). This means that puberty effects on the child and the family are best studied within the family context, ideally with genetically informative designs.

Acknowledgments I am grateful to Susan McHale for valuable discussions on issues related to the chapter and to Carolyn Scott for helpful suggestions for improving it.

References

Belsky, J., Steinberg, L., & Draper, P. (1991). Childhood experience, interpersonal development, and reproductive strategy: and evolutionary theory of socialization. *Child Development, 62,* 647–670.

Brooks-Gunn, J. (1987). Pubertal processes and girls' psychological adaptation. In R. M. Lerner & T. T. Foch (Eds.), *Biological-psychosocial interactions in early adolescence.* Hillsdale, NJ: Lawrence Erlbaum Associates.

Caspi, A., Lynam, D., Moffitt, T. E., & Silva, P. A. (1993). Unraveling girls' delinquency: biological, dispositional, and contextual contributions to adolescent misbehavior. *Developmental Psychology, 29,* 19–30.

Culbert, K. M., Burt, S. A., McGue, M, Iacono, W. G., Klump, K. L. (2009). Puberty and the genetic diathesis of disordered eating attitudes and behaviors. *Journal of Abnormal Psychology, 118,* 788–796.

Dick, D. M., Rose, R. J., Viken, R. J., & Kaprio, J. (2000). Pubertal timing and substance use: Associations between and within families across late adolescence. *Developmental Psychology, 36,* 180–189.

Dorn, L. D., Dahl, R. E., & Biro, F. (2006). Defining the boundaries of early adolescence: A user's guide to assessing pubertal status and pubertal timing in research with adolescents. *Applied Developmental Science, 10*(1), 30–56.

Ge, X., Brody, G. H., Conger, R. D., Simons, R. L., & Murry, V. M. (2002). Contextual amplification of pubertal transition effects on deviant peer affiliation and externalizing behavior among African American children. *Developmental Psychology, 38,* 42–54.

Ge, X., Conger, R. D., & Elder, G. H. (1996). Coming of age too early: pubertal influences on girls' vulnerability to psychological distress. *Child Development, 67,* 386–400.

Johnson, W., Turkheimer, E. Gottesman, I. I., & Bouchard, T. J. (2009). Beyond heritability: twin studies in behavioral research. *Current Directions in Psychological Science, 18,* 217–220.

Klump, K. L., Burt, S. A., McGue, M., & Iacono, W. G. (2007). Changes in genetic and environmental influences on disordered eating across adolescence: A longitudinal twin study. *Archives of General Psychiatry, 64,* 1409–1415.

Lenroot, R. K., & Giedd, J. G. (2006). Brain development in children and adolescents: Insights from anatomical magnetic resonance imaging. *Neuroscience and Biobehavioral Reviews, 30,* 718–729.

Lenroot, R. K., Gogtay, N., Greenstein, D. K., Wells, E. M., Wallace, G. L., Clasen, L. S., et al. (2007). Sexual dimorphism of brain developmental trajectories during childhood and adolescence. *NeuroImage, 15,* 1065–1073.

Lerner, R. M., & Steinberg, L. (Eds.).(2004). *Handbook of adolescent psychology* (3rd ed.). Hoboken, NJ: Wiley.

Mason, P., & Narad, C. (2005). Long-term growth and puberty concerns in international adoptees. *Pediatric Clinics of North America, 52,* 1351–1368.

McHale, S. M., Crouter, A. C., & Whiteman, S. D. (2003). The family contexts of gender development in childhood and adolescence. *Social Development, 12*(1), 125–148.

Petersen, A. C., Crockett, L., Richards, M., & Boxer, A. (1988). A self-report measure of pubertal status: Reliability, validity, and initial norms. *Journal of Youth and Adolescence, 17,* 117–133.

Rutter, M. (2007). Proceeding from observed correlation to causal inference: The use of natural experiments. *Perspectives on Psychological Science, 2,* 377–395.

Schulz, K. M., Molenda–Figueira, H. A., Sisk, C. L. (2009). Back to the future: The organizational-activational hypothesis adapted to puberty and adolescence. *Hormones and Behavior, 55,* 597–604.

Shirtcliff, E. A., Dahl, R. E., & Pollak, S. D. (2009). Pubertal development: correspondence between hormonal and physical development. *Child Development, 80,* 327–337.

Sisk, C. L., & Zehr, J. L. (2005). Pubertal hormones organize the adolescent brain and behavior. *Frontiers in Neuroendocrinology, 26,* 163–174.

Steinberg, L. (2008). A social neuroscience perspective on adolescent risk-taking. *Developmental Review, 28*, 78–106.

Tanner, J. M. (1978). *Foetus into man: Physical growth from conception to maturity*. Cambridge, MA: Harvard University Press.

Tither, J. M., & Ellis, B. J. (2008). Impact of fathers on daughters' age at menarche: A genetically and environmentally controlled sibling study. *Developmental Psychology, 44*, 1409–1422.

Van Hulle C. A., Waldman, I. D., D'Onofrio, B. M., Rodgers, J. L., Rathouz, P. J., Lahey, B. B. (2009). Developmental structure of genetic influences on antisocial behavior across childhood and adolescence. *Journal of Abnormal Psychology, 118*, 711–721.

Weichold, K., Silbereisen, R. K., & Schmitt-Rodermund, E. (2003). Short- and long-term consequences of early versus late physical maturation in adolescents. In C. Hayward (Ed.), *Puberty and psychopathology* (pp. 241–276). Cambridge, MA: Cambridge University Press.

Whiteman, S. D., McHale, S. M., & Crouter, A. C. (2007). Longitudinal changes in marital relationships: The role of offspring's pubertal development. *Journal of Marriage and Family, 69*, 1005–1020.

Chapter 8
Genes, Hormones, and Family Behavior: What Makes Adolescence Unique?

Sally I. Powers

Abstract Many of the most devastating mental illnesses typically have their onset during adolescence. This chapter discusses the ways in which the interplay of genetic and environmental vulnerabilities revealed in Neiderhiser's work may be *specific* to adolescence and therefore have critical relevance to psychological outcomes first expressed in adolescence. The particular functions of family conflict, gender, and epigenetic regulation in adolescence are emphasized. A second focus of the chapter is to discuss the potential value of integrating neuroscience approaches to link gene/environment relationships to adolescent mental health outcomes through mediating neuroendocrine processes. Illustrations focus on studies of hypothalamic–pituitary–adrenal axis functioning as an endophenotype linking genes, submissive behavior during family conflicts, and adolescent depression.

Introduction

Developmental psychopathologists know adolescence as a very special phase of life. Many of the most devastating mental illnesses typically have their onset during adolescence, notably depression, schizophrenia, conduct disorder, eating disorders, and substance abuse. For this reason, the life phase of adolescence can be used by researchers as a unique window through which to shed light on causal factors precipitating the emergence of these disorders. What makes adolescence special? Which elements change from childhood to adolescence to create or critically catalyze an existing vulnerability for mental disorder? A primary aim of this chapter is to push us to consider the ways in which the interplay of genetic and environmental vulnerabilities revealed by Neiderhiser (Chap. 5) are specific to adolescence and therefore have critical relevance to psychological outcomes first

S.I. Powers (✉)
Department of Psychology and Neuroscience and Behavior Program,
University of Massachusetts at Amherst, MA, USA
e-mail: powers@psych.umass.edu

A. Booth et al. (eds.), *Biosocial Foundations of Family Processes*,
National Symposium on Family Issues, DOI 10.1007/978-1-4419-7361-0_8,
© Springer Science+Business Media, LLC 2011

expressed in adolescence. The particular functions of family conflict, gender, and epigenetic regulation in adolescence are emphasized. My second aim is to build on Neiderhiser's remarkable contributions to our knowledge of gene–environment interplay in adolescence by illustrating, with examples from my own work, the potential value of integrating neuroscience approaches to link gene–environment relationships to adolescent mental health outcomes through mediating neuroendocrine processes.

I make these points from the standpoint of a nongenetic researcher. In my own lab, we have only approximated genetic effects through collecting family histories of psychopathology. (We have the typical drawback of most family studies: no variation in genetic relatedness within families.) Instead, my remarks are based on the perspective of a developmental–clinical psychologist and neuroscience researcher focused on understanding family behaviors that influence endocrine, autonomic and neural processes, which then contribute to adolescent psychopathology. Neiderhiser's work has convinced me that findings from quantitative genetics can help steer my own nongenetic work and the work of other researchers who combine family behavioral research and neuroscience. Her findings uncover specific family behavior–mental health outcome relationships for us that are not direct effect relationships. Quantitative genetic approaches reveal family behavior–mental health outcome relationships that could *only* be revealed as predictors of adolescent problems *after* accounting for the moderating influence of genes. Thus, nongenetic researchers gain insight into family behaviors that are important to adolescent outcomes that they might otherwise have ignored. In turn, I hope that spotlighting a consideration of the unique aspects of the adolescent life phase and how endocrine processes might profitably link gene–environment results to adolescent outcomes may be of interest to quantitative genetic researchers.

Which Aspects of Gene and Environment Interplay are Unique to Adolescence?

Neiderhiser (Chap. 5) gives an illustrative overview of the powerful methods of quantitative genetics. She clarifies a range of methods for discriminating gene–environment correlation (rGE) and gene–environment interaction (G × E), helping nongenetic researchers review standard quantitative genetic designs (twin, sibling, adoption, and combination studies) as well as introducing us to innovative designs, such as the extended children of twins design (ECOT), which distinguishes passive and evocative rGE (Narusyte et al., 2008).

In addition, Neiderhiser identifies a variety of gene–behavior relationships that predict adolescent mental health outcomes (Neiderhiser, Chapter 5). For example, when parental conflict is high (Feinberg, Button, Neiderhiser, Reiss, & Hetherington, 2007), monitoring of adolescent behaviors is low (Tuvblad, Grann, & Lichtenstein, 2006), or when family socioeconomic status (SES) is high (Dick et al., 2007), genetic influences on adolescents' antisocial problems become more pronounced. Within this body of rGE and G × E findings, however, it will be especially useful to carefully identify elements of the identified environmental effects (particularly family behaviors) and genetic effects that are phase-specific for adolescence. While all identified gene–environment effects are interesting and valuable, the subset of effects that are unique to adolescence may have particular power in helping us to understand disorders with *onset* in adolescence.

Environment: Family conflict in adolescence. The strengths of quantitative genetic research are magnified in much of Neiderhiser's work because of her careful attention to the measurement of complex environmental variables. This is especially true with regard to family environment (Feinberg et al., 2007; Neiderhiser et al., 2004). Much of Neiderhiser's work is distinguished by combining estimates of genetic contribution with the careful measurement of family behaviors that are more common to studies that exclusively focus on the role of family behaviors (e.g., videos of family conflict discussions, as well as multiple family informants' self-reports of family behaviors).

So how can we identify family behaviors that are particularly influential during adolescence? We suspect that some family behaviors are important in every phase of family life: A good example is Neiderhiser's assessment of *positive* family behaviors, derived from mother and child reports of affection and closeness and observer ratings of warmth and positivity (Neiderhiser et al., 2004). For behaviors that are likely to be uniformly important across all life phases, we need theoretical models and linked analyses that clarify how they may now *trigger new outcomes* in adolescence. Research must seek to clarify how nonphase-specific behaviors produce phase-specific results. One way this may happen is if there is a significant change in the amount of these family behaviors from childhood to adolescence. For example, the *amount* of a family's positive behaviors may drop dramatically when the teenager begins to wrest more autonomy from parents. A second way in which nonphase-specific positive behaviors can affect phase-specific outcomes is that consistently low positive behaviors throughout childhood and adolescence can finally reach a critical threshold, triggering the emergence of adolescent problems.

An alternative way of understanding how family behaviors may predict adolescent phase-specific outcomes is to identify behaviors that are themselves phase specific. That is, we can choose to assess behaviors that are particularly important in the context of the key developmental tasks of adolescence, such as individuation from parents. Individuation requires that the adolescent negotiate increasing levels of autonomy, often causing phase-specific family conflict. To assess the aspects of family conflict that are unique to adolescence, we must ground our behavioral assessment on theories of why conflict is important in adolescent development. Conflict is usually assessed with exclusively linear measurement and analysis strategies, in dimensions from low to high. Studies of family conflict most often seem to implicitly hypothesize that conflict is bad (less is more) and that conflict represents aggression. Perhaps the function of the experimental conflict tasks so many researchers use is to provoke aggression in order to observe it and assess variability in family aggression. At face value, if 'high conflict' signifies nonnormative aggression (e.g., verbal or physical violence), conflict should be analyzed as a constant negative factor across all life phases and not understood as a phase-specific catalyst. But I want to suggest that often family researchers have not thought as carefully as we should about the functions of conflict that may be specific to adolescence.

The positive functions of family conflict are not often fully considered, despite our widely held theoretical notions that a defining task of adolescence is negotiating increasing autonomy from parents and that the forum for this task is often situations of family conflict. Are there conditions under which family conflict is good? Perhaps parent–adolescent conflict is not something to wholly avoid or always conceptualize as less is better. In our lab, we have hypothesized that these family conflict situations are actually quite valuable for adolescents because they enable adolescents to practice and learn the normative task of negotiating and resolving differences with the people they love (Gunlicks-Stoessel & Powers, 2008; Powers & Welsh, 1999; Powers, Welsh, & Wright, 1994). Adolescents must learn to both maintain relationships with parents and stand up for their point of view. In our own work, a family's ability to tolerate and work through fairly intense levels of conflict turn out to be a valuable resource for adolescents – more helpful than family behaviors that ensure only low levels of conflict. We find the most consistent predictor of rises in adolescent depressive symptoms across 2 years of high school is adolescents' nonassertive, submissive behavior during family conflict tasks (Powers, Battle, Dorta, & Welsh, 2010; Powers & Welsh, 1999).

Thus, measuring conflict on a low–high dimension is a useful way to examine conflict if we expect (a) to see change from childhood to adolescence, (b) an accumulation threshold to be reached at adolescence, or (c) high conflict to be a specific stimulus for specific adolescent outcomes, such as aggressive delinquency. However, assessing conflict as linear and negative may obscure the protective nature of assertive conflict behaviors for other critically important internalizing adolescent outcomes, such as depression, eating disorders, and anxiety. In these cases, we need to consider the developmentally healthy function of family conflict. With such a lens, excessive submission and low tolerance of conflict are seen as adolescent-specific environmental vulnerabilities. It also may be useful to empirically examine whether families' tolerance of nonviolent, but vigorous conflict is as important for reducing delinquency and unregulated adolescent violence as it is for protecting adolescents from internalizing problems. Ignoring the positive aspects of family conflict may obscure our understanding of the full interplay of gene–environment correlations and interactions. In sum, the innovative quantitative genetic designs that Neiderhiser has pioneered gain a good deal of their power because these designs are paired with nuanced, theory-based measurement of family behavior (Feinberg et al., 2007).

Genes: Epigenetics in adolescence. Quantitative genetics' G × E findings have enabled tremendous advances in identifying adolescent-specific catalysts for the emergence of problems in adolescence. An additional, complementary method of understanding how genetic factors may operate uniquely during the adolescent life phase is to focus on how genes might be epigenetically activated at adolescence. Epigenetic actions modify gene expression by heritable, but potentially reversible, changes in DNA methylation and/or chromatin structure, which direct the quantity, location, and timing of genetic expression (Henikoff & Matzke, 1997). Epigenetic effects are not the focus of Neiderhiser's quantitative genetics work, but again her work and that of other quantitative genetic researchers can pinpoint which environmental and genetic effects are specific to adolescence and are therefore most important to explore for epigenetic mechanisms. Relevant to our focus on identifying adolescent phase-specific gene–environment influences, it is notable that epigenetic processes can be developmentally regulated (Mill & Petronis, 2007). It is also increasingly clear that social behaviors of family members can lead to long-lasting alterations in epigenetic regulation of gene expression (Mileva & Fleming, in press; Sunderland & Costa, 2003).

Hormones as Mediators of Gene–Behavior Interactions and Adolescent Outcomes

Neiderhiser's work is continually pursuing new ways to expand the gene–environment models she helped to pioneer. In pointing out new directions for future research, Neiderhiser states that "what is still unclear in this work is *why* (G × E findings) are the case" (Neiderhiser, Chap. 5). She notes that "additional work, especially work combining neuroscience with genetics, is needed to better specify how G × E is operating" (p. 7). One way in which neuroscience is now actively integrating with genetics is through the use of the construct of *endophenotypes*. An endophenotype is defined as a measureable physiological, biochemical, psychological, or cognitive factor that mediates or explains genetic influence on a clinical phenotype of a disease or disorder (Gottesman & Gould, 2003). The usefulness of this construct has gained immensely in popularity as an aid to discerning internal processes that provide more graduated links between G × E effects and disease outcomes. I would like to illustrate the usefulness of this construct (with some modification) to specifically address the outcome of adolescent-onset depression, using findings about family behavior and neuroendocrine functioning from our longitudinal studies of middle and late adolescents.

Hypothalamic–pituitary–adrenal (HPA) axis functioning as an endophenotype in adolescence. One of the most consistent findings in the psychopathology literature is that excessive or chronic stress predicts depression (Kendler, Gardner, & Prescott, 2002). Studies of life events reveal a connection of depression to trauma and accumulated stress (Kessler & Magee, 1993), and G × E studies reveal that the effects of these life-event stressors are moderated by genes; one much-studied example being the 5HTTLPR polymorphism (Caspi & Moffitt, 2006). But less is understood at present about the processes that explain why stressful life experiences for genetically vulnerable individuals result in depression, and why their depression typically surfaces during adolescence. It is possible that as new studies begin to link stressful life experiences to depression through intermediate explanatory endophenotypes, we will be able to discern why these processes are particularly potent at adolescence. An additional hope is that understanding a variety of endophenotypes will help us begin to clarify why depression is so widespread in adolescence. Depression is not a disorder that affects only the severely traumatized. We need to identify less extreme processes that arise in a much wider range of families in order to understand the rise of significant levels of subclinical as well as clinical levels of depression in adolescents. For these reasons, examining stress associated with the normative processes of family conflict is important.

As previously discussed by Fleming (Mileva & Fleming, Chap. 1), the HPA axis is one of the body's major systems for handling stress. In reaction to perceived stress, the HPA system activates a cascade of hormonal responses that culminate in the release of cortisol into the bloodstream, inhibiting nonemergency vegetative processes such as sleep, sexual activity, and growth. There is mounting evidence that HPA dysfunction is a productive endophenotype that is beginning to provide a link between a number of gene polymorphisms, such as 5HTTLPR and 9betaA/G, and depression (Gotlib, Joormann, Minor, & Hallmayer, 2008; Otte et al., 2009).

Our lab is interested in whether the endophenotype of HPA functioning may be further connected to variation in the stressful, but normative experience of interpersonal conflict, particularly within families. I now return to our finding that family intolerance of conflict and adolescents' submissive behaviors predict rises in depression for adolescents aged 14–16 years. This finding piqued our lab's interest in understanding why some adolescents submit so readily in situations of family conflict and why submissive behavior corresponds to a significant rise in depressive symptoms. We knew from primate studies conducted both in the wild and in experimental paradigms that cortisol levels of submissive baboons and monkeys were higher than dominant baboons and monkeys (Shively, Laber-Laird, & Anton, 1997). Perhaps our depressed adolescents had overly sensitive HPA responses when faced with interpersonal conflict, which then provoked submissive behavior as a way of coping with the threat? We hypothesized that excessive submission to normative conflict may be a result of the adolescent's heightened sensitivity to threat in conflict situations and a corresponding heightened HPA reaction. Moreover, because submissive behaviors do not usually lead to goal attainment, submissive behavior, in turn, is likely to maintain physiological stress after the actual conflict. Thus, we hypothesized that coping with conflict through submissive behaviors could be both a marker of high stress sensitivity and also a generator of low-level chronic stress, increasing the risk for depression.

We designed a new study to examine adolescent's stress sensitivity to conflict by assessing a trajectory of cortisol levels at seven points before, during, and after a conflict (Powers, Pietromonaco, Gunlicks, & Sayer, 2006). With a new sample of 400 older adolescents, we found that older adolescent males' depressive symptoms were predicted by their submissive behavior with their girlfriends, echoing prior findings with younger adolescent males during conflict with their mothers. By examining HPA reactions to the conflict, we found additionally that this submissive style of coping with interpersonal conflict was significantly associated with HPA reactions to adolescents' anticipation of the conflict, the actual conflict task, and to speed of recovery after the conflict, and that those HPA reactions to conflict predicted increased depressive symptoms and diagnoses (Powers, 2009). Additionally, the depression-related constructs of insecure attachment (Powers et al., 2006), excessive reliance on social support (Gunlicks-Stoessel & Powers, 2009), off-time puberty (Smith & Powers, 2009), and temperamental emotionality were related to HPA reactions before, during, and after interpersonal conflict (Laurent & Powers, 2007). Thus, we believe that HPA functioning in reaction to interpersonal conflict in close relationships is a particularly useful endophenotype that may link adolescent onset of depression to a variety of genetic influences; i.e., genes that influence interpersonal behavior such as inhibition (Fox et al., 2005) or harm avoidance (Yuh et al., 2008), genes that directly influence HPA functioning (Kumsta et al., 2007; Otte et al., 2009), or genes that moderate the effects of HPA functioning (Gotlib et al., 2008).

Gender in Gene–Behavior Interplay and Endophenotypes

Gender has a starring role in adolescence, although it has not yet been mentioned in this discussion. Just as I argue for the value of deriving our primary targets of investigation from firmly based theoretical notions of what is unique to the adolescent phase, I argue that ignoring gender, particularly in adolescence, may impede our search for understanding rGE, G × E, and putative endophenotypes. Striking gender differences accompany the emerging psychopathologies of adolescence. In our own work, gender is fundamental to the specific types of submissive behavior connected to depression in middle adolescence. We find that females' submissive behaviors serve to connect and repair family relations, whereas males' submissive behaviors are used to disengage from relationships (Powers et al., 2010). In addition, the type of HPA response to conflict that is linked to depression is dramatically different for older adolescent males and females in our studies. Females show attenuated HPA responses indicative of chronic stress, whereas males show hyperreactive HPA responses typical of acute stress. Given the remarkable gender differences in so many adolescent mental health disorders, it is imperative that gene–environment and the endophenotypes that may link gene–environment interplay to adolescent mental health outcomes include gender as a central component of their theoretical models and empirical tests of those models.

In conclusion, Neiderhiser's work has provided a rich foundation to build upon, not only for quantitative genetic researchers but also for family researchers from a broad array of disciplines. By carefully examining the myriad of findings from rGE and G × E studies, both genetic and environmental effects unique to the adolescent phase of life can be identified, eventually helping to clarify why so many disorders emerge in this life phase. Researchers who do not specialize in quantitative genetics may, in turn, be able to supply findings of biochemical, neuroendocrine, and psychological endophenotypes that help to illuminate the internal mechanisms that link gene and family environment interactions to adolescent outcomes.

Acknowledgments Research supported by grants from the National Science Foundation and the National Institute of Mental Health (R01-MH60228-01A1).

References

Caspi, A., & Moffitt, T. E. (2006). Gene–environment interactions in psychiatry: Joining forces with neuroscience. *Nature Reviews Neuroscience, 7*(7), 583–590.

Dick, D. M., Viken, R., Pucell, S., Kaprio, J., Pulkkinen, L., & Rose, R. J. (2007). Parental monitoring moderates the importance of genetic and environmental influences on adolescent smoking. *Journal of Abnormal Psychology, 116*, 213–218.

Feinberg, M. E., Button, T. M. M., Neiderhiser, J. M., Reiss, D., & Hetherington, E. M. (2007). Parenting and adolescent antisocial behavior and depression: Evidence of genotype × parenting environment interaction. *Archives of General Psychiatry, 64*(4), 457–465.

Fox, N. A., Nichols, K. E., Henderson, H. A., Rubin, K., Schmidt, L., Hamer, D., et al. (2005). Evidence for a gene–environment interaction in predicting behavioral inhibition in middle childhood. *Psychological Science, 16*(12), 921–926.

Gotlib, I. H., Joormann, J., Minor, K. L., & Hallmayer, J. (2008). HPA axis reactivity: A mechanism underlying the associations among 5-HTTLPR, stress, and depression. *Biological Psychiatry, 63*(9), 847–851.

Gottesman, I. I., & Gould, T. D. (2003). The endophenotype concept in psychiatry: Etymology and strategic intentions. *American Journal of Psychiatry, 160*(4), 636–645.

Gunlicks-Stoessel, M., & Powers, S. I. (2008). Adolescents' emotional experiences of mother-adolescent conflict predict internalizing and externalizing symptoms. *Journal of Research in Adolescence, 18*(4), 621–642.

Gunlicks-Stoessel, M., & Powers, S. I. (2009). Romantic partners' coping strategies and patterns of cortisol reactivity and recovery in response to relationship conflict. *Journal of Social and Clinical Psychology, 18*(4), 621–642.

Henikoff, S., & Matzke, M. A. (1997). Exploring and explaining epigenetic effects. *Trends in Genetics, 13*, 293–295.

Kendler, K. S., Gardner, C. O., & Prescott, C. A. (2002). Toward a comprehensive developmental model for major depression in women. *American Journal of Psychiatry, 159*(7), 1133–1145.

Kessler, R. C., & Magee, W. J. (1993). Childhood adversities and adult depression: Basic patterns of association in a U.S. national survey. *Psychological Medicine, 23*, 679–690.

Kumsta, R., Entringer, S., Koper, J. W., van Rossum, E. F. C., Hellhammer, D. H., & Wust, S. (2007). Sex specific associations between common glucocorticoid receptor gene variants and hypothalamus-pituitary-adrenal axis responses to psychosocial stress. *Biological Psychiatry, 62*(8), 863–869.

Laurent, H., & Powers, S. (2007). Emotion regulation in emerging adult couples: Temperament, attachment, and HPA response to conflict. *Biological Psychology, 76*(1–2), 61–71.

Mileva, V., & Fleming, A. (2010). How mothers are born: A psychobiological analysis of mothering. In A. Booth, S. McHale, & N. Landale (Eds.), *Biosocial research contributions to understanding family processes and problems*. New York: Springer.

Mill, J., & Petronis, A. (2007). Molecular studies of major depressive disorder: The epigenetic perspective. *Molecular Psychiatry, 12*(9), 799–814.

Narusyte, J., Neiderhiser, J. M., D'Onofrio, B. M., Reiss, D., Spotts, E. L., Ganiban, J., et al. (2008). Testing different types of genotype-environment correlation: An extended children-of-twins model. *Developmental Psychology, 44*(6), 1591–1603.

Neiderhiser, J. M. (2010). Gene–environment interplay helps to explain influences of family relationships on adolescent adjustment and development. In A. Booth, S. McHale, & N. Landale (Eds.), *Biosocial foundations of family processes* (pp. 71–84). New York: Springer.

Neiderhiser, J. M., Reiss, D., Pedersen, N. L., Lichtenstein, P., Spotts, E. L., Hansson, K., et al. (2004). Genetic and environmental influences on mothering of adolescents: A comparison of two samples. *Developmental Psychology*, *40*(3), 335–351.

Otte, C., Wüst, S., Zhao, S., Pawlikowska, L., Kwok, P.-Y., & Whooley, M. A. (2009). Glucocorticoid receptor gene and depression in patients with coronary heart disease: The Heart and Soul Study—2009 Curt Richter Award Winner. *Psychoneuroendocrinology*, *34*(10), 1574–1581.

Powers, S. I. (2009). *Hormones and lovers' quarrels: How stress translates into depression.* Paper presented at the Distinguished Faculty Lecture, University of Massachusetts: Amherst.

Powers, S. I., Battle, C. L., Dorta, K., & Welsh, D. P. (2010). Adolescents' submission and conflict behaviors with mothers predicts current and future internalizing problems. *Research in Human Development*, *7*(1).

Powers, S. I., Pietromonaco, P. R., Gunlicks, M., & Sayer, A. (2006). Dating couples' attachment styles and patterns of cortisol reactivity and recovery in response to a relationship conflict. *Journal of Personality and Social Psychology*, *90*(4), 613–628.

Powers, S. I., & Welsh, D. P. (1999). Mother-daughter interactions and adolescent girls' depression. In M. Cox & J. Brooks-Gunn (Eds.), *Conflict and cohesion in families: Causes and consequences* (pp. 243–281). Mahwah, NJ: Lawrence Erlbaum Associates.

Powers, S. I., Welsh, D. P., & Wright, V. (1994). Adolescents' affective experience of family behaviors: The role of subjective understanding. *Journal of Research on Adolescence*, *4*(4), 585–600.

Shively, C. A., Laber-Laird, K., & Anton, R. F. (1997). Behavior and physiology of social stress and depression in female cynomolgus monkeys. *Biological Psychiatry*, *41*(8), 871–882.

Smith, A. E., & Powers, S. I. (2009). Off-time pubertal timing predicts physiological reactivity to post-puberty interpersonal stress. *Journal of Research in Adolescence*, *19*(3), 441–458.

Sunderland, J. E., & Costa, M. (2003). Epigenetics and the environment. *Annuals of the New York Academy of Sciences*, *983*, 151–160.

Tuvblad, C., Grann, M., & Lichtenstein, P. (2006). Heritability for adolescent antisocial behavior differs with socioeconomic status: Gene–environment interaction. *Journal of Child Psychology and Psychiatry*, *47*(7), 734–743.

Yuh, J., Neiderhiser, J. M., Spotts, E. L., Pedersen, N. L., Lichtenstein, P., Hansson, K., et al. (2008). The role of temperament and social support in depressive symptoms: A twin study of mid-aged women. *Journal of Affective Disorders*, *106*(1–2), 99–105.

Part III
Mate Selection, Family Formation, and Fertility

Chapter 9
Human Adaptations for Mating: Frameworks for Understanding Patterns of Family Formation and Fertility

Steven W. Gangestad

Abstract Reproductive and mating systems vary substantially across modern and traditional human societies. A variety of conceptual tools may be required to explain this variation. This chapter discusses an explanatory framework based on the notion of evoked culture. Evoked cultural differences emerge when behavioral expression of an adaptation is contingent on environmental conditions, such that the behavior of groups exposed to different conditions consequently differs. This chapter has a number of components. First, it offers a brief primer of adaptation-ist concepts and methodologies within evolutionary biology. Second, it discusses how these methodologies have been used to infer particular adaptations underlying human mating. Third, it examines how some adaptations may have been shaped by selection to be expressed contingently, giving rise to variation. Finally, limitations and potentially useful applications of the evoked culture concept (e.g., illustrated by effects of the contraceptive pill on women's mate choice) are discussed.

Introduction

Modern Western patterns of mating and reproduction contrast sharply with what can be observed in human forager populations and has, presumably, existed throughout most of human history. In typical foraging populations, women's mean total fertility rate is about 5.28 (with nearly half of all offspring dying before age 17; Marlowe, 2001), whereas in the USA, it is about 1.80 – below replacement (e.g., http://www.census.gov). And in some Westernized countries, such as Italy and Japan, the rate is even lower: close to 1, despite the fact that women's reproductive potential has increased in Western societies, as a result of menarche occurring several years earlier [e.g., about 16 in the Ache, a traditional forager in Paraguay (Hill & Hurtado, 1996) vs. about 12.5 currently in the USA].

S.W. Gangestad (✉)
Department of Psychology, University of New Mexico, Albuquerque, NM, USA
e-mail: sgangest@unm.edu

A. Booth et al. (eds.), *Biosocial Foundations of Family Processes*,
National Symposium on Family Issues, DOI 10.1007/978-1-4419-7361-0_9,
© Springer Science+Business Media, LLC 2011

Patterns of mating and reproduction in traditional foraging societies, however, are not all similar. Reproductive skew reflects the extent to which some individuals outreproduce others and is typically measured by the variance in total fertility. The sex difference in the skew can reveal, for instance, the extent to which some males monopolize matings, with many males completely unsuccessful. As Brown, Laland, and Borgerhoff Mulder (2009) recently emphasized, this sex difference varies incredibly across traditional human societies, with men having 4+ times the variance in some societies, but not much over 1 in others. This difference is not merely due to gross differences in mating system. Both the Dogon and the Aka, for instance, are largely polygynous, the Ache and the Pimbwe serial monogamists, yet the Ache are much more similar to the Dogon than the Pimbwe, and the Aka are comparable to the Pimbwe, not the Dogon.

Why Have Patterns of Human Mating and Reproduction Changed Dramatically?

Throughout thousands of years of existence as foragers, people likely exhibited patterns of mating and reproduction drastically different from what we observe in contemporary Western societies. More generally, across human groups distributed in time and space, patterns of mating and reproduction differ remarkably (e.g., with regard to sex differences in reproductive skew). Why is this the case?

One answer to this question may seem obvious: At least part of the variation is due to the social and other factors that discriminate human groups. No doubt, this answer is true. At the same time, it is incomplete at a deep conceptual level. It does not specify processes whereby individuals respond differently to factors varying across groups.

In this chapter, I explore one avenue of thinking about the reasons for patterns of human mating and reproduction varying across temporally and spatially distributed human groups: That humans adapt in order to mate and reproduce in manners that predispose them to make contingent responses to factors that differentiate groups, leading human groups to vary in systematic ways. This concept has been captured by the term "evoked culture" (Tooby & Cosmides, 1992), which can be illustrated by a simple example. Humans possess adaptations to form calluses on the soles of their feet in response to friction. Suppose two groups differ in the extent to which they wear shoes when walking outside – one does, whereas the other rarely does. Members of the former group form thick calluses on their feet; members of the latter group do not. This difference owes to different experiences in the two groups. But the effect of these experiences cannot be explained without reference to a human adaptation leading to differential expression of callous formation, depending on friction (see also Gangestad, Haselton, & Buss, 2006).

I flesh out several themes.

1. I offer a brief primer of adaptationist thinking in evolutionary biology. Adaptations are features that were selected for their enhancement of fitness ancestrally.

A variety of human adaptations for mating and reproduction may, despite changes in overt behavior, perhaps remain little changed in contemporary Western societies. These adaptations include basic physiological systems for reproduction but may also include adaptations for adjustment of behavior.

2. Adaptations can, in theory, be identified through the application of methodological adaptationism. These methods not only identify adaptations; they also lead to an understanding of the selective pressures that gave rise to the adaptations and, hence, give shape to the nature of the effective selective environments in which humans evolved. Phylogenetic analysis of adaptations can help place these selective environments in a sequenced historical context.

3. Application of adaptationist methodologies has given rise to a variety of inferences about the nature of human mating systems and how humans evolved to operate within them. I discuss some of these inferences.

4. Through interaction with prevailing circumstances, adaptations may produce variable outcomes ("evoked culture"). I discuss possible examples.

5. The "evoked culture" approach offers potential understandings of variations across groups. It also has limitations and may be of minimal utility in explaining some differences, as I briefly discuss. Indeed, by no means do I claim that evoked culture provides an explanation of all cultural variability in reproductive and mating systems. With regard to some specific contrasts, it may play virtually no role. My aims here are fairly modest: To argue that evoked culture is a useful element in a broader set of conceptual tools to explain variations.

Evolutionary Analysis: Adaptationism and Phylogenetic Analysis

I begin with a basic primer on adaptationist and phylogenetic approaches to reconstructing evolutionary histories.

Adaptation, Function, Adaptiveness, and Exaptation

Adaptation. In evolutionary biology, *adaptation* refers to two related phenomena: first, a *process* whereby organisms are shaped through natural selection to be adapted to their environments; and second, a *feature* that evolved through selection because it enhanced the fitness of its carriers. The process of adaptation occurs through the evolution of adaptations.

Function. Evolutionary biologists use the term *function* in a special way, one tied to the concept of adaptation. Through an organism's interactions with the world, a trait has effects. One or more of the trait's effects may lead its beholder to have greater fitness than others lacking the trait. A beneficial effect that led selection to favor the trait is a trait's function.

Simple examples illustrate. Simply put, bird wings are adaptations *for* the function of flight. Eyes are adaptations *for* the function of seeing. Release of gonadotropins by human fetuses into the bloodstream of their mothers appears to be an adaptation *for* the function of increasing the likelihood fetuses will be retained by the mother (Haig, 1993).

Evolutionary biology's special concept of function is distinct from a more general concept used by physiologists and psychologists. Causal role functional analysis (Godfrey-Smith, 1993) examines processes through which an organism performs various activities. Some psychologists, for instance, address the question of how people read by examining the roles of various psychological capacities, and thereby perform causal role functional analysis. But that analysis does not reveal *evolutionary* functions. The evolutionary concept of function explicitly refers to historical selection. Though psychological processes function in reading in a causal role sense, their *evolutionary functions* do not directly pertain to reading (see also Millikan, 1989).

Adaptiveness. The concept of adaptiveness is distinct from adaptation. A trait is adaptive if it offers its beholders fitness benefits in a current context (or specific referenced context). Because adaptation is explicitly defined with reference to *historical*, not contemporary, events, current adaptiveness is neither a necessary nor a sufficient feature of an adaptation.

Current adaptiveness is not necessary to adaptation because features that evolved due to past adaptiveness (and hence favored by natural selection) need not remain adaptive. The human appendix arguably evolved (in the distant ancestry of the lineage leading to humans) for the function of breaking down cellulose (via symbiotic bacteria housed there). Humans, however, no longer benefit from this function. The human appendix is an adaptation (albeit in vestigial form); it was selected for its benefits. But it is not currently adaptive (see Sterelny & Griffiths, 1999).

Exaptation. Current adaptiveness is not sufficient to define a trait as an adaptation because a trait's adaptiveness may not have the historical depth to have affected trait evolution. Gould and Vrba (1982) introduced the concept of *exaptation* to highlight the difference between adaptiveness that, historically, did play a role in the evolution of a trait, and adaptiveness that has not. A trait is an exaptation to a particular beneficial effect if the trait gives rise to that beneficial effect, but the beneficial effect had no impact on the shaping of the trait historically. An example is the way the black heron uses its wing to shade water (Gould & Vrba, 1982). When foraging for fish, the heron may raise its wing to reduce glare of the sun's light off the water and increase visibility of prey under the water's surface. The wing itself evolved through selection for flight. There is no evidence that the wing was modified through selection for water shading. The wing is therefore an adaptation for flight and exapted to water shading. (Water shading may have involved adaptation, as selection may have favored variations in the heron's *brain* that led it to use its wing for shading. But the *wing itself* is not an adaptation *for water shading*.)

Another example is reading. We can read (and reading might currently yield fitness benefits) but not because selection favored traits for their effects on reading.

Reading is possible because traits evolved for reasons unrelated to the benefits of reading became used for reading.

Sometimes, however, a trait becomes adaptive after it has evolved, and though its beneficial effects do not explain why the trait evolved in the first place, they have persisted long enough to explain why the trait has been maintained. Mutations and other perturbations may lead to the degradation of traits. Selection against these perturbations that disturb a trait's development – that is, selection that maintains the trait because of its benefits – qualifies as natural selection for the trait. Is this selective history for the trait sufficient to qualify the trait as an adaptation? This question has been and continues to be debated. Gould and Vrba (1982) claimed that the answer is "no." Two different forms of selection are distinct: *positive* selection responsible for the shaping of an adaptive trait that, historically, did not exist, and *negative* or *purifying* selection against perturbations maintaining an adaptive trait. Gould and Vrba (1982) argued that positive selection for a benefit leading to trait evolution is necessary to concepts of adaptation and function. Others (e.g., Sterelny & Griffiths, 1999) disagree. In my view, Gould and Vrba's definitional distinction is useful, but the matter of whether exaptation is restricted to cases of no positive selection largely definitional.

Secondary adaptation. Often, a trait that acquires a new benefit undergoes subsequent modification that improves its proficiency in delivering the benefit. Gould and Vrba (1982) referred to this process as secondary adaptation. Adaptation (vs. exaptation) is the proper term, they claimed, because (positive) selection for the benefit led to change. From a historical standpoint, a trait that evolved for one function but is later adapted for a different benefit underwent primary adaptation for the first function, was exapted to a new benefit, and then was secondarily adapted for the new benefit. Bird feathers originally evolved for thermoregulation. They were later exapted to, and then secondarily adapted for, enhancement of flight. Feathers may retain some details (e.g., soft plumacious barbs near the skin's surface) that were never secondarily adapted.

By-Products

When selection occurs due to the beneficial effect of a particular trait, it inevitably modifies the phenotype in many ways. A trait that has a selected beneficial effect is an adaptation. Other traits also modified but with no beneficial effects themselves are *by-products* of selection (also referred to as *incidental effects* or *spandrels*; Gould & Lewontin, 1979). Vertebrate bones are composed of calcium phosphate. Bones are adaptations that enable effective movement. Calcium phosphate is white and, hence, so too are bones. The whiteness of bones has no beneficial effect itself, however; it is a byproduct of selection.

Selection for a single adaptation may potentially lead to a multitude of by-products. The precise distance between the eyes in humans may be partly due to selection for effective binocular vision. But it also affects the precise distance between each eye and any other morphological structure (e.g., the right and left kneecaps, each metatarsal bone, the appendix, and so on). In all likelihood, virtually all of these distances are mere by-products of selection; they have no gene-propagating effects themselves.

How Evolutionary Biologists Identify Adaptation

Evolutionary biologists are interested in understanding the selective forces that shaped an organism. Adaptationism has been described as a methodology for "carving" the organism into those aspects of its phenotype that have evolved due to net fitness benefits historically and nonfunctional by-products (e.g., Thornhill, 1997; see Sterelny & Griffiths, 1999, for other types of adaptationism). In doing so, the researcher not only comes to understand what aspects of the phenotype are functional, but the researcher also infers the specific nature of important selective forces that shaped the organism and thereby appreciates important evolutionary events that led to the organism we now observe. That is, a researcher not only identifies adaptations but also identifies biological function, what those adaptations are *for*.

Williams (1966) often credited with offering the first systematic statements that gave direction to the modern approach of adaptationism, noted that, as already discussed, it is not sufficient to show that a trait is beneficial. Exaptations have utility but need not have evolved as a result of selection for those beneficial effects. Williams (1966) argued that the biological concept of adaptation is an onerous one and required stringent standards of evidence, ones captured by the concept of *functional* or *special design*.

Arguments of Design

A trait or constellation of traits exhibits special design for a particular function if it performs a particular function effectively and, furthermore, it is difficult to imagine another scenario that would have led to the evolution of the trait or constellation of traits. The classic example is the vertebrate eye (see, e.g., Williams, 1992). The eye and its detailed features are effective for seeing. Moreover, it is difficult to imagine an evolutionary scenario through which the eye would have evolved other than one in which its details were selected for their optical properties and thereby the function of sight. A special design argument is an argument to the best explanation, (provisional) acceptance of one explanation over competitors if the preferred explanation explains the facts better than the competitors do (see, e.g., Sterelny & Griffiths, 1999).

How Is "Good Design" Assessed?

As Williams (1992) explained, "Adaptation is demonstrated by observed conformity to a priori design specifications" (Williams, 1992, p. 40). But as he further noted, "Unfortunately those who wish to ascertain whether some attribute of an organism does or does not conform to design specifications are left largely to their own intuitions, with little help from established methodology" (p. 41). There exist no formal rules by which to evaluate claims of fit. Ultimately, a special design argument is one about probabilities: "whether a presumed function is served with sufficient precision, economy, efficiency, etc., to rule out pure chance (i.e., any possibility other than adaptation for a particular effect) as an adequate explanation" (Williams, 1966, p. 10, bracketed information added). But the rules by which investigators evaluate these possibilities are not spelled out. Does that mean that adaptationist arguments lack scientific rigor? Not at all. As theoretical claims in science go, special design arguments are in no way exceptional. Scientific hypotheses are often accepted on the basis of informal arguments of probabilities (e.g., Salmon, 1984). Arguments for special design rely on the same: They claim that exceptional fits between a trait's forms and purported functions would have to be extraordinarily strange coincidences *if* selection had not shaped the traits for their purported functions.

Of course, that is not to say that arguments for design are all equally strong. Some fits of form to function – e.g., the details of the eye to the function of seeing – are very difficult to deny. Others are merely suggestive. Again, however, that is generally true of evaluation of scientific hypotheses: Arguments for some hypotheses are compelling; others need further bolstering. (For further readings, see Andrews, Gangestad, & Matthews, 2003; Thornhill, 1997; Williams, 1966, 1992).

Phylogenetic Analysis

Each trait of a species, whether adaptation or byproduct, has a point of origin: At some time within the lineage leading to the modern species, the trait emerged. It was then maintained through some evolutionary force. Selection is a force that maintains traits, but it cannot directly give rise to *origins*. It favors *existing* variants over others. When a trait arises, then, it can have no function. It acquires function by being selected. Typically, traits originate through perturbations in developmental processes (e.g., caused by mutations) giving rise to new variants.

Although adaptationism can inform understanding of selection, it cannot yield inferences about origins. For that task, phylogenetic analyses are needed. A phylogenetic analysis yields inferences about when a trait originated based on the distribution of a trait amongst extant species (and, where applicable, species found in the fossil record). A simple illustration is the mammary gland. All extant mammals (including monotremes and marsupials) possess mammary glands. The parsimonious explanation of this distribution is that mammary glands originated in the species ancestral to all mammals and were maintained in all mammalian lineages.

Origins are trait- and lineage-specific. Some human traits, such as a functional estrogen receptor, are common to all vertebrates and hence arose very deep in evolutionary time (approximately 450 million years ago). Others, such as the mammary gland, are common to mammals and arose about 200 million years ago. Yet others (e.g., an opposable thumb) are common to primates, and some are shared by no other extant species and, in all likelihood, arose since humans and our closest living relatives diverged, within the past eight million years.

Some human traits that emerged very recently are shared with other species, but ones distantly related to us. Those who argue that humans have evolved to engage in biparental care believe that qualities promoting paternal investment in offspring emerged recently in our lineage, as close relatives do not share them. Many bird species do share them. The parsimonious phylogenetic inference in this instance is that these paternal qualities evolved independently in humans and birds; they had multiple distinct origins.

I have thus far referred to a "trait," such as a mammary gland, as though it is a single thing. At some level, mammary glands in general do share features. (For one, they permit extraction of a nutritious supplement to young.) Mammary glands can be distinguished from one another, however, at more detailed levels of description. (Indeed, the mammary glands of monotremes appear very similar to sweat glands, leading to the inference that mammary glands first originated through perturbed development of a sweat gland. As well, the precise constituents [e.g., fat content] of milk yielded by mammary glands differ across species.) One must specify the level at which a particular trait is defined. Human mammary glands writ large originated in the species ancestral to all mammals. Particular features of human mammary glands have more recent origins, and some no doubt originated in hominins. Darwin's term "descent with modification" aptly captures the idea that individual details of features that evolve within a lineage have their own points of origin.

Evolutionary Analyses of Ancestral Patterns of Mating and Reproduction: The Question of Adaptation for Paternal Care

I now turn to the question of what we can infer about the evolution of adaptations and by-products involved in human mating using adaptationist and phylogenetic analyses. What was the nature of the human mating system (or systems) to which humans adapted? Are adaptations arising from these systems expressed similarly today, and in what ways? In what ways are they expressed differently in modern contexts? These questions are very big and broad, and I do not pretend to answer them in any way approaching completeness. But I will address some basic, fundamental components of answers here, at least in outline form. Perhaps the most fundamental question concerning human mating adaptations is the question of whether and to what extent humans have adaptations evolved in the context of biparental care. That is, are humans adapted to mating and reproduction systems in which biparental care occurs, or not?

The Evolution of Biparental Care

In theory, selection could favor any mixture of parental care by mothers and fathers. Empirically, however, an evolved solution to parenting that characterizes many species is one in which members of one sex – usually females – are fully responsible for *parental effort*. (Parental effort is defined as all effort expended by an individual to improve the quality [viability and competitiveness] of the offspring that could have been expended on other fitness-enhancing activities: e.g., gestation, lactation, feeding, defense, teaching, and so on.) The other sex – typically males – incurs by far the greatest costs of *mating effort*, costs to seek and compete for mates. This parenting solution characterizes most mammals (~97%).

Many exceptions exist, of course. Biparental care characterizes most bird species, some rodents, and some primates, among other species. (In most teleost fish species, males actually invest greater effort into care than do females.) And indeed, recent theoretical modeling and analysis suggests that male as well as female care *should be expected* to evolve in many circumstances. Several factors promote the evolution of male as well as female care.

Complementarity of efforts. Complementarity of the sexes' parental efforts exists when the total beneficial effect of the sexes' efforts exceeds the sum of the individual beneficial effects of males and females were they investing in offspring separately. (That is, complementarity entails nonadditive effects of each parent's investments.) It favors the evolution of biparental care because, with complementarity, a father's investment not only has its own fitness benefits; it ratchets up the fitness benefits of the mother's investment as well (e.g., Kokko & Johnstone, 2002). Within the aerial niche occupied by most bird species, complementarity may partly exist because, while one parent gathers food for offspring, the other guards the nest. If one parent alone were to leave the chicks in order to forage, the offspring could be easy prey for predators.

The relative costs of care and competition and the adult sex ratio. When many males die as a result of competition (whether immediately or as a result of persistent stresses due to competition, resulting in lower viability), surviving males do better in the mating market, as there is less competition. (Costly competition, that is, leads to a female-biased sex ratio.) When caring leads to mortality, such that females die as a result of it, males face stiffer competition in the mating market, as there are fewer mates to compete for. Though one might think, intuitively, that selection would favor doing the less dangerous activity (competing vs. caring), modeling and simulation show that the indirect effects of danger through effects on the sex ratio can override its direct effects. Hence, males may evolve to compete more when male competition is dangerous and evolve to care more when female care is particularly dangerous (Kokko & Jennions, 2008). Consistent with these predictions, male intrasexual competition in many mammalian species tends to be costly, leading adult sex ratios to become female-biased, whereas in birds care is often more costly, leading to male-biased adult sex ratios.

Low parentage. Females typically can discern which offspring are their own. To the extent that males cannot detect which offspring are their own, the value of male care is reduced (as a function of the nonpaternity rate) and males will be selected to care less (Kokko & Jennions, 2008). Males should care more when paternity can be validly assessed.

Sexual selection. When nonrandom (that is, phenotype-dependent) variance in male mating success (not due to selection for advertisements of ability to care) is large, males are selected to care less (Kokko & Jennions, 2008). When females particularly prefer a small subset of males (often for their "good genes"), the cost of caring for young is great for those males; they give up precious mating opportunities if they exert effort to invest in offspring. The large cost of women's loss evidence parental effort that the most desired males pay leads them not to care for offspring in most cases, leaving females alone responsible for parental care.

These factors and perhaps others influence the evolution of so-called sex roles – typical patterns of sexual divisions in competition for mates and care – observed in species. Within species, however, these factors can also influence the expression of adaptations for reproduction. For instance, males in a species may evolve adaptations that lead them to be sensitive to particular cues that affect the value of care (e.g., the adult sex ratio), and care more or less depending on the presence or absence of that cue (e.g., care more when sex ratios are male-biased and care less when they are female-biased). That is, some adaptations lead to contingent expression of behavioral tendencies that is adaptive in an ancestral context.

Was Biparental Care Favored by Selection on Ancestral Humans?

Obviously, fathers are active participants in parenting in modern human settings. But that observation does not directly address whether men possess *adaptations* for exerting parental effort – that is, whether ancestral selection has *favored* biparental care. The latter can only be decided through adaptationist analyses. In fact, issues of whether humans evolved adaptations to cooperatively parent offspring have been hotly debated by evolutionary anthropologists.

Hunting-as-Parental-Effort Views

In most primate species (including our close relatives), individuals of both sexes are largely responsible for their own subsistence after at most a few years of care following birth. Though males may provide a variety of material services to females (e.g., sharing food in exchange for sex; e.g., Dunbar, 1987), mothers harvest the overwhelming majority of calories consumed by offspring during pregnancy and lactation. By contrast, in most human foraging populations, the average adult male generates more calories than he consumes: 64% of the total calories produced in the 95 foraging societies on which sufficient information is available (Marlowe, 2001; see also Kaplan, Hill, Lancaster, & Hurtado, 2000). The primary activity through which men generate surplus calories in foraging societies is hunting (broadly defined to include any activity aimed to harvest animal meat, including fishing). Though women forage and extract roots (and, in a meaningful minority of societies, produce more calories than men), only rarely do they hunt to a substantial degree (for an exception, see Hart, Pilling, & Goodale, 1987, on the Tiwi of Australia). Human foragers appear to be adapted to a diet consisting of high-quality, calorie-rich foods. Whereas chimpanzees obtain about 95% of their calories from collected foods requiring no extraction (e.g., fruits, leaves), only about 8% of calories consumed by modern hunter-gatherers are from foods requiring no extraction. Vertebrate meat accounts for, on average, 30–80% of human hunter-gatherer caloric intake but just 2% of chimpanzee diets (Kaplan et al., 2000).

Women reproductively benefit from the male-generated surplus. The degree of male contribution to the diet varies considerably across foraging societies (~: 40-90+%). As expected if women and offspring directly benefit from male subsidies, women's fertility covaries positively with male contribution to subsistence (Marlowe, 2001). This effect is partly mediated through the interbirth interval: Men's contribution to subsistence negatively covaries with the delay between the birth of one offspring and the same woman's next offspring. (For reviews of the energetics of human pregnancy and lactation, see Dufour & Sauther, 2002; Ellison, 2001.)

A traditional anthropological view is that male surplus food production evolved as paternal care (e.g., Lancaster & Lancaster, 1983; Lovejoy, 1981; Westermarck, 1929). According to this view, the nuclear family is a key economic unit in the evolution of human mating relations. For subsidies generated by male hunting to function as parental effort, nutrients that men generate must flow from them to mates (and then to offspring) or directly to offspring.

Hunting-as-Mating-Effort Views

The male-hunting-as-parental-effort theory, critics claim, faces a fundamental difficulty: Nuclear families are not, in fact, potent economic units in foraging societies (Hawkes, 1991, 2004; Hawkes, O'Connell, & Blurton Jones, 1991; Hawkes, O'Connell, & Blurton Jones, 2001). In the Hadza of Tanzania and the Ache of Paraguay, for instance, hunters have little control over the distribution of meat they generate. Instead, meat (particularly from large game) is shared widely across community members. A Hadza hunter's own family receives no more meat from his large game kills than what they receive from the same-sized animal a neighbor killed. In one analysis, offspring nutritional status covaried with Hadza women's foraging returns but not men's (Hawkes, 2004). Large game hunting does not function as parental effort if it does not preferentially advantage a man's own offspring.

According to Hawkes (2004), men's hunting functions as (that is, evolved for) mating effort – effort to compete for access to mates through "showing off" (Hawkes et al., 1991) – rather than as parental effort. Men garner prestige through successful hunting exploits, particularly big-game hunting. Ultimately, prestige translates into mating opportunities (including mating with other men's wives) (see Kaplan & Hill, 1985; Marlowe, 2003a).

Of course, male hunting subsidizes the diets of women and their offspring. But these subsidies, in the male-hunting-as-mating-effort view, are not generated directly by women's own mates or by children's own fathers. Rather, they are generated through the efforts of men in general to gain mates. In economists' terms, the surplus calories generated by male hunting that benefit women and offspring are "positive externalities" of men's showing off – windfalls they enjoy, not benefits men's efforts were designed to achieve. In adaptationist terms, the surplus calories men's hunting generates for their community are fortuitous by-products.

Hawkes et al. (2001) did argue that the diets of women and their children are subsidized through the efforts of family members but not primarily husbands. Rather, maternal kin – most importantly, mothers' mothers (i.e., children's grandmothers) – work to directly subsidize the diets of women of reproductive age and their offspring (Hawkes, 2004; see also Hrdy, 2009).

A Blended View

The hunting-as-parental-effort and the hunting-as-mating-effort theories can be and, at times, have been presented in extreme forms. But a blend is possible: Historically, men may have benefited from hunting in currencies of enhanced viability of offspring *and* mating opportunities.

Patterns of Hadza foraging rates and activities support this view (Marlowe, 2003a). Overall, married Hadza women produce as many calories as married Hadza men. Women with young children, however, do not, as their childcare interferes with effective foraging. Women with an infant (<1 year of age), for instance, harvest about half as much as the mean of all married women. In such instances, however, their husbands forage more. In couples without a child 8 years of age or younger, wives produce more calories than husbands do (~3,300 vs. 2,900), but in couples with an infant less than 1 year of age men produce almost 70% of the calories (~1,700 by wives vs. 3,800 by husbands). Hadza men adjust their work efforts (and perhaps the prey items they target) in response to the direct food production of wives, as it varies with the presence or absence of young children. The view that men's work functions solely as mating effort cannot readily explain this pattern. (Additionally, about 30% of Hadza children have stepfathers. In contrast to genetic fathers, stepfathers do not enhance food production in response to the presence of young stepchildren in the household; see also Marlowe, 1999.)

Other data too suggest that male foraging efforts function as parental effort. Across societies of the standard cross-cultural sample (SCCS), pair-bond stability (low divorce rate) associates with older ages at weaning (Quinlan & Quinlan, 2008; see also Quinlan, Quinlan, & Flinn, 2003). As lactation interferes with women's ability to produce food, male subsidy purportedly permits women to invest in young offspring through nursing. Jointly with findings that male contributions to subsistence predict shorter interbirth intervals in foraging societies (Marlowe, 2001), these results imply that male subsidies increase the total amount of time a woman allocates to reproductive effort through both gestation and lactation.

But Is There Design Evidence for Adaptations for Parental Effort?

Once again, compelling evidence that particular selection pressures effectively shaped an organism's phenotype historically is to be found in the nature of the organism those selection pressures shaped; effective selection on an organism leaves its signature in the design of the organism. The most compelling evidence that men were historically shaped to allocate effort to parenting, then, should be found in evidence that men possess design features that function to allocate effort to parenting. Studies showing that men respond to circumstances that, in theory, affect the payoffs to parenting and mating effort (e.g., their partner having small children) suggest that men possess design to engage in parental effort. But are there specific physiological or psychological features, the design of which can be analyzed? I discuss two possible examples.

Modulation of testosterone levels. Endocrine hormones may be thought of as messengers in distributed communication networks (e.g., Finch & Rose, 1995). Across vertebrate taxa, the testosterone (T) endocrine system has been shaped to have particular functions. Specifically, T appears to facilitate male mating effort by channeling energetic resources to features particularly useful in male–male competition (e.g., muscles, sensitivity to dominance ranks and cues of social hierarchy; e.g., Mazur & Booth, 1998) and, due to necessary trade-offs, away from other targets of allocation (e.g., repair, immune function; see Bribiescas, 2001; Ellison, 2003). According to this view, systems that regulate T production and receptivity may have been tuned by selection to upregulate testosterone when mating effort is particularly called for and downregulate it when other efforts are particularly needed. T may well be used in similar roles across vertebrate species because, once it evolved, its function was maintained and conserved by selection (even if, within particular species, specific elements of the T-regulatory system have been modified).

In species in which males exert parental effort, just such a modification of the T-regulation system may have often evolved. In these species, T may modulate not just relative allocations of effort to somatic effort (e.g., repair, immune function) and mating effort. It may also modulate allocation of effort to mating effort and parental effort (in shorthand, competing vs. caring). It achieves this role through modification of the T-regulatory system to be responsive to cues that indicate value to parental efforts (e.g., provisioning of young) rather than mating efforts, such as birth of a social mate's offspring. Consistent with this view, in some species in which males invest in offspring (e.g., marmosets, some birds), male T levels drop after the birth/hatching of the mates' offspring (e.g., Nunes, Fite, & French, 2000; Nunes, Fite, Patera, & French, 2001; for a review, see Muller & Wrangham, 2001). Interestingly, this feature of the T system has evolved independently several times in vertebrates (e.g., in birds at least once, in mammals several times). (This perspective implies that the T levels of males in species lacking paternal care do not drop in response to birth of an offspring to a female mated with.)

In some birds, males already mated (and perhaps fathered offspring in a season) may benefit from seeking additional mates, particularly in pair-bonding bird species in which females engage in "extra-pair copulations" (EPCs) at high rates – copulations with males other than their social partner. When females are relatively "faithful" to their social partners, there are few additional mating possibilities available, and male efforts to seek additional matings are, on average, less successful. Across bird species, male T levels covary positively with the total extra-pair paternity rate (proportion of offspring sired by males other than social partners; Garemszegi, Eens, Hurtrez-Boussès, & Møller, 2005). They do not covary strongly with overall levels of polygyny (mean number of mates per mated male). This pattern is consistent with the T system in male birds having evolved in response to conditions that affect the relative value of exerting mating vs. parental effort.

In pair-bonding birds and some mammals, then, reductions in male T following birth of their social mate's offspring may reflect *design* for exerting parental effort. Does men's T regulatory system also possess these features? Mounting evidence suggests yes. On average, men's T-levels drop when they become mated or have offspring (e.g., Berg & Wynne-Edwards, 2001; Booth & Dabbs, 1993; Burnham et al., 2003; Gray et al., 2004; Gray, Kahlenberg, Barrett, Lipson, & Ellison, 2002; Gray, Yang, & Pope, 2006; Mazur & Michalek, 1998; Storey, Walsh, Quinton, & Wynne-Edwards, 2000). In several Western studies, one Chinese sample, and a sample from Dominica, men who are mated in serious dating or marital relationships have, on average, lower T than single men do. Some evidence indicates that the association depends partly on changes in T following changes in mating or paternal status (e.g., Mazur & Michalek, 1998; cf. Van Anders & Watson, 2006). Men who have lower T levels moreover respond more prosocially to infant cries than do men with higher levels of T (Fleming, Corter, Stallings, & Steiner, 2002), which is an additional evidence that T functions to modulate mating and parental effort.

Two sets of studies further illustrate the contingent nature of men's allocation of effort to mating. As just mentioned, in Western samples, men who are mated in serious dating or marital relationships typically have lower T than single men do. In two studies, McIntyre, Gangestad, Gray, Chapman, Burnham, O'Rourke, and Thornhill (2006) found this same difference in men's T as a function of mating status. However, the effect of mating status was moderated by men's interest in pursuing extra-pair relationships with women other than primary partners. Men who claimed to have little interest in and history of extra-pair relationships revealed the typical drop in T when mated, as compared to being single. Men who claimed interest in and had a history of extra-pair relationships, by contrast, showed no difference: They had T levels just as high when they were in relationships as when single. Causal processes underlying this finding are currently unknown. (T may affect interest in mating effort, but continued mating interest may also maintain higher T levels).

Muller, Marlowe, Bugumba, and Ellison (2009) examined differences in T levels as a function of paternity in two neighboring Tanzanian groups that differ in paternal involvement. Hadza forager men engage in substantial amounts of paternal care and, as expected, Hadza fathers have lower levels of T than Hadza nonfathers. Dotoga pastoralist men rarely engage in direct paternal care, and fathers purportedly continue to invest substantially in mating effort. Accordingly, Datoga fathers had T levels no lower than those of Dotoga nonfathers.

Though these data suggest that men have adaptation shaped for the function of parental investment (trading off against mating effort), more research is needed. One study found that, when polygynously mated, Kenyan Swahili men's T levels remain high (perhaps because maintaining multiple mates requires sustained mating effort; Gray, 2003). Alternatives must be ruled out. For instance, men may have lower opportunity to engage in male–male competition when they have offspring as a result of modern social practices, leading to lower T levels.

Psychological adaptation for discriminative investment. Men should not invest in offspring unconditionally. As already noted, selection could favor adaptations that function to lead to investment in offspring likely to be men's own. As paternity is not 100% certain, men's parental efforts may be contingent on cues of paternity, such as self-resemblance. In a large Western sample, men assisted offspring they report are likely their own genetic offspring more than offspring they suspect may be the product of their mate's infidelity (Anderson, Kaplan, & Lancaster, 2007).

Ingenious behavioral studies have examined possible psychological underpinnings of discriminative parenting (DeBruine, 2004; Platek, Burch, Panyavin, Wasserman, & Gallup, 2002; Platek et al., 2003, 2004). In one design, a digital photograph is taken of a participant. The participant's own face or, alternatively, the face of another participant is digitally combined with the face of a small child to create two composite images of child faces – one that is "self-resembling" and one that is not. Participants are asked which of the two children they would be more likely to invest in (e.g., which child they would like to spend time with, which one they would spend $50 on, which one they would rather adopt). Men prefer to invest in the self-resembling "child," an effect not due to participants being able to consciously recognize self-resemblance per se (Platek et al., 2002, 2003). The evidence that men's preference for a self-resembling child is stronger than women's is mixed: In a seminal study, Platek et al. (2002) found a sex difference, but DeBruine (2004), who used a modified procedure, did not. Subsequently, Platek et al. (2004) reported not only a behavioral sex difference in response to self-resembling vs. non-self-resembling child faces; men responded to self-resembling child faces with more overall brain activation (assessed through fMRI) than women, despite women exhibiting stronger brain responses to presentations of children's faces in general (see also Platek, Keenan, & Mohamed, 2005). These results are consistent with the view that men possess adaptation to discriminate and differentially invest in offspring as a function of phenotypic paternity cues. (One might ask how individuals could assess self-resemblance ancestrally. Even lacking mirrors, individuals could assess familial resemblance.)

Mutual Mate Choice in Human Societies

In species in which females invest in offspring and males do not, females typically have more stringent criteria for mate choice than males; they are "choosier" (Trivers, 1972; cf. Hrdy, 1981, who pointed out important exceptions). In species in which males and females cooperatively parent offspring, "mutual mate choice" may well evolve: Members of both sexes are advantaged through preference for some mates over others (e.g., Kokko & Johnstone, 2002). In many instances, choice for mates that exhibit good parenting qualities should be preferred. Studies of mate preferences strongly point to mutual mate choice in modern human societies. In seeking a long-term mate, both men and women are equally "choosy" (e.g., Kenrick, Sadalla, Groth, & Trost, 1990). And in Buss's (1989) classic study of mate preferences in 39 cultures, both men and women, on average, rated "kindness and understanding" as the top preference.

Once again, we can look to specific forms of mate preference for particularly compelling examples of adaptation for mutual choice. Specific major histocompatibility complex (MHC) genes code for cell-surface markers that function to "declare" that a cell is uninfected (when the MHC molecule presents only self-peptides) or infected (when the MHC molecule binds a non-self peptide structure "visible" to the immune system). Several sites (e.g., the A, B, and DR-β loci in humans) are highly polymorphic; at these sites, many different alleles (distinct DNA sequences) are possible, and most randomly paired individuals possess different alleles. Polymorphism probably evolved partly because heterozygotes – individuals with two different alleles at a locus – are favored. Heterozygotes possess a more complex self-code and can present a greater possible array of foreign peptides (see Black & Hedrick, 1997; Hedrick, 1998; Penn & Potts, 1999; see also Geise & Hedrick, 2003). In humans, MHC heterozygotes better resist, for instance, hepatitis B infection (Thurz, Thomas, Greenwood, & Hill, 1997; see also Wegner, Reusch, & Kalbe, 2003). In addition, human couples that possess a common MHC allele produce fewer homozygotic offspring than by chance, reflecting in utero selection against homozygotes (see, e.g., Hedrick & Black, 1997).

All else equal, it pays to mate with someone who possesses alleles different from one's own, as then only heterozygotic offspring are conceived. MHC appears to be detectable through signatures in scent. In a variety of species (e.g., house mice – though not all species; see Penn & Potts, 1999), females prefer the scent males who possess different MHC from their own. Studies on humans strongly suggest that we too are most sexually attracted to scents of others who possess nonshared MHC alleles. Consistent with their being *mutual* mate choice, these preferences have been found in both sexes – 4 of 5 studies of normally ovulating women (Santos, Schinemann, Gabardo, & Bicalho, 2005; Tal, 2009; Wedekind & Füri, 1997; Wedekind, Seebeck, Bettens, & Paepke, 1995; cf. Thornhill et al., 2003) and 3 of 4 studies of men (Tal, 2009; Thornhill et al., 2003; Wedekind & Füri, 1997; cf. Santos et al., 2005). (In another study, women preferred the scent of MHC-similar men, but its preference measure may not tap sexual attraction; Jacob, McClintock, Zelano, & Ober, 20020).

Humans Possess Adaptations Underlying Long-Term Reproductive Pairings

Both sexes have the capacity for romantic love, a capacity that, to our knowledge, can be found across cultures (e.g., Jankowiak & Fischer, 1992; see also Fisher, Aron, & Brown, 2005). The precise function of romantic love is not clear. One possibility is that love functions as a signal of intent to another person of commitment to a long-term interest in a relationship with the person (see Gangestad & Thornhill, 2007; for related and other views, see also Fisher, 2004; Frank, 1988). In any case, however, it does appear that romantic love functions in some way to promote the pair-bonding process and cooperative reproduction.

Are Humans Socially Monogamous?

Marriage is a near-universal institution in human societies. (Purportedly, the Na, an ethnic minority living in the Himalayan foothills in China, lack any such institution. Rather, brothers and sisters live together for life. Siblings help women care for offspring. Fathers do not (see Hua, 2001). The SCCS is a collection of 186 modern and historical human societies selected by Murdock and White (1969) because they are, purportedly, weakly redundant representations of human culture, not closely deriving from common cultures or possessing similarities due to horizontal cultural diffusion. Within the SCCS, over 80% of societies permit polygyny. Fewer than 20% are completely monogamous, and 1% are characterized by a nonzero level of polyandry. As agriculture, herding, and other relatively recent means of production may alter mating arrangements, Marlowe (2003b) examined mating arrangements in the SCCSs 36 foraging groups (that attain <10% of their diet from cultivated foods or domesticated animals) and found that fewer than 10% (3) permit polygyny.

Even in most societies that permit polygyny, however, monogamy is the norm. In two-thirds of foraging societies, for instance, the percentage of polygynously married women was 12% or less (Marlowe, 2003b). Most marital arrangements across human foraging societies, then, are monogamous unions. Nonetheless, humans are not strictly monogamous maters.

Summary: Human Adaptations for Biparental Care

The question of whether men have been highly important contributors to offspring quality ancestrally, and whether humans possess adaptations functional within a context of biparental care, has been vigorously debated. Overall, patterns of production in foraging societies indicate that men have evolved to exert parental effort. Analyses of design features that modulate men's parental efforts – e.g., the T system, psychological adaptations to detect relatedness – represent important avenues to explore. More generally, systems underlying male psychological motivations to father (e.g., bonding to children) or pair-bond represent opportunities to identify design features that, possibly, are signatures of ancestral selection for features that promote male parental care and adaptively modulate level of care by particular circumstances.

Evolutionary Analyses of Ancestral Patterns of Mating and Reproduction: Conflicts of Interest

To say that parents engage in biparental care implies that parents possess converging interests, and each party engages in efforts to further them. All else equal, both parents value having well-nourished, healthy offspring. When both sexes exert parental effort, each parent engages in activities that foster that outcome.

The existence of converging interests, however, does not entail lack of conflicting interests. Indeed, parents' interests almost always conflict. From an evolutionary perspective, this means that the fitness of each parent is not furthered by precisely the same circumstances. Suppose, for instance, that each parent exerts a level of parental effort optimizing its own fitness, given trade-offs between parental effort and other fitness-enhancing activities. If one parent exerted one additional unit, it would do so at its own net cost. But because the other parent benefits from that unit but does not share all of its costs, the other parent's fitness likely gains from it. Parents' interests pertaining to each of their levels of parental effort, then, conflict.

Conflicts of interest typically entail inefficiencies in parties' efforts to further common interests, as illustrated by maternal–fetal conflict. Though both mother and fetus are benefited by health of the fetus, the optimal rate of transfer of nutrients to the fetus is greater from the fetus's perspective than from the mothers' perspective. As a result, both fetuses and mothers have evolved adaptations that further own interests at the expense of the other's (e.g., in the fetus's case, adaptations that increase the rate of flow of nutrients to the placenta; in the mother's case, ones to restrict that rate; see Haig, 1993). These conflicts arguably lead to many complications of pregnancy (e.g., hyperglycemia, hypertension). Each party's costly efforts are partly negated by the others; conflicts compromise efficiency to produce healthy outcomes.

Estrus

I illustrate conflicts of interest between human romantic couples with one set of examples. Estrus is a term introduced in the late 1800s 1923 to refer to the phase of the mammalian female reproductive cycle in which she is most receptive to mating (in some species, referred to as "heat"), which typically if not universally coincides with female fecundability in the cycle. The hormone estrogen (discovered by Allen & Doisy) was named for estrus; it purportedly was the "gen" or "stimulator" of estrus. As estrogen is a functional, sexually dimorphic reproductive hormone in all extant vertebrates (~400 million years old), estrus may characterize female vertebrates more generally (Thornhill & Gangestad, 2008).

During estrus, females do not indiscriminantly mate with males, even in species in which males provide no parental assistance. In theory, females prefer males that offer heritable benefits to offspring (e.g., robustness, health). Studies show that females in specific species prefer dominant males, large males, males with testosterone-facilitated traits, and males with compatible MHC genes – arguably, ones that offer heritable benefits to offspring (for a review, see Thornhill & Gangestad, 2008).

Estrus need not be the only phase of the cycle that females are receptive to mating. In some species, females are receptive outside of the fertile phase. In chimpanzees, for instance, females are receptive to mating about 10 days of the cycle, but fecund only 2–3 days (e.g., Stumpf & Boesch, 2005). In many bird species, pairs copulate many days prior to conception and rises in female estrogen levels (for a review, see Thornhill & Gangestad, 2008). Female sexual receptivity outside of the fertile phase has been referred to as "extended sexuality." It has fitness benefits (i.e., reflects adaptation), in theory, as sex is costly activity to females. But its benefits are not via conceptive sex; sex during extended sexuality is, by definition, nonconceptive. It has a different function, which need not be identical in all species. In general, however, the theory that appears to best account for the distribution of extended sexuality across taxa is that extended sexuality functions to obtain direct benefits from conspecifics, typically males.

If extended sexuality has functions differing from that of estrus, female preferences should partly differ across phases. In chimpanzees, they do. Extended sexuality in this species probably functions to confuse paternity (as males that can rule out their own paternity may harm offspring). During extended sexuality, then, female chimpanzees solicit sex indiscriminantly. At peak fertility, by contrast, females solicit sex from specific males and more often resist male attempts to copulate. During estrus, female preference purportedly favors best sires; during extended sexuality, female sexual activities dampen male violence against offspring.

Women's Loss of Estrus?

A long-standing conclusion in anthropology and human reproductive science is that women evolutionarily "lost" estrus. Purportedly, estrus was selected against and, in its place, "continuous" sexuality – that is, unchanging sexual motivations across the cycle – arose. Behaviorally, continuous sexuality is marked by near-constant rates of intercourse (with primary partners) across the cycle (aside from a dip at menses; e.g., Brewis & Meyer, 2005). Physiologically, women's sexual motivations purportedly were released from hormonal control. As Symons (1979), quoting Beach (1974), noted "[Women's] sexual *arousability* does not depend on ovarian hormones. This relaxation of endocrine control contributes to the occurrence of coitis at any stage of the menstrual cycle"; he added, "I believe that this is the clearest available statement about what 'loss of estrus' means" (p. 106; emphasis in original).

Theorists asked why women lost estrus. One leading theory is that loss of estrus functions to facilitate pair-bonding and paternal investment. When males can discern females' fertile phase, it pays them to attend to fertile females. When they cannot, many males may benefit from attending primarily to one female and investing in her offspring. Loss of estrus and continuous sexuality hence may have nudged males toward parental care (Alexander & Noonan, 1979).

As chimpanzees illustrate, however, females are not necessarily more interested in sex during estrus, even when estrus differs from extended sexuality in other ways. Again, female chimps solicit *more* sex during extended sexuality and become "pickier" during estrus. If loss of ovarian endocrine control of sexual interest is a key to loss of estrus, chimps lost estrus as well. Arguably, however, what distinguishes estrus is not sexual interest per se, but rather *particular patterns of preference selected for the function of sire choice.*

Evidence for Women's Estrus

If female chimpanzee preferences differ across phases of estrus and extended sexuality, perhaps women's do too. This question has been addressed extensively in research over the last decade. The answer is, unequivocally, yes. In shorthand, when heterosexual women rate men's "sexiness," they find a variety of masculine features particularly attractive when fertile: masculine faces, deeper pitched voices, muscular bodies, faces of men with high testosterone; men who display greater intrasexually competitive and socially present behavior; scents of men who are socially dominant and exhibit physical symmetry, a marker of developmental robustness. This list is functionally similar to features preferred by estrus females more generally (see above). Interestingly, however, what women prefer in long-term, investing partners does not change across the cycle; changes are specific to preferences pertaining to sexual motivation. (For a review, see Gangestad & Thornhill, 2008; Thornhill & Gangestad, 2008.)

My colleague Randy Thornhill and I argue that women have not lost estrus. Women's estrus can be discerned from preferences. Sexual receptivity and proceptivity per se are not the hallmarks of estrus. Chimpanzees illustrate this point. Women do too.

A key question concerns what physiological and endocrine factors lead women's preferences to vary across the cycle. Evidence points to roles for estrogen (Garver-Apgar, Gangestad, & Thornhill, 2008; Roney & Simmons, 2008) and testosterone (Welling et al., 2007) facilitating estrous preferences and progesterone (Garver-Apgar et al., 2008; Puts, 2005) dampening them. More research is needed to clarify how hormones regulate estrous adaptations.

The Evolution of Women's Extended Sexuality

In the chimpanzee lineage, estrus evolved first. Estrus writ large, once again, may date to ~400 million years ago (though modified in specific lineages). Extended sexuality evolved as an add-on to estrus within chimpanzees. (The common ancestor of chimpanzees, gorillas, and humans may or may not have possessed extended sexuality, but almost certainly not in the form exhibited by chimpanzees.) The same is probably true of humans. In the lineage leading to humans, females have long possessed estrus. Human females did not *lose* estrus; they *gained* extended sexuality in *addition to* estrus. Extended sexuality resulted in *continuous* sexual arousability, but *not unchanging* preferences underlying sexual motivation.

Chimpanzee extended sexuality functions to confuse paternity. Human extended sexuality certainly does not. Instead, it may function in ways similar to that "loss of estrus" theorists claimed for continuous sexuality: to enhance pair-bonding and foster biparental care. Chimp and human extended sexuality both function to obtain male-delivered direct benefits, but ones achieved in very different ways: In chimps, through paternity confusion; in humans, through male parental efforts. In fact, extended sexuality may well constitute another "design argument" for the evolution of biparental care in humans. (I note, however, that more work is needed to fully explore the nature of women's sexual motivations during extended sexuality. Most work has focused on the special nature of estrous preferences and has not specifically addressed questions about the design of preferences and interests during extended sexuality).

Implications of Estrus for Conflicts of Interest

Research exploring changes in women's sexual interests largely examined rates of intercourse in pair-bonded couples. Women's sexual interests in their partners do not change much across the cycle, on average (e.g., Brewis & Meyer, 2005; see Thornhill & Gangestad, 2008, for a review), and we can now understand why: women's find particular male features (e.g., masculine features) sexier when fertile.

Because primary partners, on average, possess average features, it makes sense that estrous women do not find partners, on average, sexier.

Estrous women, however, can see men in their social spheres who do possess favored features. Hence, women in committed relationships claim to experience attraction to men *other than* their primary partners more often when fertile than when infertile in their cycles (Gangestad, Thornhill, & Garver, 2002; Gangestad, Thornhill, & Garver-Apgar, 2005). And estrous women are particularly likely to do be attracted to "extra-pair" men when their own partners lack favored features (e.g., physical attractiveness – Haselton & Gangestad, 2006; Pillsworth & Haselton, 2006; symmetry – Gangestad et al., 2005) or possess incompatible MHC alleles (Garver-Apgar, Gangestad, Thornhill, Miller, & Olp, 2006).

Women's attraction to extra-pair men during estrus conflicts with their partners' interests, even if it never leads to extra-pair sex (and no doubt it very rarely does). Men, then, are more vigilant of their partners during estrus than the luteal phase, and particularly when their partners experience attraction to other men (Gangestad et al., 2002; Haselton & Gangestad, 2006; Pillsworth & Haselton, 2006). Whether men respond to behavioral cues of women's changes in attraction or physical cues of women's estrus (men do find estrous women's scent more attractive; e.g., Singh & Bronstad, 2001) is presently unknown (see also Miller, Tybur, & Jordan, 2007).

Modification of Women's Estrus?

Estrus did not evolve in the lineage leading to humans in the context of pair-bonding; again, estrus in the hominin lineage predates pair-bonding. In theory, *extended sexuality* evolved (or was modified) in the context of pair-bonding and biparental care. One question that remains is whether estrous adaptations have been modified in the context of pair-bonding. One possibility is that distinct estrous preferences are similar to the human appendix: adaptations that were once beneficial but not in the context of pair-bonding, as they interfere with the efficiency of pair-bonded couples to produce viable, high-quality offspring. Like the appendix, estrous preferences may be vestigial – reduced in magnitude due to maladaptation in a current context. In this view, women are evolving toward continuous sexuality through suppression of estrous preferences.

An alternative possibility is that estrous preferences retained functionality in the context of pair-bonding. Though not evolved *for* adaptive extra-pair mating (they could not be, as they evolved prior to pair-bonding and hence prior to potential *extra-pair* mating), they may have sometimes led to adaptive extra-pair mating (e.g., mating with someone offering better heritable qualities than a primary mate). As extra-pair mating carries costs (e.g., through loss of a partner), estrous adaptations may have been modified to minimize costs while still retaining benefits. For instance, detectable cues of estrus may have been suppressed. As well, women may have evolved to be sensitive to the costs of extra-pair mating or the benefits of extra-pair sex. Hassebrauck (2003) found that women reflect on qualities of their relationships more during estrus than other phases. And, again, women who share incompatible MHC alleles with their partners are particularly likely to be attracted to men other than partners at estrus (Garver-Apgar et al., 2006).

Conflicts of Interest

Whether estrous adaptations are vestigial, have been adaptively modified in the context of pair-bonding, or are unmodified, they illustrate a broader theme: Pair-bonded couples not only have shared interests; their interests also conflict (here, owing to potential cuckoldry). Other conflicts of interest revolve around men's extra-pair sexual interests (taking away from paternal care) and allocation of time to other pursuits that benefit self more than partner.

Human mating, then, must be understood as outcomes of both shared and conflicting interests between partners. Shifts in conditions altering the extent to which interests are shared or conflicting can lead to shifts in patterns of mating and care. For instance, under conditions increasing chances of nonpaternity, the value and extent of male care may be reduced.

Variability in Reproductive Systems Across Traditional and Modern Cultures

In summary, (a) humans appear to have adaptations for biparental care, albeit variable male care as regulated by physiological and psychological adaptations; (b) mating systems widely vary across societies; most foraging cultures permit polygyny, though monogamy is the modal arrangement and degrees of polygyny are highly variable; (c) conflicts of interests as well as shared interests exist in reproductive pairs; and (d) historically, a variety of conditions may have affected the relative benefits of male care (see also Brown et al., 2009).

As noted repeatedly, factors that influence the relative value of various fitness-enhancing activities may have shaped adaptations that modulate reproductively relevant behaviors in response to evolutionarily recurrent cues. Again, examples include factors that influence paternity certainty; when opportunities for extra-pair mating (due to forms of male production) increase, the value of male care may decrease. Another example may be the adult sex ratio. When adult men outnumber women, male competition for mates increases and the value of male care accordingly increases (Kokko & Jennions, 2008). By contrast, when women outnumber men, the value of male care decreases. Finally, the value of male provisioning and hence the durability of male–female pair-bonds may depend on the extent to which female productivity is compromised by childcare, given available resources.

This leads to specific questions pertaining to "evoked culture." Across human groups (as a function of ecological and socioecological factors), conditions that modulate the expression of mating and reproductive adaptations vary (e.g., paternity certainty, sex ratio, added value of male provisioning). Just as conditions that affect the formation of calluses across groups lead to differences in callous formation via adaptations to form calluses, might these conditions lead to variable mating and reproductive behaviors via adaptations for mating and reproduction?

In fact, researchers have explored examples based on precisely this line of thinking.

Paternity certainty. Paternity certainty across traditional cultures varies with forms of male and female production. It is low in coastal regions, perhaps owing to dispersion of men to fish, as well as where women engage in horticulture, perhaps owing to diminished interference of women's childcare with foraging. Accordingly, certain forms of male investment in offspring (e.g., transfer of wealth to sons as opposed to matrilineal relatives) are diminished in these cultures (e.g., Gaulin & Schlegel, 1980; see also Hartung, 1985).

Adult sex ratio. Schmitt (2005) examined men's and women's propensities to restrict mating to committed, long-term relationships across 48 nations as a function of the sex ratio. Consistent with the idea that female-biased sex ratios lead men to tend to invest more in competition and less in committed relationships in countries in which sex ratios are female-biased (see Pedersen, 1991), men express less interest in being committed to long-term mates, as do women. Pollet and Nettle (2008) examined sex ratios across the 50 US states in 1910 and, using census data, found that in states in which sex ratios were heavily male-biased (largely due to differential male-to-female migration), the ratio of the socioeconomic status of married men to that of unmarried men was relatively large, consistent with the idea that men became particularly valued for assets brought to the household in such circumstances. These same authors examined rates of polygyny across 56 districts in Uganda as a function of sex ratios. As ratios became more female-biased, more men were polygynous and land-owning became a particularly important key to being polygynous (Pollet & Nettle, 2009). Across 67 nations in the WHO database, those with female-biased sex ratios experience higher rates of violent crimes (e.g., murders per 100,000 population, controlling for drug trafficking, population density, and wealth disparity), despite males committing the overwhelming majority of these crimes (Barber, 2009). Violent crime may be a downstream effect of increased male mating competition (and diminished paternal care).

An important future avenue of research may be investigation of physiological factors that account for these variations. In human groups with low paternity certainty and female-biased sex ratios, are male testosterone levels higher than in groups with high paternity certainty and male-biased sex ratios? Are T levels less sensitive to changes in paternity in these groups? To date, little data comparing male testosterone levels across human groups is available (for an exception, see Ellison et al., 2002, who compared levels across three traditional human groups and men from Boston). At the same time, are female changes in preferences and sexual interests (e.g., during estrus and extended sexuality) sensitive to changes in factors influencing paternal care vs. mating competition?

Applications to Understanding Major Changes in Family Formation and Fertility in the Contemporary USA

Are Components of U.S. Demographic Trends Owing to "Evoked Culture?"

As noted at the outset of this chapter, throughout thousands of years of existence as foragers, people likely exhibited patterns of mating and reproduction drastically different from what we observe in contemporary Western societies. It may one thing to account for variation in patterns of mating across traditional or even historical Western populations with ideas about "evoked culture," and quite another to apply this approach to account for the dramatic reductions in fertility we observe in the contemporary USA. In modern Western countries, people have available technologies never available to people in traditional human groups, such as the contraceptive pill, permitting women and couples to effectively control fertility and engage in family planning. How could people have previously-evolved adaptations that respond to such novelties? And do novelties such as the pill (or, alternatively, unprecedented changes in women's ability to pursue education, independent careers, and creations of wealth) not account for current mating and reproductive patterns much more so than do variations to which humans do possess evolved, adaptively contingent responses?

Though I suspect that, in fact, much of the causes of the decline in reproduction does have much to do with novelties, responses to which are not a function of adaptations for mating and reproduction per se (as opposed to other, more general psychological features, such as some involved in explicit family planning), it may nonetheless be worthwhile to entertain the possibility that notions of "evoked culture" can partly, even if not fully, explain current patterns. I briefly discuss two possible effects via contingent expression owing to mating adaptations.

The size of modern mating markets. Humans may be adapted to make mate choices in small mating markets. Lack of effective "stop" rules (choose this partner over others, given possibilities) in very large markets may lead individuals to typically search for long periods of time, leading to delay of family formation and the start of reproduction. This may be particularly true in densely populated segments of the population that experience high rates of interaction with novel potential partners (such as college students).

Female-biased operational sex ratios. The operational sex ratio (OSR) is defined as the ratio of males to females in a mating market. When many females are pregnant or lactating in a population, the OSR is often highly male-biased. When females delay reproduction, for whatever reason, the OSR remains relatively close to one, which, compared to historical periods, is relatively female-biased. This situation potentially fuels male competition and lowers male interest in long-term pair-bonding, possibly further delaying family formation. Female-biased sex ratios may also lead women to expect lower levels of male investment in committed relationships, with concomitant effects on bases of female preference.

Women's pursuit of education has led to increased biasing of the sex ratio on college campuses, many of which, once again, constitute large mating markets. Women's pursuit of education has direct effects on delay of reproduction, but it may also have indirect effects on patterns of family formation via effects on mating markets and OSRs.

Limitations of the "Evoked Culture" Approach

Despite suggestions that we may well fruitfully entertain the possibility that some components of modern mating phenomena and patterns of family formation are owing to evoked culture, I once again note that the approach is limited in its ability to explain all changes. And again, an example is effects of the contraceptive pill. The pill permits women and couples to make reliable choices about family planning that were not previously possible. It furthermore has led to an unprecedented level of uncoupling of formation of a romantic, sexually involved couple and reproduction. Contingent expression owing to adaptations for mating, sex, and reproduction per se is unlikely to explain its full effects. More generally, I suspect that the evoked culture framework is likely to be more useful in explaining differences between systems of mating and reproduction within traditional cultures than explaining, for instance, the incredible reduction in fertility in modern Western cultures, with which it may offer relatively little understanding.

Even in contexts in which the evoked culture approach is limited in its ability to explain changes in fertility, however, it may offer insights into modern mating phenomena. For instance, studies have shown that the contraceptive pill disrupts estrus. Women using the pill tend to respond similar to how women in general respond during extended sexuality (see Thornhill & Gangestad, 2008, for a review). Recently, Alvergne and Lummaa (2009) drew attention to an important set of questions that follow: What are the implications for mating phenomena? How does pill use affect female choice? How does it affect how women view their relationships? How are women's perceptions of their partners affected in cases in which they met their partner while on the pill, but then go off the pill (e.g., to conceive)? How is their ability to conceive with their partners affected? Only very recently have researchers even begun to address these questions.

Conclusion

I have argued that humans possess adaptations for mating and reproduction partly evolved in the context of biparental care. The value of men's care ancestrally varied across time and place, however, with factors such as paternity certainty, adult sex ratios (as affected, e.g., by sex-specific mortality rates), and complementarity of male and female contributions to care. Selection may well have shaped in men adaptations that lead them to allocate effort to care vs. competition for mates to an extent contingent on conditions modulating the value of these efforts (ancestrally). Female adaptations for mating and reproduction may similarly have been shaped to be contingently expressed as a function of these conditions. The nature of patterns of mating, family formation, and fertility in traditional foraging groups may be at least partly explained by these adaptations. But furthermore, the nature of patterns of mating, family formation, and fertility in modern Western groups too may be partly explained by these adaptations. This approach has recently been fruitfully applied to understand these variations. But both empirical and theoretical work in this regard has only just begun.

Modulation of male efforts and female responses to men may importantly be regulated by endocrine systems: in men, testosterone, and in women, a variety of reproductive hormones (estrogen, testosterone, progesterone). Efforts to better understand, both theoretically and empirically, how conditions affect expression of these systems, how, in turn, these systems specifically modulate behavior and other components of physiology, and how these psychological and physiological effects result in patterns of mating, family formation, and fertility, are important avenues of research. The explicit evolutionary biological framework that I have emphasized has productively guided efforts in this regard in the past, and I strongly suspect can do so in the future.

References

Alexander, R. D., & Noonan, K. M. (1979). Concealment of ovulation, parental care, and human social evolution. In N. A. Chagnon & W. G. Irons (Eds.), *Evolutionary biology and human social behavior: An anthropological perspective* (pp. 436–453). Scituate: North Duxbury Press.

Allen, E. V., & Doisy, E. A. (1923). An ovarian hormone: Preliminary reports of its localization, extraction and partial purification and action in test animals. *Journal of the American Medical Association, 81*, 819–821.

Alvergne, A., & Lummaa, V. (2009). Does the contraceptive pill alter mate choice in humans? *Trends in Ecology and Evolution, 25*, 171–179.

Anderson, K. G., Kaplan, H., & Lancaster, J. (2007). Confidence of paternity, divorce, and investment in children by Albuquerque men. *Evolution and Human Behavior, 28*, 1–10.

Andrews, P. W., Gangestad, S. W., & Matthews, D. (2002). Adaptationism – How to carry out an exaptationist program. *Behavioral and Brain Sciences, 25*, 489–504.

Barber, N. (2009). Countries with fewer males have more violent crimes: Marriage markets and mating aggression. *Aggressive and Violent Behavior, 13*, 237–250.

Beach, F. A. (1974). Human sexuality and evolution. In W. Montagna & W. A. Sadler (Eds.), *Reproductive behavior*. New York: Plenum. pp. 333–366.

Berg, S. J., & Wynne-Edwards, K. E. (2001). Changes in testosterone, cortisol, and estradiol levels in men becoming fathers. *Mayo Clinic Proceedings, 76*, 582–592.

Black, F. L., & Hedrick, P. W. (1997). Strong balancing selection at HLA loci: Evidence from segregation in South American families. *Proceedings of the National Academy of Sciences USA, 94*, 12452–12456.

Booth, A., & Dabbs, J. M. (1993). Testosterone and mens' marriages. *Social Forces, 72*, 463–477.

Brewis, A., & Meyer, M. (2005). Demographic evidence that human ovulation is undetectable (at least in pair bonds). *Current Anthropology, 46*, 465–471.

Bribiescas, R. G. (2001). Reproductive ecology and life history of the human male. *Yearbook of Physical Anthropology, 44*, 148–176.

Brown, G. R., Laland, K. N., & Borgerhoff Mulder, M. (2009). Bateman's principles and human sex roles. *Trends in Ecology and Evolution, 24*, 297–304.

Burnham, J. C., Chapman, J. F., Gray, P. B., McIntyre, M. H., Lipson, S. F., & Ellison, P. T. (2003). Men in committed, romantic relationships have lower testosterone. *Hormones and Behavior, 44*, 119–122.

Buss, D. M. (1989). Sex differences in human mate preferences: Evolutionary hypotheses tested in 37 cultures. *Behavioral and Brain Sciences, 12*, 1–49.

DeBruine, L. M. (2004). Resemblance to self increases the appeal of child faces to both men and women. *Evolution and Human Behavior, 25*, 142–154.

Dufour, S. L., & Sauther, M. L. (2002). Comparative and evolutionary dimensions of the energetics of human pregnancy and lactation. *American Journal of Human Biology, 14*, 584–602.

Dunbar, R. I. M. (1987). *Primate social systems*. Ithaca, NY: Comstock.

Ellison, P. T. (2001). *On fertile ground: A natural history of reproduction*. Cambridge: Harvard University Press.

Ellison, P. T. (2003). Energetics and reproductive effort. *American Journal of Human Biology, 15*, 342–351.

Ellison, P. T., Bribiescas, R. G., Bentley, G. R., Campbell, B. C., Lipson, S. F., Panter-Brick, C., et al. (2002) Population variation in age-related decline in male salivary testosterone. *Human Reproduction, 17*, 3251–3253.

Finch, C. E., & Rose, M. R. (1995). Hormones and the physiological architecture of life history evolution. *Quarterly Review of Biology, 70*, 1–52.

Fisher, H. (2004). *Why we love: The nature and chemistry of romantic love*. New York: Henry Holt.

Fisher, H., Aron, A., & Brown, L. L. (2005). Romantic love: An fMRI study of a neural mechanism for mate choice. *Journal of Comparative Neurology, 493*, 58–62.

Fleming, A. S., Corter, C., Stallings, J., & Steiner, M. (2002). Testosterone and prolactin are associated with emotional responses to infant cries in new fathers. *Hormones and Behavior, 42*, 399–413.

Frank, R. H. (1988). *Passions within reason: The strategic role of the emotions*. New York: Norton.

Gangestad, S. W., Haselton, M. G., & Buss, D. M. (2006). Evolutionary foundations of cultural variation: Evoked culture and mate preferences. *Psychological Inquiry, 17*, 75–95.

Gangestad, S. W., & Thornhill, R. (2007). The evolution of social inference processes: The importance of signaling theory. In J. P. Forgas, M. G. Haselton, & W. von Hippel (Eds.), *Evolutionary psychology and social cognition* (pp. 33–48). New York: Psychology Press.

Gangestad, S. W., & Thornhill, R. (2008). Human oestrus. *Proceedings of the Royal Society of London B, 275*, 991–1000.

Gangestad, S. W., Thornhill, R., & Garver, C. E. (2002). Changes in women's sexual interests and their partners' mate retention tactics across the menstrual cycle: Evidence for shifting conflicts of interest. *Proceedings of the Royal Society of London B, 269*, 975–982.

Gangestad, S. W., Thornhill, R., & Garver-Apgar, C. E. (2005). Women's sexual interests across the ovulatory cycle depend on primary partner fluctuating asymmetry. *Proceedings of the Royal Society of London B, 272*, 2023–2027.

Garemszegi, L. Z., Eens, M., Hurtrez-Boussès, S., & Møller, A. P. (2005). Testosterone, testes size and mating success in birds: A comparative study. *Hormones and Behavior, 47*, 389–409.

Garver-Apgar, C. E., Gangestad, S. W., & Thornhill, R. (2008). Hormonal correlates of women's mid–cycle preference for the scent of symmetry. *Evolution and Human Behavior, 29*, 223–232.

Garver-Apgar, C. E., Gangestad, S. W., Thornhill, R., Miller, R. D., & Olp, J. (2006). MHC alleles, sexually responsivity, and unfaithfulness in romantic couples. *Psychological Science, 17*, 830–835.

Gaulin, S. J. C., & Schlegel, A. (1980). Paternal confidence and paternal investment: A cross-cultural test of a sociobiological hypothesis. *Ethology and Sociobiology, 1*, 301–309.

Geise, A. R., & Hedrick, P. W. (2003). Genetic variation and resistance to a bacterial infection in endangered Gila topminnow. *Animal Conservation, 6*, 369–377.

Godfrey-Smith, P. (1993). Functions: Consensus without unity. *Pacific Philosophical Quarterly, 74*, 196–208.

Gould, S. J., & Lewontin, R. C. (1979). The spandrels of San Marco and the panglossian paradigm: A critique of the adaptationist program. *Proceedings of the Royal Society of London B, 205*, 581–598.

Gould, S. J., & Vrba, E. S. (1982) Exaptation: A missing term in the science of form. *Paleobiology, 8*, 4–15.

Gray, P. B. (2003). Marriage, parenting, and testosterone variation among Kenyan Swahili men. *American Journal of Physical Anthropology, 122*, 279–286.

Gray, P. B., Chapman, J. F., Burnham, T. C., McIntyre, M. H., Lipson, S. F., & Ellison, P. T. (2004). Human male pairbonding and testosterone. *Human Nature, 15*, 119–131.

Gray, P. B., Kahlenberg, S. M., Barrett, E. S., Lipson, S. F., & Ellison, P. T. (2002). Marriage and fatherhood are associated with lower testosterone in males. *Evolution and Human Behavior, 23*, 193–201.

Gray, P. B., Yang, C. F. J., & Pope, H. G. (2006). Fathers have lower salivary testosterone levels than unmarried men and married non-fathers in Beijing, China. *Proceedings of the Royal Society of London B, 273*, 333–339.

Haig, D. (1993). Genetic conflicts in human pregnancy. *Quarterly Review of Biology, 68*, 495–532.

Hart, C. W. M., Pilling, A. R., & Goodale, J. C. (1987). *The Tiwi of north Australia* (3rd ed.). New York: Holt, Rinehart, and Winston.

Hartung, J. (1985). Matrilineal inheritance: New theory and analysis. *Behavioral and Brain Sciences, 8*, 661–670.

Haselton, M. G., & Gangestad, S. W. (2006). Conditional expression of women's desires and male mate retention efforts across the ovulatory cycle. *Hormones and Behavior, 49*, 509–518.

Hassebrauck, M. (2003). The effect of fertility risk on relationship scrutiny. *Evolution and Cognition, 9*, 116–122.

Hawkes, K. (1991). Showing off: Tests of an hypothesis about men's foraging goals. *Ethology and Sociobiology, 12*, 29–54.

Hawkes, K. (2004). Mating, parenting, and the evolution of human pairbonds. In B. Chapais & C. M. Berman (Eds.), *Kinship and behavior in primates* (pp. 443–473). Oxford: Oxford University Press.

Hawkes, K., O'Connell, J. F., & Blurton Jones, N. G. (1991). Hunting patterns among the Hadza: Big game, common goals, foraging goals and the evolution of the human diet. *Philosophical Transactions of the Royal Society of London B, 334*, 243–251.

Hawkes, K., O'Connell, J. F., & Blurton Jones, N. G. (2001). Hunting and nuclear families – Some lessons from the Hadza about men's work. *Current Anthropology, 42*, 681–709.

Hedrick, P. W. (1998). Balancing selection and the MHC. *Genetica, 104*, 207–214.

Hedrick, P. W., & Black, F. L. (1997). Random mating and selection within families against homozygotes for HLA in South Amerindians. *Hereditas, 127*, 51–58.

Hill, K. R., & Hurtado, A. M. (1996). *Ache life history: The ecology and demography of a forest people*. New York: Aldine de Gruyter.

Hrdy, S. B. (1981). *The woman that never evolved*. Cambridge: Harvard University Press.

Hrdy, S. B. (2009). *Mothers and others*. Cambridge: Harvard University Press.

Hua, C. (2001). *A society without fathers or husbands: The Na of China*. Cambridge: MIT Press.

Jacob, S., McClintock, M. K., Zelano, B., & Ober, C. (2002). Paternally inherited HLA alleles are associated with male choice of male odor. *Nature Genetics, 30*, 175–179.

Jankowiak, W. R., & Fischer, E. F. (1992). A cross-cultural perspective on romantic love. *Ethnology, 31*, 148–155.

146   S.W. Gangestad

Kaplan, H., & Hill, K. (1985). Hunting ability and reproductive success among male Ache foragers: Preliminary tests. *Current Anthropology, 26*, 131–133.

Kaplan, H., Hill, K., Lancaster, J., & Hurtado, A. M. (2000). A theory of human life history evolution: Diet, intelligence, and longevity. *Evolutionary Anthropology, 9*, 156–185.

Kenrick, D. T., Sadalla, E. K., Groth, G., & Trost, M. R. (1990). Evolution, traits, and the stages of human courtship: Qualifying the parental investment model. *Journal of Personality, 58*, 97–116.

Kokko, H., & Jennions, M. D. (2008). Parental investment, sexual selection and sex ratios. *Journal of Evolutionary Biology, 21*, 919–948.

Kokko, H., & Johnstone, R. A. (2002). Why is mutual mate choice not the norm? Operational sex ratios, sex roles and the evolution of sexually dimorphic and monomorphic signalling. *Philosophical Transactions of the Royal Society of London B, 357*, 319–330.

Lancaster, J. B., & Lancaster, C. S. (1983). Parental investment: The hominid adaptation. In D. Ortner (Ed.), *Parental care in mammals* (pp. 347–387). New York: Plenum.

Lovejoy, C. O. (1981). The origins of man. *Science, 211*, 341–350.

Marlowe, F. (1999). Male care and mating effort among Hadza foragers. *Behavioral Ecology and Sociobiology, 46*, 57–64.

Marlowe, F. (2001). Male contribution to diet and female reproductive success among foragers. *Current Anthropology, 42*, 755–760.

Marlowe, F. W. (2003a). A critical period for provisioning by Hadza men: Implications for pair bonding. *Evolution and Human Behavior, 24*, 217–229.

Marlowe, F. W. (2003b). The mating system of foragers in the standard cross-cultural sample. *Cross-Cultural Research, 37*, 282–306.

Mazur, A., & Booth, A. (1998). Testosterone and dominance in men. *Behavioral and Brain Sciences, 21*, 353–397.

Mazur, A., & Michalek, J. (1998). Marriage, divorce, and male testosterone. *Social Forces, 77*, 315–330.

McIntyre, M., Gangestad, S. W., Gray, P. B., Chapman, J. F., Burnham, T. C., O'Rourke, M. T., & Thornhill, R. (2006). Romantic involvement often reduces men's testosterone levels-but not always: The moderating role of extrapair sexual interest. *Journal of Personality and Social Psychology, 91*, 642–651.

Miller, G. F., Tybur, J., & Jordan, B. (2007). Ovulatory cycle effects on tip earnings by lap dancers: Economic evidence for human estrus? *Evolution and Human Behavior, 28*, 375–381.

Millikan, R. (1989). In defense of proper functions. *Philosophy of Science, 56*, 288–302.

Muller, M. N., Marlowe, F. W., Bugumba, R., & Ellison, P. T. (2009). Testosterone and paternal care in East African foragers and pastoralists. *Proceedings of the Royal Society B, 276*, 347–354.

Muller, M. N., & Wrangham, R. W. (2001). The reproductive ecology of male hominoids. In. P. T. Ellison (Ed.), *Reproductive ecology and human evolution* (pp. 397–427). New York: Aldine.

Murdock, G. P., & White, D. R. (1969). Standard cross-cultural sample. *Ethnology, 9*, 329–369.

Nunes, S., Fite, J. E., & French, J. A. (2000). Variation in steroid hormones associated with infant care behaviour and experience in male marmosets (*Callithrix kuhlii*). *Animal Behaviour, 60*, 1–9.

Nunes, S., Fite, J. E., Patera, K. J., & French, J. A. (2001). Interactions among paternal behavior, steroid hormones, and parental experience in male marmosets (*Callithrix kuhlii*). *Hormones and Behavior, 39*, 70–82.

Pedersen, F. A. (1991). Secular trends in human sex ratios: Their influence on individual and family behavior. *Human Nature, 2*, 271–291.

Penn, D. J., & Potts, W. K. (1999). The evolution of mating preferences and major histocompatibility complex genes. *American Naturalist, 153*, 145–164.

Pillsworth, E. G., & Haselton, M. G. (2006). Male sexual attractiveness predicts differential ovulatory shifts in female extra-pair attraction and male mate retention. *Evolution and Human Behavior, 27*, 247–258.

Platek, S. M., Burch, R. L., Panyavin, I. S., Wasserman, B. H., & Gallup, G. G., Jr. (2002). Reaction to children's faces – Resemblance affects males more than females. *Evolution and Human Behavior, 23*, 159–166.

Platek, S. M., Critton, S. R., Burch, R. L., Frederick, D. A., Myers, T. E., & Gallup, G. G., Jr. (2003). How much paternal resemblance is enough? Sex differences in hypothetical investment decisions, but not in the detection of resemblance. *Evolution and Human Behavior, 24*, 81–87.

Platek, S. M., Keenan, J. P., & Mohamed, F. B. (2005). Sex differences in the neural correlates of child facial resemblance: An event-related fMRI study. *Neuroimage, 25*, 1336–1344.

Platek, S. M., Raines, D. M., Gallup, G. G., Mohamed, F. B., Thomson, J. W., Myers, T. E., et al. (2004). Reactions to children's faces: Males are more affected by resemblance than females are, and so are their brains. *Evolution and Human Behavior, 25*, 394–405.

Pollet, T. V., & Nettle, D. (2008). Driving a hard bargain: Sex ratio and male marriage success in a historical U.S. population. *Biology Letters, 4*, 31–33.

Pollet, T. V., & Nettle, D. (2009). Market forces affect patterns of polygyny in Uganda. *Proceedings of the National Academy of Sciences USA, 106*, 2114–2117.

Puts, D. A. (2005). Mating context and menstrual phase affect women's preferences for male voice pitch. *Evolution and Human Behavior, 26*, 388–397.

Quinlan, R. J., & Quinlan, M. B. (2008). Human lactation, pair-bonds and alloparents: A cross-cultural analysis. *Human Nature, 19*, 87–102.

Quinlan, R. J., Quinlan, M. B., & Flinn, M. V. (2003). Parental investment and age of weaning in a Caribbean village. *Evolution and Human Behavior, 24*, 1–16.

Roney, J. R., & Simmons, Z. L. (2008). Women's estradiol predicts preference for facial cues of men's testosterone. *Hormones and Behavior, 53*, 14–19.

Salmon, W. C. (1984). *Scientific explanation and the causal structure of the world*. Princeton: Princeton University Press.

Santos, P. S. C., Schinemann, J. A., Gabardo, J., & Bicalho, M. D. (2005). New evidence that the MHC influences odor perception in humans: A study with 58 southern Brazilian students. *Hormones and Behavior, 47*, 384–388.

Singh, D., & Bronstad, P. M. (2001). Female body odour is a potential cue to ovulation. *Proceedings of the Royal Society of London B, 268*, 797–801.

Schmitt, D. P. (2005). Sociosexuality from Argentina to Zimbabwe: A 48-nation study of sex, culture, and strategies of human mating. *Behavioral and Brain Sciences, 28*, 247–311.

Sterelny, K., & Griffiths, P. E. (1999). *Sex and death: An introduction to the philosophy of biology*. Chicago: University of Chicago Press.

Storey, A. E., Walsh, C. J., Quinton, R. L., & Wynne-Edwards, K. E. (2000). Hormonal correlates of paternal responsiveness in new and expectant fathers. *Evolution and Human Behavior, 21*, 79–95.

Stumpf, R. M., & Boesch, C. (2005). Does promiscuous mating preclude female choice? Female sexual strategies in chimpanzees (*Pan troglodytes verus*) of the Taï National Park, Côte d'Ivoire. *Behavioral Ecology and Sociobiology, 57*, 511–524.

Symons, D. (1979). *The evolution of human sexuality*. Oxford: Oxford University Press.

Tal, I. (2009). Unpublished dissertation data. Department of Psychology, University of New Mexico.

Thornhill, R. (1997). The concept of an evolved adaptation. In M. Daly (Ed.), *Characterizing human psychological adaptations* (pp. 4–13). London: Wiley.

Thornhill, R., & Gangestad, S. W. (2008). *The evolutionary biology of human female sexuality*. New York: Oxford University Press.

Thornhill, R., Gangestad, S. W., Miller, R., Scheyd, G., Knight, J., & Franklin, M. (2003). MHC, symmetry, and body scent attractiveness in men and women. *Behavioral Ecology, 14*, 668–678.

Thurz, M. R., Thomas, H. C., Greenwood, B. M., & Hill, A. V. S. (1997). Heterozygote advantage for HLA class-II type in hepatitis B virus infection. *Nature Genetics, 17*, 11–12.

Tooby, J., & Cosmides, L. (1992). Psychological foundations of culture. In J. Barkow, L. Cosmides, & J. Tooby (Eds.), *The adapted mind* (pp. 19–136). New York: Oxford University Press.

Trivers, R. L. (1972). Parental investment and sexual selection. In B. Campbell (Ed.), *Sexual selection and the descent of man, 1881–1971* (pp. 136–179). Chicago: Aldine.

Van Anders, S. M., & Watson, N. V. (2006). Relationship status and testosterone in North American heterosexual and non-heterosexual men and women: Cross-sectional and longitudinal data. *Psychoendocrinology, 31*, 715–723.

Wedekind, C., & Füri, S. (1997). Body odor preference in men and women: Do they aim for specific MHC combinations or simply heterozygosity? *Proceeding of the Royal Society of London B, 264*, 1471–1479.

Wedekind, C., Seebeck, T., Bettens, F., & Paepke, A. J. (1995). MHC-dependent mate preferences in humans. *Proceeding of the Royal Society of London, B, 260*, 245–249.

Wegner, K. M., Reusch, T. B. H., & Kalbe, M. (2003). Multiple parasites are driving major histocompatibility complex polymorphism in the wild. *Journal of Evolutionary Biology, 16*, 224–232.

Welling, L. L. M., Jones, B. C., DeBruine, L. M., Conway, C. A., Law Smith, M. J., Little, A. C., et al. (2007). Raised salivary testosterone in women is associated with increased attraction to masculine faces. *Hormones and Behavior, 52*, 156–161.

Westermarck, E. (1929). *Marriage*. New York: Jonathan Cape and Harrison Smith.

Williams, G. C. (1966). *Adaptation and natural selection: A critique of some current evolutionary thought*. Princeton: Princeton University Press.

Williams, G. C. (1992). *Natural selection: Domains, levels and challenges*. Oxford: Oxford University Press.

Chapter 10
The Need for Family Research Using Multiple Approaches and Methods

Brian M. D'Onofrio, Niklas Langstrom, and Paul Lichtenstein

Abstract Recent reviews by prominent researchers in many fields have called for more interdisciplinary research on family functioning using approaches that integrate biological and social considerations. Gangestad (Chap. 9) provides an important introduction to the field of evolutionary psychology and presents an overview of how the discipline approaches the study of familial processes. Here, we documents the ways in which three broad research perspectives and methods have been influenced by and can influence evolutionary psychology: (a) social neuroscience research on mate selection, (b) quasi-experimental studies that test causal inferences concerning social influences, and (c) quantitative behavior genetic research that examines whether the heritability of traits has varied across historical context.

Introduction

In this chapter, I (as the lead author) respond to Gangestad (Chap. 9) by illustrating the difficulties in conducting well-informed biosocial research on the family and the advantages of considering the insights of multiple disciplines. Recent reviews in psychology (e.g., Adele, 2009; Cacioppo, Berntson, Sheridan, & McClintock, 2000; Cicchetti, 2006; Granger & Kivlighan, 2003), psychiatry (Kendler, 2005), and sociology (Freese, 2008; Freese, Allen Li, & Wade, 2003) have urged researchers to integrate multiple levels of analysis, jointly consider biological and social factors, and incorporate insights from multiple disciplines. Family researchers have also emphasized the importance of taking an integrated biosocial perspective (Booth, Carver, & Granger, 2000; D'Onofrio & Lahey, in press). The call for more biosocial research on the family parallels recommendations from prominent

B.M. D'Onofrio (✉)
Department of Psychology, Indiana University, Bloomington, IN, USA
e-mail: bmdonofr@indiana.edu

A. Booth et al. (eds.), *Biosocial Foundations of Family Processes*,
National Symposium on Family Issues, DOI 10.1007/978-1-4419-7361-0_10,
© Springer Science+Business Media, LLC 2011

workgroups that have emphasized the importance of considering biological, behavioral, and social factors for health outcomes (Hernandez & Blazer, 2006) and the need to incorporate biological measures in large social science studies (Finch, Vaupel, & Kinsella, 2001).

The field of family research has a history of using evolutionary psychology to provide theories and explanations (e.g., Booth et al., 2000) for understanding family processes. Yet evolutionary psychology has not greatly influenced my research. Why is this the case?

First, I did not know much about evolutionary psychology before reading Gangestad's chapter. I never took a class on the subject and have only had brief exposure to the discipline. One of the difficulties in conducting research that spans several disciplines is that researchers cannot possibly integrate all relevant disciplines. And, it is important to note that integrating insights from multiple disciplines and conducting interdisciplinary research is quite difficult (for a great overview see Hernandez & Blazer, 2006). Interdisciplinary work is complicated by difficulties with basic terminology, differences in underlying assumptions, inherent biases across disciplines based on past training, and differences in research goals. It is from this perspective that I wish to first comment on Gangestad (Chap. 9). The chapter provides a didactic summary of evolutionary psychology and anthropology, as well as background definitions, research methods, approaches used by the disciplines, and examples of research in the area. The text, therefore, provides beginners (like me) with a much needed introduction to these various fields.

Second, I have never really considered evolutionary psychology to have much relevance to my work. The research methods I frequently utilize – behavior genetic approaches – are quite different from those of evolutionary psychologists. And, I thought the questions that I ask in my research program did not have much in common with those that emerge in the field of evolutionary psychology. Thus, I was pleasantly surprised by Gangestad's emphasis on understanding the specific etiological mechanisms responsible for group differences in reproduction:

> ... patterns of mating & reproduction differ remarkably ... One answer to this question may seem obvious: At least part of the variation is due to the social and other factors that discriminate human groups. No doubt, this answer is true. At the same time, it is incomplete at a deep conceptual level. It does not specify processes whereby individuals respond differently to factors varying across groups (p. 118).

Gangestad's call for research that more fully elucidates the role of individual-level factors in understanding larger social influences is, in fact, quite consistent with my research programs. My affinity for this view stems from the fact that, unfortunately, a great deal of social research is being conducted in a manner that excludes consideration of any individual-level traits, including biological influences (Freese, 2008). This lack of consideration of genetic and biological factors occurs despite the fact that every facet of psychological and family functioning is influenced in part by genetic factors (Turkheimer, 2000) and prominent reviews have highlighted the importance/necessity of family researchers taking a biosocial approach (e.g., Booth et al., 2000).

Early biosocial research on the family (i.e., traditional early behavior genetic research) was conducted from a heuristic that viewed the influences underlying characteristics as being either genetic or environmental (the fundamental nature vs. nurture debate). Certainly, the dichotomous thinking that one source of variation was more important, in a win or lose battle, was naive. But, the comfortable response that, "Of course, both genes/biology and the environment are important" is only helpful if (and only if!) that leads to research that is informed by both approaches. For too long, researchers have paid lip service to biological factors while focusing primarily (or solely) on putative social factors at the exclusion of genetics or neuroscience. And, certainly the reverse is true. Much neuroscience and genetic research, at least from my perspective, simply ignores the role of the environment. Gangestad's emphasis on etiological mechanisms is aimed at understanding the processes through which environmental influences may have systematic influences on individuals, depending on their genetic/biological makeup. This is quite consistent with calls for interdisciplinary research on the family. Thus, I now have a better appreciation for evolutionary psychology and anthropology. Yes, these disciplines use methods that are quite different from the ones that I have used to date, but the overarching goal of identifying both social- and individual-level mechanisms provides essential common ground with my research. The same is true of many other disciplines interested in study social influences (e.g., Cacioppo et al., 2000).

Along with many others, I have written that family researchers need to rely on multiple methods and incorporate insights from various disciplines to truly understand family influences (D'Onofrio & Lahey, in press). Given that I was generally quite naïve about evolutionary psychology, the question remains: how does/will Gangestad influence my thinking about biosocial research on the family? Here, I comment on three broad research perspectives that I believe are informed by and should inform evolutionary psychology approaches to family issues. These include social neuroscience studies of mate selection, quasi-experimental studies to test casual inferences, and behavior genetic studies of cohort changes in heritability.

Social Neuroscience Studies of Mate Selection

Social neuroscience is a growing field that focuses on understanding both biological and social influences through multiple research methods (Cacioppo et al., 2007; Harmon-Jones & Winkielman, 2007). The discipline uses neuroimaging techniques to understand cognitive and social processes that occur outside of conscious awareness. In fact, recent neuroimaging studies have shed great insight into the cognitive processes responsible for the changes in heterosexual women's preferences for masculine or feminine faces across the menstrual cycle (e.g., women prefer more masculinized faces during ovulation). A recent neuroimaging study of women's preferences for masculinized and feminized faces by Rupp et al. (2008) indicated that brain activation in brain areas connected to decision making and reward processing are influenced by hormonal and psychosexual factors. In a follow-up study, Rupp et al. (2009) found that some of the same brain structures and networks were activated during a sexual decision-making task after being given explicit information about sexual risks. The results suggested that cognitive processes outside of awareness that influence mate selection are quite similar to the cognitive processes involved in weighing the pros and cons of sexual risk-taking information. These two neuroimaging studies (and others) have provided great insights into the cognitive processes associated with women's evaluation of possible sexual partners.

The neuroimaging studies of mate selection are a wonderful example of interdisciplinary research. The social neuroscience research has been heavily influenced by evolutionary psychology theory and research on changes in women's preferences across the menstrual cycle. The research questions Gangestad poses at the end of his chapter concerning the influence of oral contraceptive use on mate selection are a wonderful example of how evolutionary psychology can pose critical research questions for family researchers. And, evolutionary theory can be advanced once these cognitive processes are better understood. This provides a clear example of how the questions raised by evolutionary psychologists can inform cognitive neuroscience research.

Quasi-Experimental Studies to Test Causal Inferences

Gangestad went into great detail about the process through which evolutionary psychologists make adaptationist arguments, particularly the reliance on informal arguments:

> As theoretical claims in science go, special design arguments are in no way exceptional. Scientific hypotheses are often accepted on the basis of informal arguments of probabilities (e.g., Salmon, 1984). Arguments for special design rely on the same: They claim that exceptional fits between a trait's forms and purported functions would have to be extraordinarily strange coincidences *if* selection had not shaped the traits for their purported functions (p. 123).

As one exemplar, Gangestad discussed how men's modulation of testosterone levels has adapted for "trading off" between parental investment and mating effort. Support for the special design argument rests on the fact that many studies have found correlations between paternal involvement and testosterone. Therefore, the theory makes a strong inference about causation. Yet a fundamental principle of every statistics course is that correlation does not mean causation. Gangestad acknowledges that there may be alternative explanations for the covariation between testosterone and paternal involvement, but the crux of the argument for a special design rests on a strong assumption about causation – parental involvement causes lower testosterone.

From my perspective, researchers have not adequately tested the association between social influences and testosterone. Recent reviews, in fact, suggest that the associations between behavior and testosterone are complexly bidirectional (van Anders & Watson, 2006). Although men's testosterone may influence their behavior, social context also influences men's testosterone (e.g., van der Meij, Buunk, van de Sande, & Salvador, 2008).

Given the inability to conduct a randomized controlled study of testosterone levels, researchers must rely on research methods that can identify and test alternative hypotheses for the association between paternal involvement and testosterone. Quasi-experimental designs can help test causal inferences because the approaches utilize natural experiments that can distinguish between alternative hypotheses (Rutter, 2007). For example, longitudinal studies of identical (or monozygotic) twins provide a strong test of the causal inference because the design (a) provides information about temporal ordering, (b) removes the possibility that genetic factors could account for the association, and (c) rules out environmental confounds that influence siblings within a family similarly (e.g., Caspi et al., 2004). A longitudinal study of identical twins who are discordant for having children (i.e., one co-twin has children but his or her co-twin does not) would, therefore, provide a strong test of the causal theory.

Because adaptionist arguments are based on informal probabilities, the strength of the special arguments is highly dependent on valid conclusions about the underlying basic science. If, for example, testosterone is associated with paternal investment because of shared genetic factors, representing nonrandom selection into high levels of paternal involvement, the conclusion that the modulation of testosterone is adaptive (from an evolutionary perspective) would be incorrect. Thus, the questions raised by evolutionary psychology theory and research require greater knowledge about the mechanisms through which social factors/behaviors and testosterone are associated. Such questions require the use of quasi-experimental designs (Rutter, 2007) to support or reject the underlying theory.

Behavior Genetic Studies of Cohort Changes in Heritability

Gangestad's focus on understanding social influences, as well as individual-level responses, also mirrors a burgeoning research area focused on understanding gene–environment interactions (G × E). The study of G × E focuses on whether genetic predispositions influence an individual's response to social factors. If a G × E exists, variability in responses to social factors would be based, in part, on genetic factors (reviewd in Plomin, DeFries, McClearn, & McGuffin, 2008; Rutter, Moffitt, & Caspi, 2006). Researchers have approached the study of G × E from different research approaches. For example, research has used randomized controlled studies, quantitative behavior genetic designs, and studies including measured genes and environments.

One approach to studying individual-level and social factors is conducting quantitative behavior genetic studies (e.g., twin and adoption studies) across cohorts (reviewd in Rutter et al., 2006; Shanahan & Hofer, 2005). Traditional behavior genetic twin studies have explored the degree to which genetic factors (heritability), shared environmental factors, and nonshared environmental factors influence some trait (reviewd in Plomin et al., 2008). When exploring historical context, researchers explore whether the importance of these latent (or unmeasured) factors have changed over time. The design uses historical cohorts as an index for social changes. For instance, Kendler, Thornton, & Pedersen (2000) found changes in the heritability of cigarette smoking in women throughout the 1900s, indicating that as smoking became more acceptable and prevalent cigarette use was more influenced by genetic factors. Dunne et al. (1997) found that the heritability of first sexual intercourse for individuals born between 1952 and 1965 was much higher than for individuals born between 1922 and 1952 (during a period of greater social control on sexual intercourse). These studies illustrate the importance of considering social factors (indexed by cohorts) and individual-level traits.

In the past half century, there have been enormous changes in the age at first childbearing (AFCB) for women (e.g., Casper & Bianchi, 2002). Researchers have identified many social factors to explain the historical shift, including the legalization of and greater access to abortion (Klick & Stratmann, 2003) and birth control. The question Gangestad raised in his chapter, however, remains. What are the processes (both biological and environmental) that account for variation in AFCB? Again, as Gangestad points out, a purely environmental explanation is deeply unsatisfying. What are the processes through which societal changes have influenced AFCB for women? Could, perhaps, changes in social forces have altered the degree to which genetic factors influence AFCB?

Inspired by Gangestad's chapter, I conducted some preliminary analyses of a population-based study in Sweden to begin to explore the possibility. The analyses utilized the Multigenerational Registry, a large database maintained by Statistics Sweden that contains a unique numerical identifier for each individual born in Sweden or who immigrated and became a Swedish citizen before age 18 since 1932 (Statistics Sweden, 2003). The registry also includes the numerical identification numbers of each individual's biological parents. The information allowed us to link mothers with their children and each child's father (based on maternal report). Given the information, we identified women who were either full or maternal half siblings. The data set also includes information about date of birth for each individual, enabling us to calculate AFCB for each woman in Sweden.

Based on the registry, we explored the AFCB for women born between 1945 and 1964, based on 5-year increments. Women in the earlier cohorts were raised in a very different social environment than the women born in the later cohorts because of dramatic changes in Swedish society during the 1970s. Access to legal abortion became easier for young women in the early 1970s – the Swedish parliament passed legislation making abortion free nationwide early in pregnancy. Government public health initiatives were also passed in the early 1970s that provided education programs on sexuality and birth control. These programs led to sharp reductions in the adolescent birthrate (reviewed in Danielsson, Rogala, & Sundstrom, 2001; Darroch, Frost, & Singh, 2001).

Table 10.1 presents the sample size for various comparison groups across the cohorts. The first analysis documented the historical changes in average AFCB using all women with children in these cohorts. The results are presented in

Table 10.1 Sample sizes for the analysis of maternal age at first child-bearing by cohort

Cohort	Number of women with children	Number of offspring born to full siblings[a]	Number of offspring born to half siblings[a]
1945–1949	368,254	261,103	7,867
1950–1954	325,285	228,084	9,758
1955–1959	316,044	206,335	11,233
1960–1964	330,710	241,060	12,466

[a]Based on first two women in each family

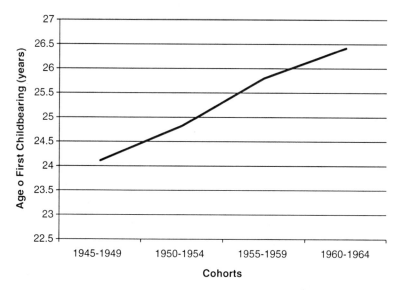

Fig. 10.1 Mean age at first childbearing by cohort

Fig. 10.1, which illustrates the dramatic rise in the average AFCB during this historical time period. On average, women born in the last cohort had their first children roughly 2 years later than the women in the first cohort.

The next set of analyses explored the variability in AFCB. Figure 10.2 illustrates that the total variability in AFCB also increased from 1945 to the late 1950s, at which point the variability decreased slightly. Therefore, the figure documents the large change in variability during across the cohorts, in addition to the dramatic change in average AFCB. Because the data set includes female siblings, the total variation could be separated into variability shared by siblings, referred to as familial variance and individual variance, the variability in AFCB that is unique to individuals after accounting for familial variance. As is frequently the case, there is greater variability within groups of siblings (the individual variance) than between families. Across the cohorts, individual variability increases, whereas familial variability remained relatively stable. The figures show how the variability in AFCB has changed throughout

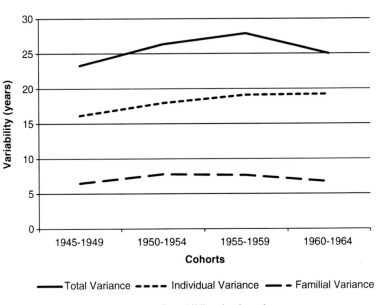

Fig. 10.2 Sources of variability in age at first childbearing by cohort

the historical time period, but the analyses do not provide great insight into the underlying mechanisms.

To help better understand the genetic and biological factors that influence variability in AFCB, we selected the first two women born to each family and identified whether they were full or half siblings. The difference in genetic relatedness between the sibling types provides the opportunity to fit behavioral genetic models that estimate the importance of genetic, shared environmental, and nonshared environmental influences (e.g., Tierney, Merikangas, & Risch, 1994). Figure 10.3 presents the intraclass correlations (an estimate of the sibling similarity) separately for full and half siblings in each historical cohort. The figure illustrates that the similarity of full and half siblings are almost identical for the first cohort, suggesting that genetic factors did not influence AFCB for women born between 1945 and 1949. The sibling correlations suggest that the heritability of AFCB for women born in the first cohort was miniscule ($h^2 = 0.04$). Because both types of sibling pairs had moderate intraclass correlations, regardless of their genetic relatedness, shared environmental factors ($c^2 = 0.28$) accounted for much greater variability in AFCB.

The results for the first cohort are in contrast to the intraclass correlations for the women in the subsequent three cohorts. Although there were some slight differences across those cohorts, the intraclass correlations for full siblings (average correlation = 0.28) were higher than the correlations for half sibling (average correlation = 0.17). The magnitude of the differences between the correlations for the two siblings types was also stable. Estimates of heritability ranged from ($h^2 = 0.33$–0.38) for women born from 1950 to 1964. Shared environmental influences were much lower ($c^2 = 0.09$–0.10) across the last three cohorts.

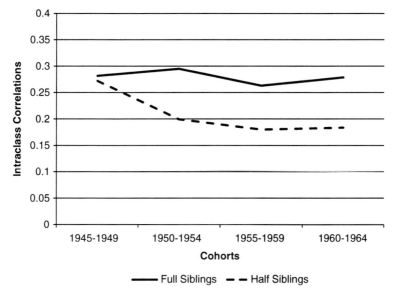

Fig. 10.3 Intraclass correlations in age at first childbearing by cohort

Certainly, more formal statistical modeling is required to test the cohort differences in heritability and shared environmental influences on AFCB (e.g., Purcell, 2002; Rathouz, Van Hulle, Rodgers, Waldman, & Lahey, 2008). These preliminary results suggest, though, that societal changes across the birth cohorts profoundly altered the genetic and environmental influences on AFCB. These findings can then direct future research aimed at identifying the individual-level factors that influence AFCB. The results suggest that genetic factors account for the similarity in AFCB among siblings. Consequently, future research should use multivariate behavior genetic models (Neale & Cardon, 1992) to more fully document and specify the traits that share genetic liability with AFCB.

Conclusion

Gangestad provides an introduction to the field of evolutionary psychology, particularly research related to the family. The focus on understanding etiological mechanisms (particularly the ways in which individual-level processes account for group-level differences) is shared with many other disciplines that also explore family functioning, highlighting the fact that evolutionary psychology can inform and be informed by family studies in other disciplines (Booth et al., 2000). From my perspective, the field of evolutionary psychology provides provocative hypotheses and theories that other disciplines can explore. As outlined in the current chapter, I also believe the social neuroscience research on mate selection, quasi-experimental research, and behavior genetic analyses across cohorts are three research methods that can greatly influence evolutionary psychology.

Acknowledgments Preparation of this chapter was supported in part by grants R01 HD061384, R01 HD056354, and R01 HD053550 from the National Institute of Child Health and Human Development and NARSAD. Special thanks to Amber Singh, Claire Coyne, and all the members of, the FRSP Program at Indiana university, the Developmental Psychopathology Lab in the Department of Psychological and Brain Sciences at Indiana University for their help in preparing this manuscript.

References

Adele, D. (2009). The interplay of biology and the environment broadly defined. *Developmental Psychology, 45,* 1–9.

Booth, A., Carver, K., & Granger, D. A. (2000). Biosocial perspectives on the family. *Journal of Marriage and the Family, 62,* 1018–1034.

Cacioppo, J. T., Amaral, D. G., Blanchard, J. J., Cameron, J. L., Carter, C. S., Crews, D., et al. (2007). Social neuroscience: Progress and implications for mental health. *Perspectives on Psychological Science, 2,* 99–123.

Cacioppo, J. T., Berntson, G. G., Sheridan, J. F., & McClintock, M. K. (2000). Multilevel integrative analyses of human behavior: Social neuroscience and the complementing nature of social and biological approaches. *Psychological Bulletin, 126,* 829–843.

Casper, L. M., & Bianchi, S. M. (2002). *Continuity and change in the American family.* Thousand Oaks, NJ: Sage.

Caspi, A., Moffitt, T. E., Morgan, J., Rutter, M., Taylor, A., Arseneault, L., et al. (2004). Maternal expressed emotion predicts childrens' antisocial behavior problems: Using monozygotic-twin differences to identify environmental effects on behavioral development. *Developmental Psychology, 50,* 149–161.

Cicchetti, D. (2006). Development and psychopathology. In D. Cicchetti & D. J. Cohen (Eds.), *Handbook of developmental psychopathology* (Vol. 1, pp. 1–18). New York: Wiley.

D'Onofrio, B. M., & Lahey, B. B. (in press). Biosocial influences on the family: A decade review. *Journal of Marriage and Family, 72* 762–782.

Danielsson, M., Rogala, C., & Sundstrom, K. (2001). *Teenage sexual and reproductive behavior in developed countries: Country report for Sweden (Occasional Report No. 7).* New York: Alan Guttmacher Institute.

Darroch, J. E., Frost, J. J., & Singh, S. (2001). *Teenage sexual and reproductive behavior in developed countries (Occasional Report No. 3).* New York: Alan Guttmacher Institute.

Dunne, M. P., Martin, N. G., Statham, D. J., Slutske, W. S., Dinwiddie, S. H., Bucholz, K. K., et al. (1997). Genetic and environmental contributions to variance in age at first sexual intercourse. *Psychological Science, 8,* 211–216.

Finch, C. E., Vaupel, J. W, & Kinsella, K. (Eds.). (2001). *Cells and surveys: Should biological measures be included in social science research?* Washington, DC: National Academy.

Freese, J. (2008). Genetics and the social science explanation of individual outcomes. *American Journal of Sociology, 114,* S1–S35.

Freese, J., Allen Li, J. C., & Wade, L. D. (2003). The potential relevances of biology to social inquiry. *Annual Review of Sociology, 29,* 233–256.

Granger, D. A., & Kivlighan, K. T. (2003). Integrating biological, behavioral, and social levels of analysis in early child development: Progress, problems, and prospects. *Child Development, 74,* 1058–1063.

Harmon-Jones, E., & Winkielman, P. (2007). *Social neuroscience: Integrating biological and psychological explanations of social behavior*. New York: Guilford Press.

Hernandez, L. M., & Blazer, D. G. (Eds.). (2006). *Gense, behavior and the social environment: Moving beyond the nature/nurture debate*. Washington, DC: National Academies Press.

Kendler, K. S. (2005). Toward a philosophical structure for psychiatry. *American Journal of Psychiatry, 162*, 433–440.

Kendler, K. S., Thornton, L. M., & Pedersen, N. L. (2000). Tobacco consumption in Swedish twins reared apart and reared together. *Archives of General Psychiatry, 57*, 886–892.

Klick, J., & Stratmann, T. (2003). The effect of abortion legalization on sexual behavior: Evidence from sexually transmitted diseases. *Journal of Legal Studies, 32*, 407–433.

Neale, M. C., & Cardon, L. R. D. (1992). *Methodology for genetic studies of twins and families*. Dordrecht, The Netherlands: Kluwer Academic.

Plomin, R., DeFries, J. C., McClearn, G. E., & McGuffin, P. (Eds.). (2008). *Behavioral genetics* (Vol. 5). New York: Worth.

Purcell, S. (2002). Variance components for gene-environment interaction in twin studies. *Twin Research, 5*, 554–571.

Rathouz, P. J., Van Hulle, C. A., Rodgers, J. L., Waldman, I. D., & Lahey, B. B. (2008). Specification, testing, and interpretation of gene-by-measured-environment interaction models in the presence of gene-environment correlation. *Behavior Genetics, 38*, 301–315.

Rupp, H. A., James, T. W., Ketterson, E. D., Sengelaub, D. R., Janssen, E., & Heiman, J. R. (2008). Neural activation in women in response to masculinized male faces: Mediation by hormones and psychosexual factors. *Evolution and Human Behavior, 30*, 1–10.

Rupp, H. A., James, T. W., Ketterson, E. D., Sengelaub, D. R., Janssen, E., & Heiman, J. R. (2009). The role of the anterior cingulate cortex in women's sexual decision making. *Neuroscience Letters, 449*, 42–47.

Rutter, M. (2007). Proceeding from observed correlation to causal inference: The use of natural experiments. *Perspectives on Psychological Science, 2*, 377–395.

Rutter, M., Moffitt, T. E., & Caspi, A. (2006). Gene-environment interplay and psychopathology: Multiple varieties but real effects. *Journal of Child Psychology and Psychiatry, 47*, 226–261.

Shanahan, M. J., & Hofer, S. M. (2005). Social context in gene-environment interactions: Retrospect and prospect. *Journals of Gerontology, 60*(B), 65–76.

Statistics Sweden. (2003). *Multi-Generation Register 2002, A description of contents and quality*. Örebro, Sweden.

Tierney, C., Merikangas, K. R., & Risch, N. (1994). Feasibility of half-sibling designs for detecting a genetic component to a disease. *Genetic Epidemiology, 11*, 523–538.

Turkheimer, E. (2000). Three laws of behavior genetics and what they mean. *Current Directions in Psychological Science, 9*, 160–164.

van Anders, S. M., & Watson, N. V. (2006). Social neuroendocrinology: Effects of social contexts and behaviors on sex steroids in humans. *Human Nature, 17*, 212–237.

van der Meij, L., Buunk, A. P., van de Sande, J. P., & Salvador, A. (2008). The presence of a woman increases testosterone in aggressive dominant men. *Hormones and Behavior, 54*, 640–644.

Chapter 11
Psychological Adaptation and Human Fertility Patterns: Some Evidence of Human Mating Strategies as Evoked Sexual Culture

David P. Schmitt

Abstract Several features of human fertility, such as age of menarche, age at first marriage, and total number of offspring, vary in significant ways across cultures. At least part of this variation may be attributable to evolved psychological adaptations designed to facultatively respond to varying local environments with different reproductive strategies. Evidence is reviewed which suggests that stressful environments appear to evoke insecure parent–child attachment, which subsequently leads to an adaptive developmental pathway that includes dismissing romantic attachment, interpersonal distrust, and the pursuit of short-term reproductive strategies. Low levels of environmental stress seem to evoke a different reproductive strategy adaptively rooted in secure attachment, heightened interpersonal trust, and long-term mating. Much of the modern variation in human fertility may result from psychological adaptations to our ancestral past differentially functioning across evoked cultures.

Introduction

Gangestad (Chap. 9) details several differences between the patterns of women's fertility observed in *foraging cultures* (the cultural form within which ancestral humans primarily evolved; Brown, 1991, Lee & Daly, 2000) and the patterns of women's fertility exhibited in *modern cultures* (especially those that are postdemographic transition; Borgerhoff Mulder, 1998). For instance, relative to women in foraging cultures, postdemographic women tend to achieve menarche much earlier (12.5 vs. 16 years), begin childbearing much later (25 vs. 17.5 years), have fewer total numbers of children (2 vs. 8 offspring), and marry much later (if at all).

D.P. Schmitt (✉)
Department of Psychology, Bradley University, Peoria, IL, USA
e-mail: dps@bradley.edu

A. Booth et al. (eds.), *Biosocial Foundations of Family Processes*,
National Symposium on Family Issues, DOI 10.1007/978-1-4419-7361-0_11,
© Springer Science+Business Media, LLC 2011

What is the source of these dramatically different patterns of human female fertility across differing cultural forms?

Obviously, several factors are likely involved when there is such massive cultural variation in human sexuality (Frayser, 1985; Kaplan & Lancaster, 2003; Low, 2000). Two evolution-relevant factors seem particularly relevant in the case of human fertility. First, features of modern cultures may be novel within the context of the evolution of our species. Certain facets of modern monotheistic religions (Keller, 1990; Reynolds & Tanner, 1983), political structures (Baumeister & Twenge, 2002; Pasternak, Ember, & Ember, 1997), and dietary nutrition (see Ellis, 2004) may not match what our evolved human nature is anticipatorily designed to experience. Modern culture, especially Western technological culture (i.e., WEIRD culture; see Henrich, Heine, & Norenzayan, 2010), may be "unnatural" in a limited sense – modern culture provides environmental stimuli that our evolved psychology does not expect, and it fails to provide certain environmental contexts that our evolutionary psychology is designed to anticipate (Alexander, 1990; Irons, 1998).

If so, various "mismatches" between the peculiarities of modern culture and our evolved psychology (i.e., a psychology specially designed to react to recurrent features of ancestral environments; Cronk, 1999; Eibl-Eibesfeldt, 1989) may account for some of the fertility variations highlighted by Gangestad (Chap. 9). A possible example is the drastic reduction in age of menarche among women in modern cultures resulting from novel features of diet and nutrition that would have been unknown among foraging women in ancestral environments (Ellis, 2004). As a result, modern culture's conspicuously prolonged period of human female adolescence (in which young fecund women are able to have children but do not, on average, become pregnant for over a decade) may represent "unnatural" human fertility variation.

The focus of this chapter is on an equally important second factor: It may be that cultural variations in patterns of human fertility are not unexpected from an evolutionary perspective (Frayser, 1985; Low, 1989; Mealey, 2000). Indeed, evolution may have built into our universal "human nature" a psychological design that anticipates that certain features of environment will be variable in critically informative ways (see Gangestad, Haselton, & Buss, 2006; Gaulin, 1997; Kenrick, Nieuweboer, & Buunk, 2010), and that different patterns of fertility may represent facultatively adaptive reactions across these varying environmental conditions. Much like our evolved callus-producing mechanisms inherent in human skin that expect physical environments to occasionally produce tactile friction (and *skin calluses* represent adaptive reactions to tactile friction that provide a protective function), there may be evolved features of our fertility and mating psychology that expect social and ecological environments to occasionally produce "emotional friction" (and features of *emotional callousness* represent adaptive reactions to this friction that also provide protective functions). As noted by Gangestad (Chap. 9), evolutionary psychologists have detailed a conceptual approach to culture that captures such anticipatory psychological variation – the concept of "evoked culture" (Tooby & Cosmides, 1992).

An Evolutionary Perspective on Attachment, Personality, and Sexuality

In 1991, Belsky, Steinberg, and Draper combined aspects of attachment theory (Bowlby, 1969) and life history theory (Low, 1998) to present an evolutionary model of adaptive variation in attachment, personality, and sexuality. In their classic paper, Belsky, Steinberg, & Draper (1991) suggested that parent–child attachment relationships might adaptively evoke individual variation in subsequent adult romantic attachment styles and the differential functional pursuit of long-term versus short-term mating strategies across adulthood (Buss & Schmitt, 1993; Gangestad & Simpson, 2000). Early social experiences, they argued, adaptively attune children to follow one of two different life history pathways.

Along one of these adaptive pathways, children who are socially exposed to high levels of stress – especially insensitive/inconsistent parenting, harsh ecological environments, and economic hardship – are channeled down a life history course that involves insecure attachment, distrustful personality traits, and short-term mating strategies (see also Chisholm, 1996). Such children also tend to physically mature earlier and be more sexually precocious than those children who are exposed to less stress (Ellis, 2004; Hoier, 2003). This pathway also appears to involve, for highly stressed females, a greater likelihood of father absence (and present stepfathers) in the home (Draper & Harpending, 1982; Ellis & Garber, 2000; Ellis et al., 2003).

According to Belsky, Steinberg, & Draper (1991), this pathway toward early attachment insecurity is an adaptive strategy that leads to the functional pursuit of "opportunistic" or short-term-oriented mating strategies in adulthood (see also Kirkpatrick, 1998; Schmitt, 2005a; Simpson, 1999). It is thought that an opportunistic strategy leads to higher levels of fitness in unreliable, high-stress reproductive environments (Cohen & Belsky, 2008; Ivan & Bereczkei, 2006). In cultures with inconsistent or stressful social relations, therefore, children may adaptively respond by developing the more viable life history strategy of high risk-taking (Quinlan & Quinlan, 2007), interpersonal distrust (Figueredo et al., 2008), high psychopathy (Mealey, 1995), low levels of pair-bonding and love (Schmitt et al., 2009), and increased pursuit of short-term mating strategies rooted in dismissing attachment (Jonason, Li, Webster, & Schmitt, 2009).

The second pathway hypothesized by Belsky, Steinberg, & Draper (1991) involves the adaptive obverse of the first. Those children exposed to low levels of stress and less environmental hardship tend to be more emotionally secure, to physically mature later, and to take less risks. These children are thought to develop a more "investing" reproductive strategy in adulthood (i.e., high levels of monogamy, love, pair-bonding, and secure romantic attachment; Schmitt et al., 2009). This pathway is thought to pay higher evolutionary dividends in low stress environments (see also Belsky, 1997; Burton, 1990; Lancaster, 1989). There may be heritable factors within and between populations that account for some of the variation along these pathways, but early experiences appear to be formative above and beyond these influences (Gillath, Shaver, Baek, & Chun, 2008).

Importantly, a particular life history pathway cannot be viewed, in an evolutionary sense, as wholly superior to the other. Although one could argue from a public health perspective (or take a moral position) that the second pathway involving attachment security, monogamy, and love is "better," from an evolutionary perspective each life history trajectory is differentially effective depending on the local levels of stress and safety (Ellis & Boyce, 2008). Just as other species have facultative mating adaptations that differentially respond to varying environmental conditions (including stress; see Bijlsma & Loeschcke, 2005), we humans may have life history strategies that functionally vary in response to environmental stress in terms of attachment security, interpersonal trust, and long-term/short-term mating strategies (Del Giudice, 2009; Huether, 1998; Muehlenbein & Bribiescas, 2005; cf. Flinn, 2006). Much work remains to be done, but discovering the precise nature of these different human life history trajectories represents one of the great challenges of modern evolutionary psychology (Figueredo et al., 2005).

Variation in Attachment, Personality, and Sexuality as "Evoked Culture"

In the view of the evolutionary perspectives outlined above, all children can be viewed as naturally equipped with the potential for developing a variety of attachment styles, personality traits, and sexual strategies (Belsky, 1999; Simpson, 1999). More specifically, we all possess context-dependent, facultative psychological adaptations that are sensitive to local environments (stressors and otherwise) and regulate our life history strategies in functional ways (Del Giudice, 2009; Gangestad & Simpson, 2000). Although many of the causal mechanisms that most prominently influence attachment are located within the family, evolutionary perspectives also suggest that certain aspects of culture may be related to attachment, personality, and sexuality variation (Schmitt, 2005a; Schmitt et al., 2004). Namely, in cultures where families are under more stress and have fewer resources, dismissing romantic attachment levels should be manifestly higher than in cultures with lower stress and more ample resources (Schmitt et al., 2003).

Chisholm (1996, 1999) argued further that local mortality rates – presumably related to high stress and inadequate resources – act as specific cues that contingently shift human attachment and mating strategies in evolutionary-adaptive ways. In cultures with high mortality rates, the optimal mating strategy is to reproduce early and often, a strategy related to dismissing attachment, short-term temporal orientations, and unrestricted sociosexuality (Ellis & Boyce, 2008; Schmitt, 2005a; Wilson & Daly, 2006). In cultures that have abundant resources, the optimal strategy is to invest heavily in fewer numbers of offspring, a strategy associated with low fertility, secure romantic attachment, monogamous mating behavior, and long-term temporal horizons. This perspective suggests that cultures with higher mortality rates, earlier reproduction, and more prolific reproduction should manifest higher levels of dismissing romantic attachment, interpersonal distrust, weak pair-bonding, and short-term mating than cultures with lower mortality, later reproduction, and relatively limited reproduction (Schmitt, 2005a; Schmitt et al., 2003, 2004).

An ecological factor that may have a special impact on dismissing romantic attachment is the amount of *ecological* stress in local environments. Some cultures possess high-stress ecologies (Chisholm, 1999; Keller, 1990). For example, cultures with high levels of pathogens and disease are thought to present high-stress environments because raising offspring in disease-prone environments is associated with higher childhood mortality (see Fincher, Thornhill, Murray, & Schaller, 2008; Gangestad & Buss, 1993; Low, 1990). Indeed, mortality rate (or low life expectancy) itself is a strong indicator of ecological stress. Reproductive environments with high fertility rates and scarce resources can also be considered stressful because human children, relative to other primate species, require heavy parental investment, and raising multiple offspring makes it more difficult to invest the necessary amounts of care in each child (Harvey & Clutton-Brock, 1985; Walker et al., 2006).

The preceding evolutionary perspectives on romantic attachment lead to several expectations concerning cultural differences in romantic attachment, personality traits, and mating strategies across cultures. First, in cultures where families are under more ecological stress and have fewer resources, dismissing romantic attachment, interpersonal distrust, and short-term mating levels should be higher than in cultures with lower stress and ample resources (Belsky, Steinberg, & Draper, 1991). Second, in cultures with higher mortality rates, earlier reproduction, and more prolific reproduction, dismissing romantic attachment, interpersonal distrust, and short-term mating levels should be higher than in cultures with low mortality, later reproduction, and limited reproduction (Chisholm, 1996, 1999).

Findings from several large cross-cultural data sets – such as the International Sexuality Description Project (ISDP) – support many of these evolutionary hypotheses (see Schmitt, 2005b, 2009; Schmitt & Allik, 2005; Schmitt et al., 2003, 2004, 2009). For example, those ISDP nations with lower human development indexes (including lower GDP per capita; United Nations Development Programme, 2001) have higher levels of dismissing attachment and psychopathic traits (including callous affect). Moreover, cross-national data confirm that national levels of dismissing attachment and psychopathic traits are related to lower life expectancy, lower adult literacy, and lower political freedom (see Schmitt, 2009). Dismissing attachment and psychopathic traits are also linked to higher fertility, higher rates of low birth weight newborns, higher tuberculosis rates, and higher average daily temperature (Schmitt, 2009). Overall, it appears that there are consistent empirical associations between indexes of stress and dismissing attachment (e.g., pathogen stress is positively correlated with dismissing romantic attachment, $r(55) = 0.39$, $p < 0.001$; see Fig. 11.1). These findings support Kirkpatrick's (1998) assertion that dismissing attachment, among the various forms of insecure attachment, is most closely associated with psychopathic traits and short-term temporal horizons (Chisholm, 1999), including short-term mating strategies (Belsky, Steinberg, & Draper, 1991; Schmitt, 2005a).

The results for short-term mating at the national level were less clear. Although indicators of "early short-term mating" (e.g., teen birthrates) were positively

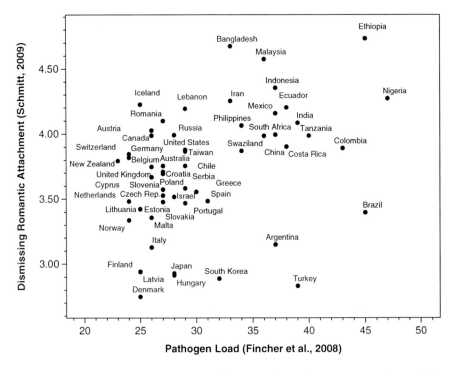

Fig. 11.1 Pathogen load related to dismissing romantic attachment across nations of the International Sexuality Description Project-2

associated as expected with cultural and ecological stress (and with insecure attachment and distrustful personality traits), various indicators of "late short-term mating" (e.g., infidelity) were negatively related to national levels of cultural and ecological stress (Schmitt, 2009). It may be that attachment, distrust, and "early short-term mating" function, as Belsky, Steinberg, & Draper (1991) predicted, as a life history response to uncertain reproductive environments (as indicated by high stress), but a separate pathway of "late short-term mating" is followed only when stress levels are low and humans are capable – given ample resources and cultural openness – to support children outside the context of monogamous marriage (see Schaller & Murray, 2008; Schmitt, 2009).

Conclusion

Cross-cultural patterns of attachment, personality, and sexuality are related to local ecologies in ways that support the view that cultural variation that stems from a human nature is designed to be "evoked" (Belsky, Steinberg, & Draper, 1991; Burton, 1990; Chisholm, 1999). It appears that high levels of ecological stress lead to attachment insecurities that precipitate an adaptive developmental pathway that involves dismissing attachment, tendencies toward interpersonal distrust, and the pursuit of short-term reproductive strategies (at least in adolescence; Ellis, McFadyen–Ketchum, Dodge, Pettit, & Bates, 1999; Schmitt, 2005a). Although ecological stress seems to evoke dismissing attachment (e.g., inconsistent/unloving parenting leads to mistrust) in ways that give rise to *early* reproduction (e.g., adolescent fertility, early age at first sexual intercourse) and associated facets of sexuality (e.g., low levels of love/pair-bonding, high levels of sexual aggression), adulthood or *later* features of short-term mating (e.g., short-term mate poaching, marital affairs, and extra-pair copulations) – while linked to dismissing attachment and psychopathy *within nations* – are not linked to ecological stress and its sequelae *across cultures* (Schmitt, 2009).

Perhaps ecological stress and lack of resources evoke dismissing attachment and distrust in individuals, from which cultures of *early* sexual permissiveness adaptively emerge. Other studies have shown that features of short-term mating emerge in high stress cultures, such as heightened mate preferences for physical attractiveness (possibly an adaptive desire for low mutation load; Gangestad, Haselton, & Buss, 2006). Low stress and ample resources may slow individual reproductive life history trajectories, in contrast, and allow for love and pair-bonding combined with permissive short-term mating in *later* adulthood (e.g., mate poaching and extra-pair copulations; Schmitt et al., 2009).

Complex models will be needed to fully chart differing human fertility trajectories. As the "early" versus "late" short-term mating findings above illustrate, it is unlikely that only a few basic evolved mechanisms explain contemporary variations in fertility across cultures. Instead, future investigators will need to integrate models of multiple psychological adaptations that likely react to local ecology and other features of culture in ways that evoke strategic mating behavior. Fertility researchers should seriously consider the possibility that much modern cultural variation in fertility is produced, at least in part, by psychological adaptations to our ancestral past differentially functioning across "evoked cultures."

References

Alexander, R. D. (1990). Epigenetic rules and Darwinian algorithms: The adaptive study of learning and development. *Ethology and Sociobiology*, *11*, 1–63.

Baumeister, R. F., & Twenge, J. M. (2002). Cultural suppression of female sexuality. *Review of General Psychology*, *6*, 166–203.

Belsky, J. (1997). Attachment, mating, and parenting: An evolutionary interpretation. *Human Nature*, *8*, 361–381.

Belsky, J. (1999). Modern evolutionary theory and patterns of attachment. In J. Cassidy & P. R. Shaver (Eds.), *Handbook of attachment* (pp. 141–161). New York: Guilford.

Belsky, J., Steinberg, L., & Draper, P. (1991). Childhood experience, interpersonal development, and reproductive strategy: An evolutionary theory of socialization. *Child Development*, *62*, 647–670.

Bijlsma, R., & Loeschcke, V. (2005). Environmental stress, adaptation and evolution: An overview. *Journal of Evolutionary Biology*, *18*, 744–749.

Borgerhoff Mulder, M. (1998). The demographic transition: Are we any closer to an evolutionary explanation? *Trends in Ecology and Evolution, 13*, 266–270.

Bowlby, J. (1969). *Attachment and loss: Vol. I. Attachment.* New York: Basic Books.

Brown, D. E. (1991). *Human universals.* New York: McGraw-Hill.

Burton, L. M. (1990). Teenage childbearing as an alternative life-course strategy in multigenerational black families. *Human Nature, 1*, 123–144.

Buss, D. M., & Schmitt, D. P. (1993). Sexual strategies theory: An evolutionary perspective on human mating. *Psychological Review, 100*, 204–232.

Chisholm, J. S. (1996). The evolutionary ecology of attachment organization. *Human Nature, 7*, 1–38.

Chisholm, J. S. (1999). Steps to an evolutionary ecology of the mind. In A. L. Hinton (Ed.), *Biocultural approaches to the emotions* (pp. 117–149). Cambridge: Cambridge University Press.

Cohen, D. L., & Belsky, J. (2008). Individual differences in female mate preferences as a function of attachment and hypothetical ecological conditions. *Journal of Evolutionary Psychology, 6*, 25–42.

Cronk, L. (1999). *That complex whole: Culture and the evolution of human behavior.* Boulder: Westview.

Del Giudice, M. (2009). Sex, attachment, and the development of reproductive strategies. *Behavioral and Brain Sciences, 32*, 1–21.

Draper, P., & Harpending, H. (1982). Father absence and reproductive strategy: An evolutionary perspective. *Journal of Anthropological Research, 38*, 255–273.

Eibl–Eibesfeldt, I. (1989). *Human ethology.* New York: Aldine de Gruyter.

Ellis, B. J. (2004). Timing of pubertal maturation in girls: An integrated life history approach. *Psychological Bulletin, 130*, 920–958.

Ellis, B. J., Bates, J. E., Dodge, K. A., Fergusson, D. M., Horwood, L. J., Pettit, G. S., & Woodward, L. (2003). Does father absence place daughters at special risk for early sexual activity and teenage pregnancy? *Child Development, 74*, 801–821.

Ellis, B. J., & Boyce, W. T. (2008). Biological sensitivity to context. *Current Directions in Psychological Science, 17*, 183–187.

Ellis, B. J., & Garber, J. (2000). Psychosocial antecedents of variation in girls' pubertal timing: Maternal depression, stepfather presence, and marital and family stress. *Child Development, 71*, 485–501.

Ellis, B. J., McFadyen–Ketchum, S., Dodge, K. A., Pettit, G. S., & Bates, J. E. (1999). Quality of early family relationships and individual differences in the timing of pubertal maturation in girls: A longitudinal test of an evolutionary model. *Journal of Personality and Social Psychology, 77*, 387–401.

Figueredo, A. J., Brumbach, B. H., Jones, D. N., Sefcek, J. A., Vásquez, G., & Jacobs, W. J. (2008). Ecological constraints on mating tactics. In G. Glenn & G. Miller (Eds.), *Mating intelligence: Sex, relationships, and the mind's reproductive system* (pp. 337–363). Mahwah: Lawrence Erlbaum.

Figueredo, A. J., Sefcek, J., Vásquez, G., Brumbach, B. H., King, J. E., & Jacobs, W. J. (2005). Evolutionary personality psychology. In D. M. Buss (Ed.), *Handbook of evolutionary psychology* (pp. 851–877). Hoboken: Wiley.

Fincher, C. L., Thornhill, R., Murray, D. R., & Schaller, M. (2008). Pathogen prevalence predicts human cross-cultural variability in individualism/collectivism. *Proceedings of the Royal Society B, 275*, 1279–1285.

Flinn, M. V. (2006). Evolution and ontogeny of stress response to social challenges in the human child. *Developmental Review, 26*, 138–174.

Frayser, S. (1985). *Varieties of sexual experience: An anthropological perspective.* New Haven: HRAF.

Gangestad S. W. (2010). Human adaptations for mating: Frameworks for understanding modern family formation and fertility? In A. Booth, S. McHale, & N. Landale (Eds.), *Biosocial foundations of family processes* (pp. 117–148). New York: Springer.

Gangestad, S. W., & Buss, D. M. (1993). Pathogen prevalence and human mate preferences. *Ethology and Sociobiology, 14*, 89–96.

Gangestad, S. W., Haselton, M. G., & Buss, D. M. (2006). Evolutionary foundations of cultural variation: Evoked culture and mate preferences. *Psychological Inquiry, 17*, 75–95.

Gangestad, S. W., & Simpson, J. A. (2000). The evolution of human mating: Trade-offs and strategic pluralism. *Behavioral and Brain Sciences, 23*, 573–587.

Gaulin, S. J. C. (1997). Cross-cultural patterns and the search for evolved psychological mechanisms. In G. R. Bock & G. Cardew (Eds.), *Characterizing human psychological adaptations* (pp. 195–207). Chichester: Wiley.

Gillath, O., Shaver, P. R., Baek, J., & Chun, D. S. (2008). Genetic correlates of adult attachment style. *Personality and Social Psychology Bulletin, 34*, 1396–1405.

Harvey, P. H., & Clutton-Brock, T. H. (1985). Life history variation in primates. *Evolution, 39*, 559–581.

Henrich, J., Heine, S. J., & Norenzayan, A. (2010). The weirdest people in the world? *Behavioral and Brain Sciences, 33*, 61–83.

Hoier, S. (2003). Father absence and age at menarche: A test of four evolutionary models. *Human Nature, 14*, 209–233.

Huether, G. (1998). Stress and the adaptive self organization of neuronal connectivity during early childhood. *International Journal of Developmental Neuroscience, 16*, 297–306.

Irons, W. (1998). Adaptively relevant environments versus the environment of evolutionary adaptedness. *Evolutionary Anthropology, 6*, 194–204.

Ivan, Z., & Bereczkei, T. (2006). Parental bonding, risk-taking behavior and life history theory. *Journal of Cultural and Evolutionary Psychology, 4*, 267–275.

Jonason, P. K., Li, N. P., Webster, G. D., & Schmitt, D. P. (2009). The dark triad: Facilitating short–term mating in men. *European Journal of Personality, 23*, 5–18.

Kaplan H., & Lancaster J. B. (2003). An evolutionary and ecological analysis of human fertility, mating patterns, and parental investment. In K. W. Wachter & R. A. Bulatao (Eds.), *Offspring: Human fertility behavior in biodemographic perspective* (pp. 170–223). Washington: National Academy.

Keller, H. (1990). Evolutionary approaches. In J. W. Berry, Y. H. Poortinga, & J. Pandey (Eds.), *Handbook of cross–cultural psychology* (2nd ed.) (Vol. 1, pp. 215–255). Boston: Allyn and Bacon.

Kenrick, D. T., Nieuweboer, S., & Buunk, A. P. (2010). Universal mechanisms and cultural diversity: Replacing the Blank Slate with a coloring book. In M. Schaller et al. (Eds.), *Evolution, culture, and the human mind* (pp. 257–272). New York: Psychology Press.

Kirkpatrick, L. A. (1998). Evolution, pair–bonding, and reproductive strategies: A reconceptualization of adult attachment. In J. A. Simpson & W. S. Rholes (Eds.), *Attachment theory and close relationships* (pp. 353–393). New York: Guilford.

Lancaster, J.B. (1989). Evolutionary and cross–cultural perspectives on single–parenthood. In R. W. Bell & N. J. Bell (Eds.), *Interfaces in psychology* (pp. 63–72). Lubbock: Texas Tech University Press.

Lee, R. B., & Daly, R. (Eds.). (2000). *The Cambridge encyclopedia of hunters and gatherers*. Cambridge: Cambridge University Press.

Low, B. S. (1989). Cross–cultural patterns in the training of children: An evolutionary perspective. *Journal of Comparative Psychology, 103*, 311–319.

Low, B. S. (1990). Marriage systems and pathogen stress in human societies. *American Zoologist, 30*, 325–339.

Low, B. S. (1998). The evolution of human life histories. In C. Crawford & D. L. Krebs (Eds.), *Handbook of evolutionary psychology: Ideas, issues, and applications* (pp. 131–161). Mahwah: Lawrence Erlbaum.

Low, B. S. (2000). *Why sex matters*. Princeton: Princeton University Press.

Mealey, L. (1995). The sociobiology of sociopathy: An integrated evolutionary model. *Behavioral & Brain Sciences, 8*, 523–599.

Mealey, L. (2000). *Sex differences: Developmental and evolutionary strategies*. San Diego: Academic.

Muehlenbein, M. P., & Bribiescas, R. G. (2005). Testosterone-mediated immune functions and male life histories. *American Journal of Human Biology, 17*, 527–558.

Pasternak, B., Ember, C., & Ember, M. (1997). *Sex, gender, and kinship: A cross-cultural perspective.* Upper Saddle: Prentice Hall.

Quinlan, R. J., & Quinlan, M.B. (2007). Parenting and cultures of risk: A comparative analysis of infidelity, aggression, and witchcraft. *American Anthropologist, 109,* 164–179.

Reynolds, V., & Tanner, R. E. S. (1983). *The biology of religion.* London: Longman.

Schaller, M., & Murray, D. R. (2008). Pathogens, personality, and culture: Disease prevalence predicts worldwide variability in sociosexuality, extraversion, and openness to experience. *Journal of Personality and Social Psychology, 95,* 212–221.

Schmitt, D. P. (2005a). Is short-term mating the maladaptive result of insecure attachment? A test of competing evolutionary perspectives. *Personality and Social Psychology Bulletin, 31,* 747–768.

Schmitt, D. P. (2005b). Sociosexuality from Argentina to Zimbabwe: A 48-nation study of sex, culture, and strategies of human mating. *Behavioral and Brain Sciences, 28,* 247–275.

Schmitt, D. P. (2009). *Self-reported psychopathy across 58 nations: On the evolution of sex differences and cultural variations in anti-sociality.* Manuscript in preparation.

Schmitt, D. P., Alcalay, L., Allensworth, M., Allik, J., Ault, L., Austers, I., et al. (2003). Are men universally more dismissing than women? Gender differences in romantic attachment across 62 cultural regions. *Personal Relationships, 10,* 307–331.

Schmitt, D. P., Alcalay, L., Allensworth, M., Allik, J., Ault, L., Austers, I., et al. (2004). Patterns and universals of adult romantic attachment across 62 cultural regions: Are models of self and of other pancultural constructs? *Journal of Cross-Cultural Psychology, 35,* 367–402.

Schmitt, D. P., & Allik, J. (2005). Simultaneous administration of the Rosenberg Self–Esteem Scale across 53 nations: Exploring the universal and culture-specific features of global self-esteem. *Journal of Personality and Social Psychology, 89,* 623–642.

Schmitt, D.P., Youn, G., Bond, B., Brooks, S., Frye, H., Johnson, S., Klesman, J., Peplinski, C., Sampias, J., Sherrill, M., & Stoka, C. (2009). When will I feel love? The effects of personality, culture, and gender on the psychological tendency to love. *Journal of Research in Personality, 43,* 830–846.

Simpson, J. A. (1999). Attachment theory in modern evolutionary perspective. In J. Cassidy & P. R. Shaver (Eds.), *Handbook of attachment* (pp. 115–140). New York: Guilford.

Tooby, J., & Cosmides, L. (1992). The psychological foundations of culture. In J. Barkow, L. Cosmides, & J. Tooby (Eds.), *The adapted mind: Evolutionary psychology and the generation of culture.* New York: Oxford University Press.

United Nations Development Programme. (2001). *Human development report 2001.* New York: Oxford University Press.

Walker, R., Gurven, M., Hill, K., Migliano, A., Chagnon, N., De Souza, R., Djurovic, G., Hames, R., Hurtado, A. M., Kaplan, H., Kramer, K., Oliver, W. J., Valeggia, C., & Yamauchi, T. (2006). Growth rates and life histories in twenty-two small-scale societies. *American Journal of Human Biology, 18,* 295–311.

Wilson, M., & Daly, M. (2006). Are juvenile offenders extreme future discounters? *Psychological Science, 17,* 989–994.

Chapter 12
Comments on Consilience Efforts

S. Philip Morgan

Abstract In questioning the usefulness of Gangestad's concept of *evoked culture* as an explanation for major shifts in family and fertility behavior, I offer an alternative way to conceptualize the role of biological predispositions and potential that focuses on the human brain. Brain evolution, brain development, and brain functioning are the keys to understanding broad sweeps of family change and variation. More specifically, I develop a very broad conception of schema that locates them both "in the mind" and "in the world"; that is, schema can be codified in the brain's neural circuits, and they can also be widely shared by a community of interacting individuals. At the macro-level schemas also can be embodied in *materials* – tangible aspects of our culture. The schemas "in the mind" and "in the world" produce Sewell's (1992, 2005) "duality of structure" that can account for continuity as well as the dramatic, pervasive, and rapid change that are observed in aspects of family/ fertility behavior.

Introduction

The time is right for a consilient effort to understand family change and variation. Consilience, a term popularized by Wilson (1998), refers to a jumping together of knowledge across the sciences to produce a more unified explanation. It is clear that any consilient effort must incorporate the key theories/concepts that have unified the physical sciences – evolution and genetics. But key insights from the social sciences are crucial too if we are to bridge the levels of analyses from "cells to society" or "genes to globalization." As a final note on my perspective in this chapter, I am interested in major changes: the decline in fertility from high to

S.P. Morgan (✉)
Department of Sociology, Duke University, Durham, NC, USA
e-mail: pmorgan@soc.duke.edu

A. Booth et al. (eds.), *Biosocial Foundations of Family Processes*,
National Symposium on Family Issues, DOI 10.1007/978-1-4419-7361-0_12,
© Springer Science+Business Media, LLC 2011

low levels, persistently low fertility in some societies, pervasive shifts toward later ages at childbearing, increases in cohabitation and postponed or reduced marriage. These changes cannot be "effects of genes" which have not changed in the relevant time span or even effects of gene environment interactions since the changes mentioned above are remarkably pervasive within the relevant populations. But an environmental/social explanation must still be consilient with other knowledge. Evolution and genetics are thus, for me, about human predispositions and potentials (not about individual variation within the population).

Evoked Culture

I read Gangestad (Chap. 9), asking how it contributes to this consilience effort. How useful are the key ideas for thinking about family/fertility change/variation? First, Gangestad's goals are limited. Gangestad is offering concepts from anthropology and evolutionary thinking that might be part of a consilient effort. He is clear:

> Though I suspect that, in fact, much of the causes of the decline in reproduction does have much to do with novelties, responses to which are not a function of adaptations for mating and reproduction per se ..., it may nonetheless be worthwhile to entertain the possibility that notions of "evoked culture" can partly, even if not fully, explain current patterns (p. 141).

So Gangestad is not claiming to have the tiger by the tail – he claims only to have a piece of the tiger, and he is not sure of its anatomical location or how big a tiger chunk he has.

The key concept Gangestad offers for incorporation into a consilient theory of family/fertility change is *evoked culture*. This evoked culture is not a gene environment interaction; it is an environmental additive effect. Using Gangestad's metaphor, all people have the ability to develop calluses on their feet (a universal feature of humans); certain experiences (walking without shoes) produce this structure. Gangestad says this cannot be fully understood without knowing about the biological structures (which is true), but we can explain/predict precisely real world patterns of foot calluses from the environmental data alone.

How useful is this metaphor (foot calluses) or its associated, more complex concept of evoked culture? I am unsure because neither of the two examples are developed sufficiently. In one page, Gangestad discusses two examples: *the size of modern mating markets* and *female-biased operational sex ratios*. These are environmental conditions that somehow elicit identical responses across all human populations – unless the populations "wear" the fundamental equivalent of shoes. For example, Gangestad says that modern mating markets are large, and if "(h)umans (are) adapted to make mate choices in small mating markets ... (, then) ... (l)ack of effective 'stop' rules (e.g., choose this partner over others, given possibilities) ... may lead individuals to typically search for long periods of time, leading to delay of family formation and the start of reproduction."

Certainly, postponed family formation is a pervasive global phenomena and a major part of the story of low and very low fertility. But the mechanisms by which humans were "adapted to make mate choices in small mating markets" are not specified. We are also not told how these "wired" tendencies promote pervasive postponement of family formation and fertility. Examples of search "stop" rules (functional equivalents of shoes?) are not described and instances of "stop rules" in practice are not identified.

So I am unconvinced that evoked culture is very useful, and I will offer an alternative way to conceptualize the role of biological predispositions and potential. While a full explanation would include many factors, I am convinced that a consilient explanation of human family change and difference must focus on the human brain. I *am* claiming to have the "tiger by the tail"; we should be focusing on brain modularity and malleability as distinctive features of humans. Seventy-five percent of the human genome codes for brain development. We are linked to biology – to evolution and genetics – by a malleable, modular brain that permits the biological tether to be quite long. Much longer than (my current understanding) of what evoked culture implies. Brain evolution, brain development, and brain functioning are the keys to understanding broad sweeps of family change and variation.

Schemas and the Evolved Brain

A subgroup of colleagues working on an NIH project (Models of Family Change and Variation: Johnson-Hanks, Bachrach, Morgan, & Kohler, forthcoming; Morgan, 2008) is proposing a consilient theory of family change and behavior. My comments reflect our joint work but my colleagues should not be blamed for shortcomings in the current exposition.

The evolutionary success of humans is fact; our number, dispersion across environments, and power over other species are dramatic. The key junctures in our evolutionary path are less clear, although all accounts point to upright posture, opposable thumbs, and, always most importantly, the evolved human brain. Linden (2007) disputed the common characterization of the brain as "the pinnacle of biological design" (p. 5). Instead, he stresses the "inelegant design of the brain" produced by evolution; that is, understanding much of human behavior requires us to reject the notion of optimized design and to acknowledge the "quirky engineering" of evolution. To use Linden's metaphor, the human brain is really three brains – one overlaid on the next like scoops of ice cream on a cone. "Through evolutionary time, as higher functions were added, a new scoop was placed on top, but the lower scoops were left largely unchanged" (p. 21).

Traditional psychological research and the explosion of results from neuroscience indicate multiple types of information processing and locate these processes in different parts or circuits of the brain (see LeDoux, 2002; Liberman, 2007). Common to all areas are basic processes of learning, involving the creation, alteration, and pruning of synapses, and memory, or the stabilization and maintenance of such changes over time (LeDoux, 2002).

My colleagues and I have developed a very broad conception of schema that locates them both "in the mind" and "in the world." In the psychological literature, schemas are "in the mind," i.e,

A **schema** (pl. *schemata*), in psychology and cognitive science, is a mental structure that represents some aspect of the world. People use schemata to organize current knowledge and provide a framework for future understanding. Examples of schemata include rubrics, stereotypes, social roles, scripts, worldviews, and archetypes. (http://en.wikipedia.org/wiki/Schema_(psychology)).

Schemas can also become widely shared by a community of interacting individuals and in this sense they exist at the macro-level ("in the world" separate from any individual) as the elements of a language, widely known scripts, or world views. At this level, they can also be embodied in *materials* – tangible aspects of our culture. Schemas specify that good dads care for their children; courts and laws that can award child support are "materials." The schemas "in the mind" and "in the world" produce Sewell's (1992, 2005) "duality of structure."

Schema is only one concept in our meta theory, but it is a crucial one and one closely linked to fertility change and variation. Although referred to by other names and frequently underspecified, the import of schemas in explanations of fertility decline is widely accepted. Cleland and Wilson (1989, p. 30) argued that "explanations of the initial (fertility) decline must give fuller recognition to the role played by ideational forces." Mason (1997, p. 450) stated that causal models of fertility transition "need to be ideational in that they must recognize that changing perceptions ultimately drive fertility change." This emphasis can be traced to Coale's (1973, p. 65) classic preconditions for a fertility decline: (1) fertility must be "within the calculus of conscious choice," (2) people must be motivated to have fewer children, and (3) the means of fertility control must be available and acceptable. The second and third preconditions are linked to material structures (referred to above). I focus here on the first precondition. Coale (1973, p. 65) stated:

Fertility must be within the calculus of conscious choice. Potential parents must consider it an acceptable mode of thought and form of behavior to balance advantages and disadvantages before deciding to have another child....

In elaborating on this precondition, Van de Walle (1992) argued that some past societies (including many in the West) were characterized by "innumeracy in children," and that new schemas were required for people to think explicitly about child numbers in the abstract and to link family size to child and family well being. In fact, family size (i.e., seven vs. four vs. two) was not conceptualized as a family variable of great import or one under significant individual control. As a result, the number of children was left "up to God" or to chance. Van de Walle said:

Numeracy about children – that is, the perception of a particular family size as a goal in the long-term strategy of couples – may be a cultural trait present in some places and times and not in others; and that without this perception, it is unlikely that family limitation could exist.

Numeracy about children and the norm of an ideal family size appeared not long before the fertility transition. A fertility decline is not very far away when people start conceptualizing their family size, and it cannot take place without such conceptualizing. (pp. 489, 501).

As a schema, this "numeracy about children" (i.e., the linking of a particular number of children to long-term family welfare) is general and underspecified. However, additional social historical work could elaborate these schemas by specifying the cultural logic linking number of children and family welfare. Other work suggests that although people in many settings may have ignored child numbers, other aspects of reproductive practice were of great interest. For instance, Bledsoe's ethnographic work in Africa during the 1980s and 1990s described fertility-related schemas that link the timing of births and the health of the mother and the child.

In sum, brain modularity and brain malleability link what we know about evolution, genetics, and family/fertility change. Evolution did not create the human brain as a "blank slate" – there are many schemas (much neural wiring) in the brain at birth and many more that are programed to accompany aspects of development. But other schemas can be encoded in neural structures from "scratch" – the result of learning and from experience in the world. The amount of such learning in humans exceeds the amount in other species by several factors. In short, new schemas allow for rapid, dramatic, and pervasive period change – the patterns of change of interest to many demographers. The import of evolution, and genetics, here is not to explain individual variation but to identify common predispositions and potentials. The notion of "schemas in the world" (shared with others) and codified in material culture and institutions places the brain as the "meeting place" or "integration nexus" of biological and social forces.

Love, Emotion, and Family

It is interesting that scholars interested in the family can meet for days without mentioning "love." Gangestad (Chap. 9) devotes a full paragraph to love. I reproduce it here:

> Both sexes have the capacity for romantic love, a capacity that, to our knowledge, can be found across cultures (e.g., Jankowiak & Fischer, 1992; see also Fisher et al., 2005). The precise function of romantic love is not clear. One possibility is that love functions as a signal of intent to another person of commitment to a long-term interest in a relationship with the person (see Gangestad & Thornhill, 2007; for related and other views, see also Fisher, 2004; Frank, 1988). In any case, however, it does appear that romantic love functions in some way to promote the pair-bonding process and cooperative reproduction (p. 133).

This paragraph implies that, like the ability to develop calluses on our feet, we have the innate hardware to fall in love. I think this is true, but the usefulness of the calluses example and evoked couture is modest, or at least seriously undeveloped. How might the notion of schemas be used?

Let's begin with the "hardware"; love is at its base a "warm glow," or euphoria, with biological foundations. (Maybe warm glow is too subtle, as suggested by Johnny Cash's famous song, "Ring of Fire"). My thinking here relies on what we have learned from voles (see Young, 2003). In a fascinating set of studies, two species of voles are compared. Members of the first species are usually monogamous and in the second they are not. "Monogamy" is measured by separating "coupled moles" in two cages connected by tubing. Coupled moles have (1) had sex and spent 4 h together or (2) spent 8 h together. The experimental design places the mate and an alternative mate in equidistant cages that can be reached via tubing. Thus, the vole can "choose" his mate or a new partner. In repeated trials, species 1 (both males and females) show strong monogamous tendencies; species 2 does not.

Prior research suggested some candidate hormones that might help promote this pair bonding. Consistent with this hypothesis, an "antagonist" drug that neutralizes these hormones eliminates the monogamous tendencies. So perhaps species 1 releases more of these hormones in mating/cohabitation (than does species 2). Interestingly, this hypothesis receives only modest support. A stronger explanation links the pair bonding to the number/density of brain receptors for the candidate hormones. In fact, the species 1 voles have more receptors, and examination of the vole species genomes allows researchers to trace convincingly these receptor differences to one of the few genome sequences that differentiate species 1 and 2. Thus, in voles we have a template for what pair-bonding hardware might look like.

Are these "warm glows" an example of Gangestad's evoked culture? Perhaps, but what is left to be explained is the variability of love and its expression. The similarity of foot calluses across space and time seem to be a poor metaphor to capture the various manifestations of love. In our theory, the biological basis of these "warm glows" (or euphoria) can be linked through learning to schemas that interpret these feelings and provide "mental maps" of how to respond to them. For instance, in the US context "falling in love" is highly desired. So one might embrace a schema for being in love as a way to interpret or respond to "warm glows." But additional schema could compete for interpretation of these warm glows. One can be "too young" to fall in love because schooling and training have not been completed. Or one can fall in love with "the wrong person" (by ego's or other's definition) producing pressures against continuing the relationship. Further, tensions between such schema can be resolved by new ones that legitimate romantic love without the commitments that make one "too young" or lower concerns about the current partner's long-term appropriateness. The rise of cohabitation can be seen as a cultural resolution to the conflicting concerns about current intense love and relationship sustainability.

In short, humans certainly have biological predispositions and potentials that can produce "warm glows." These warm glows are the raw materials on which various cultural conceptions of romantic love can be built. These cultural conceptions are the "materials" (norms and institutions that surround love) that individuals experience in their environment. Individual behavior is influenced both by these biologically generated warm glows and socially constructed notions of "what to do with them." This type of explanation seems highly consistent with what we know and borrows heavily from a range of sciences that focus on levels of analysis from cells to societies.

References

Cleland, J., & Wilson, C. (1989). Demand theories of the fertility transition: An iconoclastic view. *Population Studies, 41*, 5–30.

Coale, A. (1973). The demographic transition reconsidered. *Proceedings of the International Union for the Scientific Study of Population Conference, 1*, 53–72.

Gangestad, S. W. (2010). Human adaptations for mating: Frameworks for understanding modern family formation and fertility? In A. Booth, S. McHale, & N. Landale (Eds.), *Biosocial foundations of family processes* (pp. 117–148). New York: Springer.

Johnson-Hanks, J., Bachrach, C., Morgan, S. P., & Kohler, H.-P. (Forthcoming) *Understanding family change and variation: Structure, conjuncture, and action*. New York: Springer.

LeDoux, J. (2002). *Synaptic self: How our brains become who we are*. New York: Penguin.

Liberman, M. D. (2007). Social cognitive neuroscience: A review of core processes. *Annual Review of Psychology, 58*, 259–289.

Linden, D. J. (2007). *The accidental mind*. Cambridge: Harvard University Press.

Mason, K. O. (1997). Explaining fertility transitions. *Demography, 34*(4), 443–454.

Morgan, S. P. (2008). *Explaining Family Change – Final Report*. http://www.soc.duke.edu/~/efc/

Sewell, W. H. (1992). A theory of structure: Duality, agency, and transformation. *American Journal of Sociology, 98*(1), 1–29.

Sewell, W. H. (2005). *Logics of history*. Chicago: University of Chicago Press.

Van de Walle, E. (1992). Fertility transition, conscious choice and numeracy. *Demography, 29*, 487–502.

Wilson, E. O. (1998). *Consilience: The unity of knowledge*. New York: Knopf.

Young, L. J. (2003). The neural basis of pair bonding in a monogamous species: A model for understanding the biological basis of human behavior. In K. W. Wachter & R. A. Bulatao (Eds.), *Offspring: Human fertility behavior in biodemographic perspective* (pp. 91–103). Washington: National Academies Press.

Part IV
Family Adaptations to Resource Disparities

Chapter 13
Family Influences on Children's Well-Being: Potential Roles of Molecular Genetics and Epigenetics

Guang Guo

Abstract We address a number of questions related to the potential roles of molecular genetics and epigenetics in estimating family effects on children's well-being. What is the nature of family effects? Where do we need genetics? What is our best evidence? What could we do at the moment and in the next 10 years? We review relevant advances in molecular genetics over the past few decades and discuss what these advances may contribute to social sciences. We focus on gene–environment interactions for delinquency. We define the concept and describe an empirical study. We also review an earlier animal gene–environment/experience study to understand the prospects of human gene–environment studies. Very soon, we may create a gigantic amount of genetic and epigenetic data, but appropriate ways of analyzing these data and proper interpretations of the findings remain enormously challenging.

Introduction

In this article, we address a number of questions related to the potential roles of molecular genetics and epigenetics in estimating family effects on children's well-being. What is the nature of family effects? Where do we need genetics? What is our best evidence? What could we do at the moment and in the next 10 years?

Family influences are considered important for a host of individual outcomes, such as binge drinking, smoking, marijuana use, delinquency, dietary patterns, mental health, education, occupation, and income. Family has long been thought a place where social/cultural and genetic influences meet, that is, some of family influences may be social/cultural and some may be biological. Family does not only transmit social/cultural influences; it also transmits genetic influences. Popular traditional approaches included fixed effects models and sibling studies. Fixed effects models could use identical twins to difference out shared effects between an

G. Guo (✉)
Department of Sociology, University of North Carolina, Chapel Hill, NC, USA
e-mail: guang_guo@unc.edu

A. Booth et al. (eds.), *Biosocial Foundations of Family Processes*,
National Symposium on Family Issues, DOI 10.1007/978-1-4419-7361-0_13,
© Springer Science+Business Media, LLC 2011

identical twin pair including shared environmental and shared genetic effects while estimating the effects of individual-level variables. Variance decomposition analysis based on identical twins and fraternal twins could be used to estimate aggregate variances due to genetic factors, shared environmental factors, and unshared environmental factors (including measure errors). Traditional approaches for separating social/cultural from genetic influences treat the genetic influences as a black box because genetics effects were not observed.

Recent Advances in Molecular Genetics

Until recently, while studying individual traits and behaviors such as cognitive development, educational achievement, occupational attainment, mental health, binge drinking, smoking, and illegal drug use, most social scientists either assume that individuals are the same at birth or treat the differences across individuals at birth as a black box. When treated as a black box, intrinsic individual differences are typically subsumed by unobserved heterogeneity. Though it is possible to exercise some control over it via statistical methods (e.g., fixed effect models), unobserved heterogeneity is considered generally impenetrable and incomprehensible.

The spectacular advances in molecular genetics over the past few decades have made it possible to begin to decipher the black box. Evidence is mounting up that substantial genetic variation exist across individuals. The year 2007 saw an unparalleled succession of discoveries in the genomics of complex traits (e.g., Frayling et al., 2007; Scott et al., 2007; Sladek et al., 2007; Steinthorsdottir et al., 2007; Zeggini et al., 2007). These studies identified genetic variants associated with acute lymphoblastic leukemia, obesity, type 2 diabetes mellitus, prostate cancer, breast cancer, and coronary heart disease.

The scientific community is experiencing such newly found confidence in genetic findings for complex human traits that the American Association for the Advancement of Science (AAAS) chose human genetic variation as *Science*'s breakthrough of the year in 2007 (Pennisi, 2007). If individuals do differ in genetic propensities for human diseases, it would be logical to predict that individuals also differ in genetic propensities for other human traits and behaviors. If individuals do have differential genetic propensities for cognitive development, educational achievement, occupational attainment, mental health, binge drinking, smoking, and illegal drug, sociologists will be compelled to reevaluate their long-standing-related assumptions and strategies.

Genetics-Informed Social Sciences

For much of the social sciences in which the emphasis is on understanding the influences of social context, these developments are challenges as well as opportunities. Social scientists are challenged to re-examine relevant areas in light of the new developments, which, on the other hand, have given rise to opportunities to enhance sociology. By whether they primarily interested geneticists/medical researchers or social scientists, the opportunities and challenges are of two types: The first type focuses on understanding the effects of genes; in this context, the focus of a gene–environment interaction could still be on effects of genes, that is, on how environmental effects moderate genetic effects. The focal point of the second is to advance social science models. It is in the context of the second type of challenges and opportunities that we propound the approach of genetics-informed social sciences.

Geneticists and medical researchers have increasingly recognized that social scientists' expertise in social context is essential for understanding many complex human diseases. The success of the Human Genome Project (Collins, Morgan, & Patrinos, 2003) and the HapMap Project[1] (The_International_HapMap_Consortium, 2005) is improving the design and effectiveness of genetic studies of complex outcomes. However, these advances do not lessen the need for understanding the social/environmental component of the puzzles. On the contrary, inadequate understanding of social environments has increasingly become a bottleneck for the rapid technological advances in molecular genetics. Recently, the HapMap project (The_International_HapMap_Consortium, 2005), the National Human Genome Research Institute (Collins et al., 2003), and the Committee on Gene-Environment Interactions for Health Outcomes at the Institute of Medicine in the National Academies of Sciences (Hernandez & Blazer, 2006) called for heavy investment in information on social/cultural exposures and in longitudinal studies of adequate size that could obtain such information.

Our theoretical concept is inspired by personalized medicine – a new major health care approach that has been accumulating evidence rapidly and that may become a major component of health care in the next 2–3 decades (Bottinger, 2007; Guttmacher & Collins, 2003; Guttmacher & Collins, 2005). Personalized medicine uses genetic tests to divide individuals into subcategories in which the individuals are similar in genetic makeup with respect to susceptibility to a disease, adverse reaction to drug dosage, and efficacy to a medical treatment. The information is then used to develop personalized strategies for disease prevention and "designer" drugs to reduce adverse reactions and increase efficacy.

So far, cancer research has produced the most evidence. The best-known genetic test for disease susceptibility on the market is a test for the *BRCA1* and *BRCA2* variants (Nelson, Huffman, Fu, & Harris 2005). The test identifies increased susceptibility for breast cancer and provides a basis for preventive measures such as earlier and more frequent mammography, prophylactic surgery, and chemoprevention.

The following example of tests for drug efficacy is also from cancer research. A substantial proportion of breast cancers (25%) are marked by overexpression of

---

[1]The International HapMap Project is a multi-country endeavor to identify and catalog genetic similarities and differences in human beings. The project is a collaboration among scientists and funding agencies from Japan, the United Kingdom, Canada, China, Nigeria, and the United States.

a cell surface protein called HER2. The overexpression of the *HER2* gene leads to more rapid tumor growth, higher risk of recurrence after surgery, and poorer response to standard chemotherapy (Ross & Fletcher, 1998). The development of the trastuzumab (Herceptin) therapy specifically targeted for tumors overexpressing the HER2 protein has greatly improved the survival rate of women with this deadly form of cancer. To determine HER2 status, molecular diagnostic tests have been developed to identify HER2-positive patients by measuring either HER2 protein levels or gene copy numbers (Dendukuri, Khetani, McIsaac, & Brophy, 2007).

Although there seems to be little doubt that the scientific foundation of personalized medicine will accrue rapidly pointing to its growing weight in heath care, many potential economic, ethical, legal, and social complications remain. For example, many may be reluctant to take beneficial genetic tests because of potential genetic discrimination in health insurance and the workplace.

Genetics-informed social sciences take advantage of the information on genetic propensity to advance the understanding of effects of social context. The primary motivation for the approach is that individuals with different genetic propensity may respond to the same social context differently. In such a case, a social theory that assumes a uniform social influence on all individuals would be unable to measure up against empirical data. Genetics-informed social sciences do not make a prediction in the direction of a social influence; it sophisticates and rarifies a social-context effect. The direction depends on a particular genotype and/or a particular social influence.

There are at least two specific ways through which genetics can advance social sciences: (1) isolating purer effects of social context from genetic confounders and (2) understanding how effects of social context are conditioned by genetic propensities through gene–environment interaction analysis.

Many effects of social context yielded by conventionally sociological models may be overestimated because of genetic confounding. For example, conventionally estimated effects of parental education on children's educational attainment may not be "purely" environmental since parents and children share 50% of genetic material. "Purer" effects of parental education can be estimated to the extent that genetic measures are included in analyses that are correlated with parental education. The current difficulty with this strategy is that many of these genetic measures are still not discovered. For this reason, gene–environment interaction analysis will likely remain the most fruitful vehicle for some time to come for social scientists whose primary interest is to understand the effects of social context.

Gene by Environment Interactions

Gene–environment interaction refers to the principle that an environment may influence how sensitive we are to the effects of a genotype and vice versa (Hunter, 2005). A classic example is that of phenylketonuria (PKU), an autosomal recessive disease that could potentially cause hopeless mental and physical degeneration. However, only individuals who have recessive mutations in the phenylalanine hydroxylase gene and who are exposed to phenylalanine in the diet are susceptible to PKU (Khoury, Adams, & Flanders, 1988). The disease or the gene expression can be effectively controlled by restricting the dietary intake of phenylalanine starting within the first month after birth.

An influential social-science example comes from recent work by Caspi and colleagues (2002). Their study found that a functional polymorphism in *MAOA* modifies the effect of maltreatment. Only maltreated children with a genotype generating low levels of *MAOA* expression tended to develop a violent behavior problem. Maltreated children with a genotype that produces high levels of *MAOA* activity were less affected.

Two recent studies using twins and siblings reported evidence for gene–environment interactions for educational performance. Guo and Stearns (2002) showed that heritability for a cognitive measure is much lower among those growing up in disadvantaged social environments than those living in "normal" environments, suggesting genetic potential's dependence on social environments. Turkheimer, Haley, Waldron, D'Onofrio, and Gottesman (2003) analyzed scores on the Wechsler Intelligence Scale in a sample of 7-year-old twins from the National Collaborative Perinatal Project. Results demonstrated that the proportions of IQ variance attributable to genes and environment vary with SES. These models suggest that in impoverished families, 60% of the variance in IQ is accounted for by the shared environment and the contribution of genes is close to zero; in affluent families, the result is almost exactly the opposite.

Environmental measures used in a gene–environment interaction study may not be purely environmental; they may be partially determined by genetic influences. In this regard, animal models are often in a position to create genuine environmental conditions by manipulation. Suomi and colleagues assigned rhesus monkeys into one of two groups at birth: mother-reared (MR) and nursery- and peer-reared (NPR). MR infants were reared in the first 6 months in a group that consists of 8–12 adult females including their mothers. NPR infants were separated from their mothers at birth and reared in a neonatal nursery. From the 37th day on, each NPR monkey was placed with three other monkeys of similar ages; no adult was included in the group. Using these experimental monkeys, a number of studies demonstrated interactions between the 5-HTTLPR polymorphism in the serotonin transporter gene (5-HTT) and rearing type. Among nursery- and peer-reared monkeys, compared with the 5-HTT*l/l genotype, the 5-HTT*l/s genotype had lower cerebrospinal fluid concentrations, an indicator of CNS function (Bennett et al., 2002); higher adrenocorticotropic hormone (ACTH) levels during a separation/stress experiment [interpreted as exaggerated limbic-hypothalamic-pituitary-adrenal (LHPA) responses to stress] (Barr et al., 2004); lower visual orientation scores assessed on days 7, 14, 21, and 30 of life (Bennett et al., 2002); and increased level of alcohol consumption among females (Barr et al., 2004).

The mechanisms of gene–environment interaction are only understood in a few isolated cases. A particularly interesting case is the interplay between maternal behavior of mother rats and the glucorticoid receptor gene for offspring's responses to stress (Meaney, Szyf, & Seckl, 2007). Mother rats are classified into low or high licking/grooming (LG) and arched back nursing (ABN). The latter is characterized by a mother rat nursing her offspring with her back arched and legs splayed outward. The offspring of low LG-ABN mothers were found grow up more fearful and abnormally sensitive to stress than offspring of high LG-ABN mothers. Cross-fostering studies, in which pups born to low LG-ABN mothers and high LG-ABN mothers were switched at birth, exclude the possibility of a direct transmission of maternal care to offspring stress responses (Francis, Diorio, Liu, & Meaney, 1999).

One mechanism for gene–environment interaction is methylation, a process in which DNA sequences are chemically modified by acquiring methyl groups to cytosine bases. DNA methylation plays an important part in the regulation of gene expression. Mounting evidence shows that the silencing of tumor suppressor genes by DNA methylation is a typical process in cancer development (Baylin et al., 2001). Methylation is a main component of epigenetics, which are chemical instructions for gene activity and which do not alter DNA sequences (Tsankova, Renthal, Kumar, & Nestler, 2007). Epigenetics promises to be the key to revealing the mechanisms of how gene expression is regulated in response to environment.

Meaney and colleagues (Weaver et al., 2004) discovered that rats' maternal behavior alters the dynamics of methylation and demethylation of the promoter in offspring's glucorticoid receptor genes. In response to stress, this receptor protein helps bring about gene expression in the brain. Methylation is only observed in the gene promoter shortly after birth (not before birth) and among offspring of low LG-ABN mothers. It is hypothesized that low LG-ABN nursing causes the methylation, which leads to lowered levels of gene expression and produces more stressful animals. These biochemical and behavioral changes are stable and tend to last for the remainder of an animal's life.

Examples of Gene–Environment Interactions

Data Source

The data source for our analysis is the DNA subsample in the National Longitudinal Study of Adolescent Health (Add Health), which started as a nationally representative sample of about 20,000 adolescents in grades 7–12 in 1994–1995 (Wave I) in the USA (Harris et al., 2003). Add Health is longitudinal; initial interviews with respondents were followed by two additional in-home interviews in 1996 (Wave II) and 2001–2002 (Wave III). Our analysis uses the sibling sample of Add Health because DNA measures collected at Wave III in 2002 are available only for this subset of the respondents. The subset consists of about 2,500 MZ twins, DZ twins, full biological siblings, and singletons. This study is based on approximately 1,100 males whose DNA and social control measures are available in Add Health.

Serious and Violent Delinquency

We constructed a serious delinquency scale and a violent delinquency scale using 12 questions asked to all the Add Health respondents at Waves I–III. The questions and scaling weights used to create the scales are given in Appendix 1. These two scales are variations of a type of scale widely used in contemporary research on delinquency and criminal behavior (Thornberry & Krohn, 2000). Our scales are closely related to the scales used by, for example, Hagan and Foster (2003) and Haynie (2001, 2003) in the analysis of Add Health data and by Hannon (2003) in the analysis of data from the 1979 National Longitudinal Study of Youth.

Following the delinquency literature (Hagan & Foster, 2003; Hannon, 2003; Haynie, 2001, 2003), we divide the 12 questions/items into the nonviolent and violent categories. Nonviolent delinquency includes stealing amounts larger or smaller than $50, breaking and entering, and selling drugs. Violent delinquency includes serious physical fighting that resulted in injuries needing medical treatment, use of weapons to get something from someone, involvement in physical fighting between groups, shooting or stabbing someone, deliberately damaging property, and pulling a knife or gun on someone. The serious delinquency scale is based on the entire 12 items and the violence scale is based on a subset (8) of the 12 items.

The Cronbach's alpha values for the serious delinquency scale for Waves I, II, and III, respectively, are 0.81, 0.79, and 0.73. Our serious delinquency scale overlaps with Hagan and Foster's (2003) delinquency scale to a substantial extent. The serious delinquency scale is designed to capture a wide range of serious delinquent behavior that could result in state sanction of arrest, conviction, and incarceration. Hagan and Foster (2003) utilized a 15-item scale that included most of the 12 items used for our scale as well as a number of items on acts more typically viewed as common adolescent deviance such as lying to parents/guardians about where they had been, minor vandalism, being loud in a public place, and driving a car without its owner's permission. As the name suggests, our violent delinquency scale focuses on an array of violent delinquent behavior that could potentially be classified as violent offenses by the criminal justice system. For Waves I, II, and III, the Cronbach's alpha values for the violent delinquency scale are 0.75, 0.74, and 0.66, respectively.

Measuring delinquency and crime is challenging. Official measures based on police reports and the prison and court system have long been known to substantially underestimate delinquency and crime (Hood & Sparks, 1970; Murphy, Shirly, & Witmer, 1946; Robison, 1936; Thornberry & Krohn, 2000) because official measures reflect not only the behavior of offenders, but also the political processes in the justice system. For these reasons, many criminologists have turned to self-reports in recent decades (Hindelang, 1981; Hindelang, Hirschi, & Weis, 1979; Thornberry & Krohn, 2000). Self-reports are now a fundamental method of measuring criminality and capable of yielding reliable and valid data (Hindelang, Hirschi, &Weiss, 2001; Hindelang, 2001; Thornberry & Krohn, 2000).

As with any survey of sensitive private information, reporting accuracy is a concern. To protect confidentiality, reduce nonresponses, and increase reporting accuracy, this section of the interview in Add Health was self-administered by audio-Computer-Assisted Self-Interview (CASI). Sensitive questions were read to respondents by means of audio headphones. Respondents were given instructions by the computer on how to complete their answers. Self-reported rates of illegal and embarrassing behavior are higher when computer-assisted techniques, particularly self-administered techniques, are used (Tourangeau & Smith, 1996; Wright, Aquilino, & Supple, 1998).

The percent of the US adult population that has ever been incarcerated in a state or federal prison increases sharply in ages 25–34 over ages 18–24 (Bonczar, 2003), pointing to a likely heavier sample attrition among more chronic offenders because of incarceration at Wave III than at Waves I–II. Add Health Wave III recorded the specific causes of why some Wave I and Wave II respondents were not interviewed at Wave III; approximately one dozen individuals from the sibling sample were not interviewed due to incarceration. Chantala, Kalsbeek, and Andraca (2004) estimated the extent of underreporting at Wave III relative to Wave I, using the respondents and the reports at Wave I and taking advantage of the observation that some of the respondents at Wave I were nonresponders at Wave III. These estimates indicate that most of the delinquent and violently delinquent activities could be underrepresented by 1–2.5% in the Wave III data relative to the Wave I population and that selling drugs, carrying a weapon, and shooting or stabbing someone could be underrepresented by about 5%. To reduce the potential impact of disproportional sample attrition at Wave III, we have removed observations of serious and violent delinquency measured at ages 24 or older.

Social Control: Structural and Demographic Variables

Table 13.1 provides the description, mean, and standard deviation for the variables used in our analysis. The declining delinquency scores from Wave I to Wave III reflect the underlying age patterns of delinquency. PVT is a slightly abridged version of the Peabody Picture Vocabulary Test (Lubin, Larsen, & Matarazzo, 1984; Rice & Brown, 1967) usually considered as a verbal IQ test. About 4% of the participants are missing on PVT. The original religiosity, measured by church attendance at all three Waves, has four categories: never, less than monthly, less than weekly, and weekly or more. Our exploratory data analysis showed that the main distinction is between "weekly or more" and the other three categories. We created a dummy variable to reflect this result.

"Household size" measuring household crowding includes all individuals living in the household at Wave I. "Parent Jobless" measures parental unemployment, which is coded as one if one or two parents were unemployed at Wave I and zero otherwise. "Education" refers to the education level of the adult interviewed at

Table 13.1 Variable description, means, and standard deviations

Variable name	Description	Mean	SD
Serious and violent delinquency			
Wave I	Serious delinquency scale, Wave I	2.43	4.32
Wave II	Serious delinquency scale, Wave II	1.65	3.45
Wave III	Serious delinquency scale, Wave III	1.18	2.35
Wave I	Violent delinquency scale, Wave I	1.68	3.13
Wave II	Violent delinquency scale, Wave II	1.05	2.36
Wave III	Violent delinquency scale, Wave III	0.69	1.62
Structural/demographic			
Age/ethnicity			
Age	Respondent's age at the time of interview at Wave I	17.6	2.89
White	Respondent's race reported as White at Wave I	0.603	0.48
Black	Respondent's race reported as Black at Wave I	0.167	0.372
Hispanic	Respondent's race reported as Hispanic at Wave I	0.149	0.357
Asian	Respondent's race reported as Asian at Wave I	0.081	0.271
Cognitive development			
PVT < 90	Verbal IQ less than 90 at Wave I	0.247	0.431
PVT 90–110	Verbal IQ between 90 and 110 at Wave I	0.484	0.499
PVT > 110	Verbal IQ greater than 110 at Wave I	0.269	0.444
PVT missing	Missing on IQ score at Wave I	0.044	0.205
Religiosity			
Weekly or more, WI	Respondent attends church weekly or more at Wave I	0.352	0.478
Weekly or more, WII	Respondent attends church weekly or more at Wave II	0.475	0.499
Weekly or more, WIII	Respondent attends church weekly or more at Wave III	0.173	0.378
Family SES			
Household size	Number of individuals living in household Wave I	5.02	1.48
Parent jobless	Parent unemployed at Wave I	0.053	0.224
Jobless missing	Parent missing response on employment at Wave I	0.127	0.330
Less than high school	Parent interviewed has less than high school education	0.238	0.426
High school	Parent interviewed has high school education only Wave I	0.272	0.456
Greater than high school	Parent interviewed has education beyond high school	0.490	0.499
Contextual traits			
Proportion black	Proportion black in Census Tract at 1990 Census	0.128	0.245
Family process			
Daily family meals	Eating meals with parent 6 days per week at Wave I	0.479	0.50
Social services	Having been taken out of home by social services by sixth grade	0.013	0.11
Two biological parents	Living with both parents at Wave I	0.640	0.480
Parental attachment	Emotional attachment to resident parent, Wave I	4.48	0.74

(continued)

Table 13.1 (continued)

Variable name	Description	Mean	SD
Dad jailed	Biological parent having served time in jail, Wave III	0.14	0.35
School process			
Repeated a grade	Having repeated grade by Wave I	0.257	0.437
School attachment	Emotional attachment to school at Wave I	2.21	0.83
Peer problems	Problems of getting along with other students, Wave I	0.076	0.26
Truancy in last year	Having 5 or more unexcused absences from school, Wave I	0.097	0.30
Being expelled	Having been expelled from school by Wave I	0.031	0.174
Social networks Wave I			
Friends delinquency	Friends' delinquent behavior at Wave I	5.96	3.75
Centrality	Respondent's centrality in friends social network	0.81	0.67
Density	Respondent's density in friends social network	0.28	0.14
Popularity	Respondent's popularity in friends social network	4.84	4.00
Genotype			
9R/9R	Proportion of 9R/9R genotype in DAT1	0.053	0.223
10R/9R	Proportion of 10R/9R genotype in DAT1	0.348	0.476
10R/10R	Proportion of 10R/10R genotype in DAT1	0.599	0.490
178/304	Proportion of A1/A2 genotype in DRD2	0.372	0.497
178/178	Proportion of A2/A2 genotype in DRD2	0.549	0.483
304/304	Proportion of A1/A21 genotype in DRD2	0.079	0.271
2R	Proportion of 2R/other genotype in MAOA	0.008	0.089

Note: $N = 1,111$ persons; 3,071 person-observations; fewer when some family, school, and social network variables are considered

home at Wave I with categories of less than high school graduation, high school graduation, and at least some college education. We have also considered a number of contextual characteristics and, in our final analysis, focused on percent of African Americans in the census tract.

Social Control: Family Process Variables

"Two biological parents" is based on a family structure variable in Add Health that has categories of two-biological-parent, single-parent, step-parent, and other families including children from adopted families and foster homes (Harris, Duncan, & Boisjoly, 2002). A dummy variable was created for two-biological-parent families versus all others. "Daily family meals" is based on the Add Health Wave I question: On how many of the past 7 days was at least one of your parents in the room with you while you ate your evening meal? The answer was coded as a dummy variable with six or seven as one and fewer than six as zero. Wave I parental attachment is an average of two variables constructed from:

(1) "How close do you feel toward your resident mother or resident father," and
(2) "How much do your parents care about you?" Both range from 1 to 5. "Dad
jailed" coded 0 or 1 is constructed from the Wave III question of "Has your
biological father ever served time in jail or prison?" "Social services," also from
Wave III, is coded as 1 if the respondent reported having been taken out of home
by social services before the sixth grade.

Social Control: School Process Variables

"Repeating a grade" is coded as 1 if the respondent had repeated a grade by Wave I;
about 25% of Add Health respondents had repeated a grade by Wave I. "School
Attachment" (Haynie, 2001) is an average of the responses (each ranging 1–5) to
the three Wave I questions of whether in the last year the respondent felt close to
people at school, felt like being part of school, and was happy to be at school. "Peer
problems" is based on Wave I self-report of daily problems with getting along with
peers at school; the variable is coded as one if the answer is "almost everyday" or
"everyday" and zero otherwise. "Truancy" is a measure of skipping school for a full
day without an excuse last year; it is coded as one if the number of unexcused
absences is five or more.

Social Control: Friend Social Network Variables

These variables include centrality, density, popularity, and friend delinquency
(Haynie, 2001). Our centrality measure, developed by Bonacich (1987), attempts to
gage an adolescent's position within his or her friend network. It is a measure of the
number of links required to connect all other adolescents in an ego's friendship
network; the lower the number of links required, the more central the adolescent.
The measure is weighted by the centrality of those the ego nominates as friends.
This measure of centrality thus takes into consideration not only the ego's position,
but also ego's friends' social positions.

   The most dense possible network is one in which every member has ties to
every other member. Our density is measured by the observed number of ties
divided by the number of possible ties in the adolescent's friendship network
standardized by the maximum number of friends the ego can nominate. The ties
include both "send" and "receive" nominations. An average value of density of
0.28 indicates that 72% of the potential pair-wise ties in an adolescent's social
network are not nominated.

   Popularity is measured by the number of receive nominations or the number of
times the respondent is nominated by other students in school. On average, each
adolescent was nominated as a friend 4.84 times.

Friend delinquency is measured by the average number of self-reported minor delinquency items over the past 12 months per send-and-receive-friend nomination. The minor delinquency items include "smoked cigarettes," "drank alcohol," "got drunk," "skipped school without an excuse," "did dangerous things on a dare," and "raced vehicles such as cars or motorcycles." The measure is based on responses obtained directly from the friends themselves at the Add Health Wave I school interview. Almost all studies on peer influences use data based on ego's perceptions of a friend's behavior instead of the actual behavior of a friend. Perceptions of friends' behavior have been considered unreliable because the reporters tend to project their own behavior onto others (Bauman & Ennett, 1996). The perception bias can be corrected only with data that allow the measures of friends to be taken directly.

Compared with the delinquency items which were obtained from the in-home surveys at Waves I–III and used for the construction of our dependent variables, these friend delinquency items are fewer and more minor; but these are the only delinquency items available from the friends themselves. Friend delinquency has a mean value of 5.96, indicating that friends committed an average six minor delinquent activities over the past 12 months.

Genetic Variants

At Wave III, in collaboration with the Institute for Behavioral Genetics in Boulder, Colorado, Add Health collected, extracted, and quantified DNA samples from the sibling subsample. This chapter reports findings from three genetic polymorphisms in three genes: a 40-bp variable number tandem repeat (VNTR) polymorphism in the 3' region of the *DAT1* gene; a polymorphic TaqIA restriction endonuclease site about 2,500 bp downstream from the coding region of the *DRD2* gene; and the 30-bp VNTR in the promoter region of the *MAOA* gene. The additional details on these genetic polymorphisms are found in Appendix 2 and at the Add Health website.

Findings on Gene–Environment Interaction Effects

Table 13.2 presents models that investigate the GE interaction between *MAOA* and "grade retention" and the interaction between *DRD2* and "having daily family meals." All the interaction terms are statistically significant. The *P*-values for the two *MAOA* interaction terms are 0.0005 (serious delinquency) and 0.0001 (violent delinquency), respectively. The *P*-values for the two *DRD2* interaction terms are 0.023 and 0.0069, respectively. The likelihood ratio test of the model of serious delinquency *with* two interaction terms (two combined model) against the model (data not shown here) *without* the two interaction terms produced a χ^2 of 15.6 with 2 df and a

Table 13.2 Coefficients (standard errors) of random-effects models of serious and violent delinquency among male adolescents and young adults: interactions between genetic propensities and social controls (Add Health Waves I–III)

	MAOA		DRD2		Two combined	
Models	Serious delinquency	Violent delinquency	Serious delinquency	Violent delinquency	Serious delinquency	Violent delinquency
Intercept	-2.366 (2.207)	-0.639 (1.56)	-2.476 (2.209)	-0.738 (1.562)	-2.622 (2.206)	-0.867 (1.561)
Age	0.639 (0.242)**	0.318 (0.172)+	0.629 (0.242)**	0.310 (0.172)+	0.639 (0.242)**	0.319 (0.172)*
Age²	-0.022 (0.007)***	-0.012 (0.005)**	-0.022 (0.007)***	-0.012 (0.005)**	-0.022 (0.007)***	-0.012 (0.005)**
White						
Black	-0.068 (0.324)	-0.076 (0.225)	0.048 (0.325)	-0.057 (0.226)	-0.10 (0.323)	-0.104 (0.225)
Hispanic	0.548 (0.255)*	0.331 (0.178)+	0.509 (0.256)*	0.301 (0.18)+	0.531 (0.254)*	0.318 (0.178)+
Asian	0.521 (0.311)	0.267 (0.216)	0.487 (0.316)	0.235 (0.22)	0.474 (0.311)	0.224 (0.216)
School attachment						
Repeated grade	0.299 (0.190)	0.309 (0.132)*	0.306 (0.191)	0.316 (0.134)*	0.268 (0.189)	0.284 (0.133)*
PVT < 90	0.022 (0.253)	0.2 (0.178)	0.040 (0.256)	0.215 (0.179)	0.025 (0.253)	0.200 (0.177)
PVT 90–110	0.215 (0.191)	0.211 (0.134)	0.18 (0.193)	0.181 (0.136)	0.185 (0.191)	0.185 (0.134)
PVT > 110						
PVT missing	-0.358 (0.415)	-0.356 (0.292)	-0.411 (0.418)	-0.401 (0.294)	-0.370 (0.415)	-0.370 (0.291)
Religiosity						
Weekly or more	-0.761 (0.143)***	-0.462 (0.101)***	-0.779 (0.14)***	-0.477 (0.099)***	-0.772 (0.143)***	-0.471 (0.099)***
Family SES						
Two biological parents	-0.160 (0.181)	-0.078 (0.126)	-0.155 (0.183)	-0.073 (0.128)	-0.138 (0.181)	-0.059 (0.127)
Others						
Household size	0.030 (0.056)	0.027 (0.039)	0.027 (0.056)	0.025 (0.04)	0.038 (0.056)	0.033 (0.039)
Parent jobless	0.791 (0.376)*	0.355 (0.263)	0.826 (0.379)*	0.381 (0.267)	0.833 (0.376)*	0.392 (0.264)
Jobless missing	0.231 (0.322)	0.163 (0.223)	0.132 (0.322)	0.083 (0.227)	0.203 (0.320)	0.138 (0.223)
Less than high school	-0.358 (0.284)	-0.303 (0.198)	-0.280 (0.287)	-0.244 (0.201)	-0.357 (0.285)	-0.302 (0.199)
High school						
Greater than high school	0.099 (0.198)	-0.058 (0.138)	0.107 (0.201)	-0.051 (0.14)	0.090 (0.199)	-0.065 (0.138)
Daily family meals	-0.464 (0.157)***	-0.276 (0.11)**	-0.198 (0.196)	-0.067 (0.138)	-0.191 (0.194)	-0.065 (0.136)
Contextual traits						

(continued)

Table 13.2 (continued)

Models	MAOA Serious delinquency	MAOA Violent delinquency	DRD2 Serious delinquency	DRD2 Violent delinquency	Two combined Serious delinquency	Two combined Violent delinquency
Proportion black	0.708 (0.468)	0.594 (0.327)+	0.708 (0.471)	0.581 (0.332)+	0.663 (0.468)	0.553 (0.326)+
Genotype						
178/304			0.692 (0.219)**	0.602 (0.155)***	0.664 (0.219)**	0.577 (0.153)***
178/178 or 304/304						
2R	-0.213 (1.036)	-0.137 (0.739)			-0.19 (1.032)	-0.118 (0.734)
No 2R						
GxE interaction						
Repeated grade*2R	6.44 (1.84)***	5.479 (1.32)***			6.27 (1.834)***	5.323 (1.312)***
Daily meals*178/304			-0.719 (0.317)*	-0.605 (0.222)**	-0.693 (0.313)*	-0.581 (0.219)**
Random effects omitted						
LR test: two interact terms					$P = 0.0003$	$P < 0.0001$
-2Log L	15,990.5	13,865.9	15,996.9	13,873.9	15,981.2	13,851.6
Number of persons	1,111	1,111	1,111	1,111	1,111	1,111
Number of measures	3,071	3,071	3,071	3,071	3,071	3,071

+Significant at 0.10; *0.05; **0.01; ***0.001 for a two-tailed test

P-value of 0.0003. The parallel model of violent delinquency produced a χ^2 of 23.6 with 2 df and a *P*-value <0.0001.

These GE interaction findings indicate that certain genotype effects and the effects of social control are mutually dependent. For example, in the *MAOA* model of serious delinquency, the effect of repeating a grade depends on whether one has a 2-repeat in *MAOA*. Without a 2-repeat, repeating a grade only raises the serious delinquency score by 0.30; with a 2-repeat allele, repeating a grade raises the score by a large value of 6.44. The above-described interaction term is interpreted as an effect of grade retention that depends on a genotype. An interaction term can also be interpreted as a genotype effect that hinges on the level of social control. For example, in the *DRD2* model of serious delinquency, for those who do not have regular meals with parent(s), having the 178/304 genotype raises the delinquency score by 0.70 points. However, for those having daily meals with parent(s), the negative effect of 178/304 is completely suppressed (0.70–0.72 ≈ 0).

The estimates in the last two models in Table 13.2 that consider two interaction terms jointly are very similar to those models that consider one interaction term at a time. The parameter estimates in the joint model are slightly smaller and the *P*-values are slightly larger than those in the single-term models, suggesting the absence of major correlations among the two genetic polymorphisms.

Figures 13.1–13.4 illustrate the gene–environment interaction effects between the DRD2*178/304 genotype and having a regular meal with parents (Fig. 13.1), between the MAOA*2R genotype and having repeated a grade (Fig. 13.2), between the DRD2*178/*304 genotype and the presence of two biological parents (Fig. 13.3), and between the DRD2*178/304 genotype and friends' delinquent behavior (Fig. 13.4).

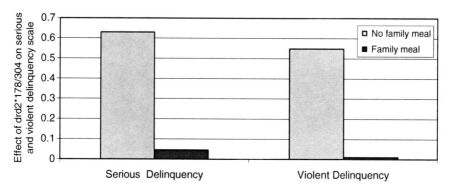

Fig. 13.1 The effect of DRD2 178/304 genotype depends on whether having regular meals with parents

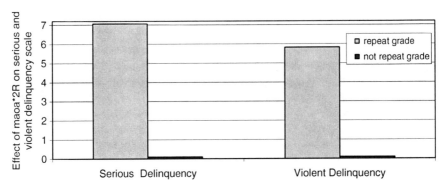

Fig. 13.2 The effect of MAOA*2R genotype depends on whether having repeated a grade

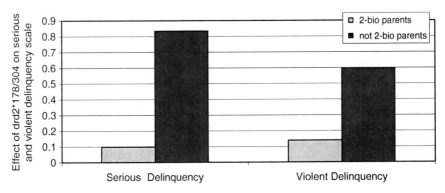

Fig. 13.3 The effect of DRD2 178/304 genotype depends on whether both biological parents are present

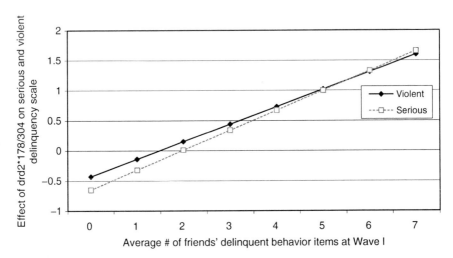

Fig. 13.4 The effect of DRD2 178/304 genotype depends on friends' delinquent behavior

Discussion and Conclusion

We begin our more general assessment of the prospect of gene–environment research by examining the findings from a 1942 study on aggression which used highly inbred strains of mice (Ginsburg & Allee, 1942). Contrasting these earlier findings with the current molecular results may enable us to better illustrate some of the difficulties facing gene–environment studies.

Before the DNA era, genetic influences could be estimated from highly inbred strains of mice – mice that had been inbred for more than ten generations of brother–sister mating. As a result, each stock of animals was nearly pure breeding. These animals were characterized by small genetic differences within a stock and by large genetic differences between stocks. Different levels and patterns of aggressive behavior across stocks were attributed to genetic influences.

When assisted by researchers, mice of a pacific strain could be rendered aggressive through winning fights. Similarly, mice of an aggressive strain could be rendered pacific by experiencing defeats. Although social hierarchy was largely determined by fighting, the hierarchy was not fixed. Assistance by researchers could move animals upward or downward. However, it was far easier to move a high-status mouse downward by engineered defeats than move a low-status mouse upward. Mice lowest in social scale showed extreme subordination. Mice with middle positions were more easily moved in either direction.

These findings were essentially gene-experience or gene–environment interactions in contemporary terminology. These findings indicate that genetic influences were not deterministic and that there should be a plenty of gene–environment interactive effects on behaviors such as aggression at least for mice. However, abundant estimates of gene–environment interactive effects from animal experiments do not necessarily suggest similar gene–environment interaction effects could be estimated from observational human studies. We discuss another major complicating factor for gene–environment interaction research before attempting to link the mice findings to current gene–environment interaction efforts.

Large-scale gene–environment studies are possible today because SNP genotyping technology has improved dramatically in the past several years (Kwok & Chen, 2003). Technology has been developed that allows many (>1,000) SNPs to be genotyped in the same reaction or multiplexed (Fan et al., 2003; Hardenbol et al., 2003). As a result, genotype costs have been reduced more than 50-fold from $1–2/genotype down to about $0.01–0.05/genotype. This increased throughput has been coupled with improved genotype accuracy and completion rates. For example, the Infinium technology available from Illumina is highly cost-effective for large-scale genotyping and its genotypes are highly accurate (>99.9%) and successful (>99.8%) (Gunderson et al., 2005; Steemers et al., 2006). Many studies published over the past few years have genotyped 300,000–1,000,000 genetic markers for each individual. Even though social sciences will directly benefit from these technological developments; for social scientists who routinely work with 10, 20, or even 30 independent variables, the sheer numbers of genetic markers present a huge methodological challenge. So far, GWAS has focused on estimating genetic main effects, which is typically done by including one SNP in a regression at a time. The resulting multiple testing for the initial analysis was addressed by setting P at an extremely low value of 5×10^{-8}.

There are two major difficulties facing gene–environment interaction analysis in the era of genome-wide association studies: (1) the issue of multiple testing for gene–environment interaction analysis is many times more daunting than main effect analysis and (2) observational data tend not to have a lot of statistical power for estimating gene–environmental effects.

In a genome-wide association study with one million SNPs, an investigation of gene–environment interaction effects could easily involve another several millions of tests. Does this mean the P-values need to be dramatically reduced further? This difficulty is likely why no serious attempt has been made in GWAS in estimating gene–environment interaction effects. While the 1942 mice study showed abundant gene–environment interaction effects, it may not bode well for gene–environment interaction analysis with observational data. The mice study has a much better control for genetic background and for environmental influences. The researchers in the mice experiment could implement one factor and only one factor at a time. In contrast, the phenotypes captured in human observational studies are results of a large number of factors in real life. Even if we could identify factors we are interested in studying, individuals who are subject to those factors and other potential confounders are likely to be quite small.

Thus, although the general consensus is that gene–environment interactions are part of the links between genetic heritage and complex human traits – especially human behaviors – the work that takes into account multiple genes, epigenetic markers, environmental factors, and the interactions among these sources remains enormously complicated.

Many authors have raised the issue of gene–environment correlation. In the delinquency example, "having regular meals with parents" may be correlated with genetic influences, that is, those whose parents did not have regular meals with the adolescent might be genetically somewhat different. Another issue is that "having regular meals with parents" may not be the causing environmental variable. It may be merely correlated with the unknown causal variable(s). Gene–environment correlation is not a new problem; it is essentially a long-standing difficulty facing social scientists because genetic effects are generally not observed.

By estimating genetic effects or illuminating genetic sources of some family effects, we are in a sense creating another black box, that is, the biochemical mechanisms behind the statistical correlation between genetic variation and outcome variables are not understood. Epigenetics could be one way to decipher the black box. There are other efforts to illuminate the underlying physiological processes that might be altered in the course of development, but the progress is understandably slow.

When we consider the question of family disparities, and the question of whether existing data and methods can and cannot tell us about the "haves" versus the "have nots" and why the divide may be getting larger, we must remember the long-standing sensitivity about genetic determinism and about social Darwinist implications of study of genes. Biological factors have historically been used to impugn disadvantaged classes in order to justify the unjust systems. Genetically or scientifically, genetic effects on poverty are much harder to verify. Animal models could be more easily created for outcomes such as type II diabetes, binge drinking, and even aggressive behavior, but for many social-science cherished outcomes such as poverty, social status, and wealth, anything beyond a statistical link is much harder to come by.

Given the dramatic advances in molecular genetics over the past 20–30 years, most social scientists may be willing to consider genetic and other biological factors as potential influences on health behaviors and other outcomes. However, as we discussed, we may be able to create a gigantic amount of genetic and epigenetic data, but appropriate ways of analyzing these data and proper interpretations of the findings remain enormously challenging.

Acknowledgments This research uses data from Add Health, a program project designed by J. Richard Udry, Peter S. Bearman, and Kathleen Mullan Harris, and funded by a grant P01-HD31921 from the National Institute of Child Health and Human Development, with cooperative funding from 17 other agencies (www.cpc.unc.edu/addhealth/contract.html). Special acknowledgment is due to Andrew Smolen and John K. Hewitt of the Institute for Behavior Genetics, University of Colorado, for DNA isolation and genotyping. We gratefully acknowledge support from NIH P01-HD31921 to Add Health; R03 HD042490-02 to G.G.; R03 HD053385-01 to G.G.; and support from NSF, SES-0210389 to G.G.

Appendix 1: The Serious Delinquency Scale and the Violent Delinquency Scale

1. In the past 12 months, how often did you hurt someone badly enough to need bandages or care from a doctor or nurse? (see Note 1)
2. In the past 12 months, how often did someone hurt you badly enough to need bandages or care from a doctor or nurse? (see Note 1)
3. In the past 12 months, how often did you use or threaten to use a weapon to get something from someone? (see Note 1)
4. In the past 12 months, how often did you take part in a fight where a group of your friends was against another group? (see Note 1)
5. In the last 12 months, how often did you deliberately damage property that did not belong to you? (see Note 1)
6. In the past 12 months how often did you carry a handgun to school or work? (see Note 1)
7. In the past 12 months, how often did you steal something worth more than $50? (see Note 1)
8. In the past 12 months, how often did you steal something worth less than $50? (see Note 1)
9. In the past 12 months, how often did you go into a house or building to steal something? (see Note 1)

10. In the past 12 months, how often did you sell marijuana or other drugs? (see Note 1)
11. In the past 12 months, have you shot or stabbed someone? (see Note 2)
12. In the past 12 months, have you pulled a knife or gun on someone? (see Note 2)

Notes

1. For this question, the score value on the scale is determined in the following manner: The score is coded as zero if the event did not occur in the past 12 months; the score is coded as one if the event occurred once or twice in the past 12 months; the score is coded as two if the event occurred three or four times in the past 12 months; the score is coded as three if the event occurred five or more times in the past 12 months.
2. For this question, the score value on the scale is determined in the following manner: the score is coded as zero if the event did not occur in the past 12 months; the score is coded as three if the event did occur once or more during the past 12 months.

Appendix 2: Measures of Genetic Polymorphisms

Genomic DNA was isolated from buccal cells using a modification of published methods (Freeman, Powell, Ball, Hill, Craig, & Plomin, 1997; Lench, Stanier, & Williamson, 1988; Meulenbelt, Droog, Trommelen, Boomsma, & Slagboom, 1995; Spitz et al., 1996). All the methods employed Applied Biosystems instruments and reagents. Microsatellite and VNTR polymorphisms were done using fluorescent primers that were analyzed on an ABI capillary electrophoresis instrument. Single nucleotide polymorphisms were analyzed using an ABI Sequence Detection System and 5'-nuclease (Taqman®) methodology. To reduce errors, two individuals independently scored all genotyping. The additional details on DNA collection and genotyping can be found at Add Health website (Smolen and Hewitt, http://www. cpc.unc.edu/projects/addhealth/).

A 40 bp variable number tandem repeat (VNTR) polymorphism in the 3'-untranslated region of the *DAT1* gene has been genotyped with a modified method of Vandenbergh et al. (1992). The primer sequences were: forward, 5'-TGTGGTGTAGGGAACGGCCTGAG-3' (fluorescently labeled) and reverse: 5'-CTTCCTGGAGGTCACGGCTCAAGG-3'. This VNTR ranges from 3 to 11 copies with the 9-repeat (9R or 440 bp) and 10-repeat (10R or 480 bp) polymorphisms being the two most common alleles in Caucasian, Hispanic, and African American populations (Doucettestamm, Blakely, Tian, Mockus, & Mao 1995). In our male analysis sample, the 9R and 10R account for about 21 and 76% of all alleles, respectively; 34.8, 59.9, and 0.053% of the respondents possess one 10R, two 10Rs, and two 9Rs, respectively. The variation across ethnic groups appears to be moderate with the 10R allele accounts for 80, 86, 80, and 90% of all alleles in Whites, Blacks, Hispanics, Asians, respectively.

The *DRD2* gene has a polymorphic *Taq*IA restriction endonuclease site about 2,500 bp downstream (3'-untranslated region) from the coding region of the gene. The A1 allele of this polymorphism has a point mutation C T (TCGA to TTGA). The *DRD2* TaqIA genotyping was performed using the fluorogenic 5' nuclease (Taqman®, Applied Biosystems, Foster City, CA) method with reagents (VIC™ and 48 FAM™ labeled probes and TaqMan® Universal PCR Master Mix without AMPerase® UNG) obtained from Applied Biosystems (ABI) (Haberstick and Smolen 2004). In our male sample, the proportions of *DRD2**A1/A2, A2/A2, and A1/A1 are 37, 55, and 8%, respectively.

The *MAOA*-uVNTR polymorphism was assayed by a modified method (Haberstick et al., 2005; Sabol, Hu, & Hamer 1998). The primer sequences for the 30 bp VNTR in the promoter region of the *MAOA* open reading frame were: forward, 5'-ACAGCCTGACCG-TGGAGAAG-3' (fluorescently labeled) and reverse, 5'-GAACGTGACGCTCCATTCGGA-3' (Sabol, Hu, & Hamer 1998). The reaction yielded five fragment sizes that included 291, 321, 336, 351, and 381 bps (2, 3, 3.5, 4, and 5 repeats, respectively). The focus allele in *MAOA* in this study is the rare 2R. A series of χ^2 tests for each polymorphism and for each self-reported ethnic group (European, African American, Hispanic, and Asian) reveals no deviation from the Hardy–Weinberg equilibrium[2].

Doucette-Stamm, L.A., Blakely, D.J., Tian, J., Mockus, S., & Mao, J.I.(1995). Population genetic-study of the human dopamine transporter gene (DAT1). *Genetic Epidemiology, 12*, 303–308.

Freeman, B, Powell, J., Ball, D., Hill, L., Craig, I., & Plomin, R. (1997). DNA by mail: An inexpensive and noninvasive method for collecting DNA samples from widely dispersed populations. *Behavior Genetics, 27*, 251–257.

Haberstick, B.C., Lessem, J.M., Hopfer, C.J., Smolen, A., Ehringer, M.A., Timberlake, D., & Hewitt, J.K. (2005). Monoamine oxidase A (MAOA) and antisocial behaviors in the presence of childhood and adolescent maltreatment. *American Journal of Medical Genetics Part B-Neuropsychiatric Genetics, 135B*, 59–64.

Haberstick, B.C., & Smolen, A. (2004). Genotyping of three single nucleotide polymorphisms following whole genome preamplification of DNA collected from buccal cells. *Behavior Genetics, 34*, 541–547.

Lench, N., Stanier, P., & Williamson, R. (1988). Simple non-invasive method to obtain DNA for gene analysis. *Lancet, 1*, 1356–1358.

Meulenbelt, I., Droog, S., Trommelen, G.J., Boomsma, D.I., & Slagboom, P.E. (1995). High-yield noninvasive human genomic DNA isolation method for genetic studies in geographically dispersed families and populations. *American Journal of Human Genetics, 57*, 1252–1254.

---

[2]The population is said to be in Hardy-Weinberg equilibrium (HWE) if the genotype frequencies are equal to the product of the allele frequencies, which indicates the absence of disturbing forces such as selection, mutation, or migration and the presence of random mating in a population.

Sabol, S.Z., Hu, S., & Hamer, D. (1998). A functional polymorphism in the monoamine oxidase A gene promoter. *Human Genetics, 103,* 273–279.

Spitz, E., Moutier, R., Reed, T., Busnel, M.C., Marchaland, C., Roubertoux, P.L., & Carlier, M. 1996. Comparative diagnoses of twin zygosity by SSLP variant analysis, questionnaire, and dermatoglyphic analysis." *Behavior Genetics, 26,* 55–63.

References

Barr, C. S., Newman, T. K., Lindell, S., Shannon, C., Champoux, M., Lesch, K. P., Suomi, S. J., Goldman, D., & Higley, J. D. (2004). Interaction between serotonin transporter gene variation and rearing condition in alcohol preference and consumption in female primates. *Archives of General Psychiatry, 61,* 1146–1152.

Barr, C. S., Newman, T. K., Shannon, C., Parker, C., Dvoskin, R. L., Becker, M. L., Schwandt, M., Champoux, M., Lesch, K. P., Goldman, D., Suomi, S. J., & Higley, J. D. (2004). Rearing condition and rh5–HTTLPR interact to influence limbic-hypothalamic-pituitary-adrenal axis response to stress in infant macaques. *Biological Psychiatry, 55,* 733–738.

Bauman, K. E., & Ennett, S. T. (1996). On the importance of peer influence for adolescent drug use: Commonly neglected considerations. *Addiction, 91,* 185–198.

Baylin, S. B., Esteller, M., Rountree, M. R., Bachman, K. E., Schuebel, K., & Herman, J. G. (2001). Aberrant patterns of DNA methylation, chromatin formation and gene expression in cancer. *Human Molecular Genetics, 10,* 687–692.

Bennett, A. J., Lesch, K. P., Heils, A., Long, J. C., Lorenz, J. G., Shoaf, S. E., Champoux, M., Suomi, S. J., Linnoila, M. V., & Higley, J. D. (2002). Early experience and serotonin transporter gene variation interact to influence primate CNS function. *Molecular Psychiatry, 7,* 118–122.

Bonacich, P. (1987). Power and centrality: A family of measures. *American Journal of Sociology, 92,* 1170–1182.

Bonczar, T. P. (2003). *Prevalence of imprisonment in the U.S. population, 1974–2001.* Washington, DC: Bureau of Justice Statistics.

Bottinger, E. P. (2007). Foundations, promises and uncertainties of personalized medicine. *Mount Sinai Journal of Medicine, 74,* 15–21.

Caspi, A., McClay, J., Moffitt, T. E., Mill, J., Martin, J., Craig, I. W., Taylor, A., & Poulton, R. (2002). Role of genotype in the cycle of violence in maltreated children. *Science, 297,* 851–854.

Chantala, K., Kalsbeek, W. D., & Andraca, E. (2004). *Non-response in wave III of the Add Health study.* Report on bias in Wave III sampling in the National Longitudinal Survey of Adolescent Health. Available online at: http://www.cpc.unc.edu/projects/addhealth/pubs/guides.

Collins, F. S., Morgan, M., & Patrinos, A. (2003). The human genome project: Lessons from large-scale biology. *Science, 300,* 286–290.

Dendukuri, N., Khetani, K., McIsaac, M., & Brophy, J. (2007). Testing for HER2-positive breast cancer: A systematic review and cost-effectiveness analysis. *Canadian Medical Association Journal, 176,* 1429–1434.

Fan, J. B., Oliphant, A., Shen, R., Kermani, B. G., Garcia, F., Gunderson, K. L., et al. (2003). Highly parallel SNP genotyping. *Cold Spring Harbor Symposia on Quantitative Biology, 68,* 69–78.

Francis, D., Diorio, J., Liu, D., & Meaney, M. J. (1999). Nongenomic transmission across generations of maternal behavior and stress responses in the rat. *Science, 286,* 1155–1158.

Frayling, T. M., Timpson, N. J., Weedon, M. N., Zeggini, E., Freathy, R. M., Lindgren, C. M., et al. (2007). A common variant in the FTO gene is associated with body mass index and predisposes to childhood and adult obesity. *Science, 316,* 889–894.

Ginsburg, B. E., & Allee, W. C. (1942). Some effects of conditioning on social dominance and subordination in inbred strains of mice. *Physiology and Zoology, 15.*

Gunderson, K. L., Stemmers, F. J., Lee, G., Mendoza, L. G., & Chee, M. S. (2005). A genome-wide scalable SNP genotyping assay using microarray technology. *Nature Genetics, 37*, 549–554.

Guo, G., & Stearns, E. (2002). The social influences on the realization of genetic potential for intellectual development. *Social Forces, 80*, 881–910.

Guttmacher, A. E., & Collins, F. S. (2003). Welcome to the genomic era. *New England Journal of Medicine, 349*, 996–998.

Guttmacher, A. E., & Collins, F. S. (2005). Realizing the promise of genomics in biomedical research. *Journal of the American Medical Association, 294*, 1399–1402.

Hagan, J., & Foster, H. (2003). S/He's a rebel: Toward a sequential stress theory of delinquency and gendered pathways to disadvantage in emerging adulthood. *Social Forces, 82*, 53–86.

Hannon, L. (2003). Poverty, delinquency, and educational attainment: Cumulative disadvantage or disadvantage saturation? *Sociological Inquiry, 73*, 575–594.

Hardenbol, P., Baner, J., Jani, M., Nilsson, M., Namsaraev, E. A., Karlin-Neumann, G. A., et al. (2003). Multiplexed genotyping with sequence-tagged molecular inversion probes. *Nature Biotechnology, 21*, 673–678.

Harris, K. M., Duncan, G. J., & Boisjoly, J. (2002). Evaluating the role of nothing to lose attitudes on risky behavior in adolescence. *Social Forces, 80*, 1005–1039.

Harris, K. M., Florey, F., Tabor, J., Bearman, P. S., Jones, J., & Udry, J. R. (2003). The National Longitudinal Study of Adolescent Health: Research design. Available online at: http://www.cpc.unc.edu/projects/addhealth/design. vol. 2005.

Haynie, D. L. (2001). Delinquent peers revisited: Does network structure matter? *American Journal of Sociology, 106*, 1013–1057.

Haynie, D. L. (2003). Contexts of risk? Explaining the link between girls' pubertal development and their delinquency involvement. *Social Forces, 82*, 355–397.

Hernandez, L. M., & Blazer, D. G. (2006). *Genes, behavior, and the social environment: Moving beyond the nature/nurture debate*. Washington, DC: National Academies Press.

Hindelang, M. J., Hirschi, T., & Weiss, J. G. (2001). *Measuring delinquency*. Thousand Oaks, CA: Sage.

Hindelang, M. J. (1981). Variations in sex-race-age-specific incidence rates of offending. *American Sociological Review, 46*, 461–474.

Hindelang, M. J., Hirschi, T., & Weis, J. G. (1979). Correlates of delinquency—Illusion of discrepancy between self-report and official measures. *American Sociological Review, 44*, 995–1014.

Hindelang, M. J., Hirschi, T., & Weis, J. G. (2001). *Measuring delinquency*. Thousand Oaks, CA: Sage.

Hood, R., & Sparks, R. (1970). *Key issues in criminology*. Wallop, NH: BAS.

Hunter, D. J. (2005). Gene–environment interactions in human diseases. *Nature Reviews Genetics, 6*, 287–298.

The_International_HapMap_Consortium. (2005). A haplotype map of the human genome. *Nature, 437*, 1299–320.

Khoury, M. J., Adams, M. J., & Flanders, W. D. (1988). An epidemiologic approach to ecogenetics. *American Journal of Human Genetics, 42*, 89–95.

Lubin, B., Larsen, R. M., & Matarazzo, J. D. (1984). Patterns of psychological test usage in the United States – 1935–1982. *American Psychologist, 39*, 451–454.

Meaney, M. J., Szyf, M., & Seckl, J. R. (2007). Epigenetic mechanisms of perinatal programming of hypothalamic-pituitary-adrenal function and health. *Trends in Molecular Medicine, 13*, 269–277.

Murphy, F. J., Shirly, M. M., & Witmer, H. L. (1946). The incidence of hidden delinquency. *American Journal of Orthopsychiatry, 16*, 686–696.

Nelson, H. D., Huffman, L. H., Fu, R. W., & Harris, E. L. (2005). Genetic risk assessment and BRCA mutation testing for breast and ovarian cancer susceptibility: Systematic evidence review for the U.S. Preventive Services Task Force. *Annals of Internal Medicine, 143*, 362–379.

Neumark-Sztainer, D., Story, S., Ackard, D., Moe, J., & Perry, C. (2000). The family meal: Views of adolescents. *Journal of Nutrition Education, 32*, 329–334.

Neumark-Sztainer, D., Wall, M., Story, M., & Fulkerson, J. A. 2004. Are family meal patterns associated with disordered eating behaviors among adolescents? *Journal of Adolescent Health, 35,* 350–359.

Pennisi, E. (2007). Breakthrough of the year – Human genetic variation. *Science, 318,* 1842–1843.

Rice, J. A., & Brown, L. F. (1967). Validity of Peabody picture vocabulary test in a sample of low IQ children. *American Journal of Mental Deficiency, 71,* 602–607.

Robison, S. M. (1936). *Can delinquency be measured?* New York: Columbia University Press.

Ross, J. S., & Fletcher, J. A. (1998). The HER-2/neu oncogene in breast cancer: Prognostic factor, predictive factor, and target for therapy. *Stem Cells, 16,* 413–428.

Scott, L. J., Mohlke, K. L., Bonnycastle, L. L., Willer, C. J., Li, Y., Duren, W. L., Erdos, M. R., et al. (2007). A genome-wide association study of type 2 diabetes in Finns detects multiple susceptibility variants. *Science, 316,* 1341–1345.

Sladek, R., Rocheleau, G., Rung, J., Dina, C., Shen, L., Serre, D., et al. (2007). A genome-wide association study identifies novel risk loci for type 2 diabetes. *Nature, 445,* 881–885.

Steemers, F. J., Chang, W., Lee, G., Barker, D. L., Shen, R., & Gunderson, K. L. (2006). Whole-genome genotyping with the single-base extension assay. *Nature Methods, 3,* 31–33.

Steinthorsdottir, V., Thorleifsson, G., Reynisdottir, I., Benediktsson, R., Jonsdottir, T., Walters, G. B., et al. (2007). A variant in CDKAL1 influences insulin response and risk of type 2 diabetes. *Nature Genetics, 39,* 770–775.

Thornberry, T. P., & Krohn, M. D. (2000). The self-report method for measuring delinquency and crime. *Criminal Justice 2000* (vol. 4, pp. 33–83). Washington, DC: National Institute of Justice.

Tourangeau, R., & Smith, T. W. (1996). Asking sensitive questions – The impact of data collection mode, question format, and question context. *Public Opinion Quarterly, 60,* 275–304.

Tsankova, N., Renthal, W., Kumar, A., & Nestler, E. J. (2007). Epigenetic regulation in psychiatric disorders. *Nature Reviews Neuroscience, 8,* 355–367.

Turkheimer, E., Haley, A., Waldron, M., D'Onofrio, B., & Gottesman, I. J. (2003). Socioeconomic status modifies heritability of IQ in young children. *Psychological Science, 14,* 623–628.

Weaver, I. C. G., Cervoni, N., Champagne, F. A., D'Alessio, A. C., Sharma, S., Seckl, J. R., Dymov, S., et al. (2004). Epigenetic programming by maternal behavior. *Nature Neuroscience, 7,* 847–854.

Wright, D. L., Aquilino, W. S., & Supple, A. J. (1998). A comparison of computer-assisted and paper-and-pencil self-administered questionnaires in a survey on smoking, alcohol, and drug use. *Public Opinion Quarterly, 62,* 331–353.

Zeggini, E., Weedon, M. N., Lindgren, C. M., Frayling, T. M., Elliott, K. S., Lango, H., et al. (2007). Replication of genome-wide association signals in UK samples reveals risk loci for type 2 diabetes. *Science, 316,* 1336–1341.

Chapter 14
Social Inequalities, Family Relationships, and Child Health

Mark V. Flinn

Abstract Humans are extraordinarily social creatures. We evolved large brains with a unique suite of abilities, including empathy, consciousness, and language. Our sociocognitive adaptations involve complex integration of neurological (brain) and neuroendocrine (hormone) systems. We are just beginning to understand the genetics that underpin these core aspects of the human psyche. In this chapter, my goal is to develop ideas from evolutionary biology about how and why family environment affects child development that can be integrated with emerging new opportunities in genetic studies. I suggest potential links with stress endocrinology, illustrated with empirical examples from my long-term study of child health in a rural community on the island of Dominica.

Introduction

The human child is highly sensitive to her social environment. Armed with an enormous brain, she is "the most powerful learning machine in the universe" (Gopnik, Meltzoff, & Kuhl, 1999, p. 1). Guided by life's most sophisticated and creative communication system (human language), she absorbs bits of knowledge from others at a phenomenal pace. Her sensitivity to social interactions is interwoven with the ontogeny of flexible cognitive skills, including empathy, consciousness, social-scenario building, mental time travel, and Theory of Mind (ToM), which are the foundation of human relationships. These socio-cognitive adaptations involve complex integration of neurological (brain) and neuroendocrine (hormone) systems.

We are just beginning to understand the genetics that underpin these core aspects of the human psyche (e.g., Frigerio et al., 2009; Gilbert, Dobyns, & Lahn, 2005). My goal here is to develop ideas from evolutionary biology about how and why family environment affects child development that hopefully can be integrated with

M.V. Flinn (✉)
Department of Anthropology, University of Missouri, Columbia, MO, USA
e-mail: FlinnM@missouri.edu

A. Booth et al. (eds.), *Biosocial Foundations of Family Processes*,
National Symposium on Family Issues, DOI 10.1007/978-1-4419-7361-0_14,
© Springer Science+Business Media, LLC 2011

emerging new opportunities in genetic studies (Chap. 13). I suggest potential links with stress endocrinology, illustrated with a few empirical examples from my long-term study of child health in a rural community on the island of Dominica.

Physiological Mechanisms Linking Genetics, Social Environment, and Health

Neuroendocrine systems may be viewed as sets of mechanisms designed by natural selection to communicate information among cells and tissues. Steroid and peptide hormones, associated neurotransmitters, and other chemical messengers guide behaviors of mammals in many important ways (Lee, Macbeth, Pagani, & Young, 2009; Panksepp, 2009). Analysis of patterns of hormone levels in naturalistic contexts can provide important insights into the evolutionary functions of the neuroendocrine mechanisms that guide human behaviors. Here, I focus on the apparent evolutionary paradox of neuroendocrine response to psychosocial stressors and the consequent relations among social inequalities, family environment, and child health.

Acute and chronic stressful experiences are associated with a variety of negative health outcomes in humans, including susceptibility to upper respiratory infections (Cohen, Doyle, Turner, Alper, & Skoner, 2003), anxiety and depression (Heim & Nemeroff, 2001), and coronary heart disease (McEwen, 2004). The effects of psychosocial stress can be substantial: in the rural community of Bwa Mawego, Dominica, where I have studied child health for the past 22 years, overall morbidity among children for the 2–7 days following an acute stress event (cortisol > 2 SD) is more than double the normal rate (Fig. 14.1; Flinn & England, 2003). Studies of U.S. populations indicate that chronic stress is similarly associated with a long-term, threefold increase in adverse health outcomes (Cohen et al., 2003). Moreover, exposure to stressful events early in development appears to have lifelong effects (Champagne, 2008; de Bellis et al., 1994; de Kloet, Sibug, Helmerhorst, & Schmidt, 2005; Flinn, 2006b; Seckl, 2008; cf. Flinn, 2009; Ader, Felten, & Cohen, 2001; Wilkinson, 2006).

Stress endocrinology is suspected to have an important role in the links between social environment and health. Chronic release of stress hormones such as cortisol in response to psychosocial challenges is posited to have incidental deleterious effects on immune and metabolic regulatory functions (Ader, 2001; Sapolsky, 2005). Release of androgens such as testosterone and DHEA/S is also influenced by social conditions (e.g., Gray & Ellison, 2009) and can affect immunocompetence (Muehlenbein, 2008). Social inequalities may be an especially important source of psychosocial challenges in modern societies because of the chronic, persistent, and novel nature of negative stressors (Barker, 1991; Farmer, 2001; Gravlee, 2009; Kleinman, 2007; Wilkinson, 2006), combined with the disruption of kin-based social support networks (Flinn & England, 1997).

The significance of the social environment for a child's physical and mental health presents an evolutionary puzzle. Why, given the apparent high cost to human

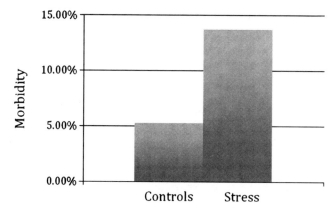

Fig. 14.1 Morbidity following a high stress event. High stress events (cortisol level >2 standard deviations above expected) are associated with morbidity (mostly "common cold" upper respiratory tract infections) during a 2–7 day period following the event. A small part of this huge effect is explained by stressful events such as the start of school and holidays that have elevated epidemiological risk. The primary reason appears to involve diminished immunity. Modified from Flinn and England (2003)

health of psychosocial stress, would natural selection have favored links (including epigenetic DNA methylation – see Murgatroyd et al., 2009; Weaver et al., 2004) between the psychological mechanisms that assess social challenges and the neuroendocrine mechanisms that regulate stress and reproductive physiology and downstream immune functions?

I approach this question from the integrative evolutionary paradigm of Tinbergen (1963), who emphasized the importance of linking proximate physiological explanations with ontogeny (development), phylogeny (ancestry), and adaptive function (natural selection). My basic argument is that a *benefit* of hormonal stress response to psychosocial challenges is the mediation of the neural remodeling and potentiation that is necessary to adapt to the dynamic informational arms race of the human sociocultural environment (Flinn, 2006b). The *costs* involve trade-offs that can become especially problematic in stressful family environments.

Why is the Human Child So Sensitive to the Social Environment?

The human child is an extraordinarily social creature, motivated by and highly sensitive to interpersonal relationships (Gopnik et al., 1999). The life history stage of human childhood appears to have evolved for the function of enabling the development of complex social skills (Bjorklund & Pelligrini, 2002; Bogin, 1999; Flinn, 2004; Geary & Bjorklund, 2000), including emotional regulation. Learning, practice, and experience are imperative for social success. The information processing capacity used for human social interactions is considerable and perhaps significantly greater than that involved with foraging, locomotion, toolmaking, and other subsistence skills (Roth & Dicke, 2005).

The child needs to master complex dynamic tasks such as learning the personalities, social biases, relationships, and so forth of peers and adults in the local community, and developing appropriate cognitive and emotional responses to these challenges (Bugental, 2000). The learning environments that facilitate and channel these astonishing aspects of human mental phenotypic plasticity appear to take on a special importance. Much of the data required for the social behavior necessary to be successful as a human cannot be "preprogrammed" into specific, detailed, fixed responses. Social cleverness in a fast-paced, cumulative cultural environment must contend with dynamic, constantly shifting strategies of friends and enemies and hence needs information from experiential social learning (Flinn, 1997, 2006a; Flinn & Alexander, 2007). The links among psychosocial stimuli, emotions, and physiological stress response may guide both the acute and long-term neurological plasticity necessary for adapting to the dynamic aspects of human sociality.

To summarize my argument to this point, human childhood is viewed as a life history stage that is necessary for acquiring the information and practice to build and refine the mental algorithms critical for negotiating the social coalitions that are key to success in our species (Flinn, Muehlenbein, & Ponzi, 2009; Geary & Flinn, 2001). Mastering the social environment presents special challenges for the human child. Social competence is difficult because the target (other children and adults) is constantly changing and similarly equipped with theory of mind and other cognitive abilities. The family environment is a primary source and mediator of the ontogeny of social competencies. Human biology has been profoundly affected by our evolutionary history as unusually social creatures, including, perhaps, a special reliance upon smart mothers, protective fathers, cooperative siblings, and helpful grandparents (Flinn, Quinlan, Ward, & Coe, 2007). Indeed, the mind of the human child may have design features that enable its development as a group project, guided by the multitudinous informational contributions of its ancestors and codescendants (Coe, 2003; Flinn & Coe, 2007; Hrdy, 2009). Studies of the genetics of hormonal responses to these complex components of human sociality may provide important clues about relations between psychosocial stress and health.

Neuroendocrine Response to the Social Environment

The constellation of behaviors associated with the human family and the dynamics of social competition described in previous sections are enabled by complex physiological regulatory systems. The genetics of these regulatory systems are just beginning to be investigated (e.g., Frigerio et al., 2009). In this section, I first briefly discuss the potential hormonal mechanisms for human pair bonding, maternal and paternal attachment to offspring (see also Chap. 1), kin attachment, and male coalitions. I then discuss how the hormonal stress response system functions to enable acquisition of social competencies during childhood in the context of the human family environment. And finally, I suggest links among these two neuroendocrine systems and social inequalities, family environments, and child health.

The chemical messenger systems that orchestrate the ontogeny and regulation of sexual differentiation, metabolism, neurogenesis, immune function, growth, and other complex somatic processes tend to be evolutionarily conservative among primates and more generally among mammals. Hence, rodent and nonhuman primate models provide important comparative information about the functions of specific human neuroendocrine systems, for which we often have little direct empirical research. It is the particular balance of human mechanisms and abilities that is unique and reflects the history of selection for complex social interactions that shaped the human lineage.

The Chemistry of Affiliation

Some of the most precious of all our human feelings are stimulated by close social relationships: a mother holding her newborn infant for the first time, brothers reunited after a long absence, or lovers entangled in each other's arms. Natural selection has designed our neurobiological mechanisms, in concert with our endocrine systems, to generate potent sensations in our interactions with these most evolutionarily salient individuals. We share with our primate relatives the same basic hormones and neurotransmitters that enable these mental states. But our unique evolutionary history has modified us to respond to different circumstances and situations; we are rewarded and punished for somewhat different stimuli than our phylogenetic cousins. Chimpanzees and humans share the delight – the neurobiological reward – when biting into a ripe, juicy mango. But the endocrine, neurological, and associated emotional responses of a human father to holding his infant child (e.g., Berg & Wynne-Edwards, 2001; Fleming, Corter, Stallings, & Steiner, 2002) are likely to be quite different from those of a chimpanzee male. Happiness for a human has many unique designs (Gilbert, 2001; Nesse & Stearns, 2008), such as romantic love (Fisher et al., 2002), that involve shared endogenous messengers from our phylogenetic heritage.

Attachments and bonding are central in the lives of the social mammals. Basic to survival and reproduction, these interdependent relationships are the fabric of the social networks that permit individuals to maintain cooperative relationships over time. Although attachments can provide security and relief from stress, close relationships also exert pressures on individuals to which they continuously respond. It should not be surprising, therefore, that the neuroendocrine mechanisms underlying attachment and stress are intimately related to one another. And although more is known about the stress response systems than the affiliative systems, some of the pieces of the puzzle are beginning to fall into place (Bridges, 2008; Curley & Keverne, 2005; Meyer-Lindenberg, 2008; Panksepp, 2004; Wynne-Edwards, 2003).

The mother–offspring relationship is at the core of mammalian life, and it appears that the biochemistry at play in the regulation of this intimate bond was also selected to serve in primary mechanisms regulating bonds between mates, paternal care, the family group, and even larger social networks (Fisher et al., 2002; Hrdy, 2009). Although a number of hormones and neurotransmitters are involved in attachment and other components of relationships, the two peptide hormones, oxytocin (OXT) and arginine-vasopressin (AVP), appear to be primary (Carter, 2002; Curtis & Wang, 2003; Lee et al., 2009; Ross & Young, 2009; Young & Insel, 2002), with dopamine, cortisol, and other hormones and neurotransmitters having mediating effects (e.g., Fleming et al., 1997).

The hypothalamus is the major brain site where OXT and AVP (closely related chains of nine amino acids) are produced. From there, they are released into the central nervous system (CNS) as well as transported to the pituitary where they are stored until secreted into the bloodstream. OXT and AVP act on a wide range of neurological systems, and their influence varies among mammalian species and stage of development. The neurological effects of OXT and AVP appear to be key mechanisms (e.g., Bartels & Zeki, 2004) involved in the evolution of human family behaviors. The effects of OXT and AVP in humans are likely to be especially context dependent, because of the variable and complex nature of family relationships.

fMRI studies of brain activity involved in maternal attachment in humans indicate that the activated regions are part of the reward system and contain a high density of receptors for OXT and AVP (Bartels & Zeki, 2004). These studies also demonstrate that the neural regions involved in attachment activated in humans are similar to those activated in nonhuman animals. Among humans, however, neural regions associated with social judgment and assessment of the intentions and emotions of others exhibited some deactivation during attachment activities, suggesting possible links between psychological mechanisms for attachment and management of social relationships. Falling in love with a mate and affective bonds with offspring may involve temporary deactivation of psychological mechanisms for maintaining an individual's social "guard" in the complex reciprocity of human social networks. Dopamine levels are likely to be important for both types of relationship but may involve some distinct neural sites (Heinrichs & Domes, 2008). It will be interesting to see what fMRI studies of attachment in human males indicate because father–offspring, male–female mating, grandparental, and male–male coalitionary relationships are where the most substantial evolved differences from other mammals would be expected. Likewise, fMRI studies of attachment to mothers, fathers, and alloparental caretakers in human children may provide important insights into the other side of parent–offspring bonding.

The challenge before human evolutionary biologists and psychologists is to understand how these general neuroendocrine systems have been modified and linked with other special human cognitive systems (e.g., Allman, 1999; Blakemore, Winston, & Frith, 2004; Fisher, Aron, & Brown, 2006; Geary & Flinn, 2002; Henry & Wang, 1998) to produce the unique suite of human family behaviors. Analysis of hormonal responses to social stimuli may provide important insights into the selective pressures that guided the evolution of these key aspects of the human mind. Identification of specific genes involved in the relevant neuroendocrine processes will not be easy. Because the sample sizes of existing studies of hormone responses to social environment are small, genome-wide association studies (GWAS) might be problematic. However, several candidate genes may give us a place to start. The serotonin transporter gene (5HTT), dopamine receptor genes (e.g., DRD4), OXT receptor genes, catecholamine metabolism genes (e.g., COMT), and HPA regulation genes (e.g., GABRA6) are involved in several important aspects of stress response and affiliation (e.g., Frigerio et al., 2009; Rodrigues & Saslow, in press).

The Chemistry of Stress, Family, and the Social Mind

The evolutionary scenario proposed in previous sections posits that the family is of paramount importance in a child's world. Throughout human evolutionary history, parents and close relatives provided calories, protection, and information necessary for survival, growth, health, social success, and eventual reproduction. The human mind, therefore, is likely to have evolved special sensitivity to interactions with family care providers, particularly during infancy and childhood (Baumeister & Leary, 1995; Belsky, 1997, 2005; Bowlby, 1969; Daly & Wilson, 1995).

The family and other kin provide important cognitive "landmarks" for the development of a child's understanding of the social environment. The reproductive interests of a child overlap with those of its parents more than with any other individuals. Information (including advice, training, and incidental observation) provided by parents is important for situating oneself in the social milieu and developing a mental model of its operations. A child's family environment may be an especially important source and mediator of stress, with consequent effects on health.

Psychosocial stressors are associated with increased risk of infectious disease (Cohen et al., 2003) and a variety of other illnesses (Ader, Felten, & Cohen, 2001). Physiological stress responses regulate the allocation of energetic and other somatic resources to different bodily functions via a complex assortment of neuroendocrine mechanisms. Changing, unpredictable environments require adjustment of priorities. Digestion, growth, immunity, and sex are irrelevant while being chased by a predator (Sapolsky, 2005). Stress hormones help shunt blood, glucose, and so on to tissues necessary for the task at hand. Chronic and traumatic stress can diminish health, evidently because resources are diverted away from important health functions. These costs can be referred to as "allostatic load" (Korte, Koolhaas, Wingfield, & McEwen, 2005). Such diversions of resources may have special significance during childhood because of the additional demands of physical and mental growth and development and possible long-term ontogenetic consequences (Nepomnaschy & Flinn, 2009).

Stress Response Mechanisms and Theory

Physiological response to environmental stimuli perceived as stressful is modulated by the limbic system (amygdala and hippocampus) and basal ganglia. These components of the CNS interact with the sympathetic and parasympathetic nervous systems and two neuroendocrine axes, the sympathetic – adrenal medullary system (SAM) and the HPA. The SAM and HPA systems affect a wide range of physiological functions in concert with other neuroendocrine mechanisms and involve complex feedback regulation. The SAM system controls the catecholamines norepinephrine and epinephrine (adrenalin). The HPA system regulates glucocorticoids, primarily cortisol (for review see Lupien, McEwen, Gunnar, & Heim, 2009; Sapolsky, 2005).

Cortisol is a key hormone produced in response to physical and psychosocial stressors. It is produced and stored in the adrenal cortex. Release into the plasma is primarily under the control of pituitary adrenocorticotropic hormone (ACTH). The free or unbound portion of the circulating cortisol may pass through the cell membrane and bind to a specific cytosolic glucocorticoid receptor. This complex may induce genes coding for at least 26 different enzymes involved with carbohydrate, fat, and amino-acid metabolism in brain, liver, muscle, and adipose tissue (Yuwiler, 1982).

Cortisol modulates a wide range of somatic functions, including: (1) energy release (e.g., stimulation of hepatic gluconeogenesis in concert with glucagon and inhibition of the effects of insulin), (2) immune activity (e.g., regulation of inflammatory response and the cytokine cascade), (3) mental activity (e.g., alertness, memory, and learning), (4) growth (e.g., inhibition of growth hormone and somatomedins), and (5) reproductive function (e.g., inhibition of gonadal steroids, including testosterone). These complex multiple effects of cortisol muddle understanding of its adaptive functions. The demands of energy regulation must orchestrate with those of immune function, attachment bonding, memory (Beylin & Shors, 2003), and so forth. Mechanisms for localized targeting (e.g., glucose uptake by active versus inactive muscle tissues and neuropeptide-directed immune response) provide fine-tuning of the preceding general physiological effects. Cortisol regulation allows the body to respond to changing environmental conditions by preparing for *specific* short-term demands.

These temporary beneficial effects of glucocorticoid stress response, however, are not without costs. Persistent activation of the HPA system is associated with immune deficiency, cognitive impairment, inhibited growth, delayed sexual maturity, damage to the hippocampus, and psychological maladjustment (Ader et al., 2001; McEwen, 2004). Chronic stress may diminish metabolic energy and produce complications from autoimmune protection. Stressful life events – such as divorce, death of a family member, change of residence, or loss of a job – are associated with infectious disease and other health problems (Maier, Watkins, & Fleschner, 1994).

Stress Response and Family Environment

Composition of the family or caretaking household may have important effects on child development (Whiting & Edwards, 1988). For example, in Western cultures, children with divorced parents may experience more emotional tension or "stress" than children living in a stable two-parent family. Investigation of physiological stress responses in the human family environment has been hampered by the lack of noninvasive techniques for measurement of stress hormones. Frequent collection of plasma samples to assess temporal changes in endocrine function is not feasible in nonclinical settings. The development of saliva immunoassay techniques, however, presents new opportunities for stress research. Saliva is relatively easy to collect and store, even in naturalistic field conditions.

In this section, I briefly review results from a longitudinal, 22-year study of child stress and health in a rural community on the island of Dominica (see Flinn, 1999, 2006b). The research design uses concomitant monitoring of a child's daily activities, stress hormones, and psychological conditions to investigate the effects of naturally occurring psychosocial events.

Associations between average cortisol levels of children and family environment indicate that children living in stable households with high quality caregiving had lower average levels of cortisol than children living in more difficult conditions (Fig. 14.2; Flinn, 1999). A further test of this hypothesis is provided by comparison of step- and genetic children residing in the same households. Stepchildren had higher average cortisol levels and higher morbidity than their half-siblings residing in the same household who were genetic offspring of both parents (Fig. 14.3a,b; Flinn & England, 1995). Family conflicts were associated with elevated cortisol levels for all ages of children more than any other factor that we examined (Fig. 14.4; Flinn, 1999).

These results suggest that family interactions were a critical psychosocial stressor in most children's lives, although the sample collection during periods of intense family interaction (early morning and late afternoon) may have exaggerated this

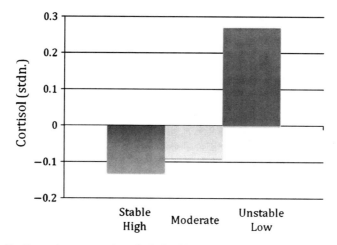

Fig. 14.2 Family environment and cortisol. Family environment and mean (average) cortisol levels of children. *Stable, high* parental care = biparental with grandparents and/or parent ratings of high levels of care. (*N* = 108 children). *Moderate* = biparental or single mom with grandparents and/or caregiver ratings of moderate levels of care (*N* = 103 children). *Unstable, low* = single parent, stepfamily, distant relatives, and/or caregiver ratings of low levels of care (includes neglect and abuse) (*N* = 53 children). Modified from Flinn (1999)

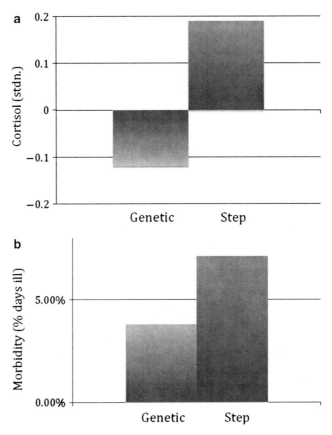

Fig. 14.3 (**a**) Mean (average) cortisol levels of genetic and step children residing in same households. Cortisol levels of maternal half-siblings living in the same households with a genetic ($N = 25$) or a stepfather ($N = 27$). Figure modified from Flinn and England (1995). (**b**) Morbidity levels of genetic and step children residing in same households. Morbidity levels of maternal half-siblings living in the same households with a genetic ($N = 25$) or a stepfather ($N = 27$). Figure modified from Flinn and England (2003)

association. Although elevated cortisol levels are associated with traumatic events such as family arguments, long-term stress may result in diminished cortisol response. In some cases, chronically stressed children had blunted response to physical activities that normally evoked cortisol elevation. Comparison of cortisol levels during "nonstressful" periods (no reported or observed crying, punishment, anxiety, residence change, family conflict, or health problem during 24-h period before saliva collection) indicates a striking reduction and, in many cases, reversal of the family environment-stress association (Flinn, Quinlan, Turner, Decker, & England, 1996). Chronically stressed children sometimes had subnormal cortisol levels when they were not in stressful situations. For example, cortisol levels immediately after school (walking home from school) and during noncompetitive play were lower among some chronically stressed children. Some chronically stressed

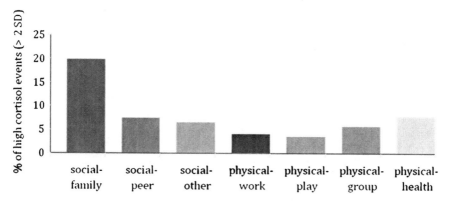

Fig. 14.4 Proportion (%) of high cortisol events (>2 SD) linked to reported or observed stressors. Observed or reported context of high cortisol (stressful) events. Modified from Flinn et al (1996)

children appeared socially "tough" or withdrawn and exhibited little or no arousal to the novelty of the first few days of the saliva collection procedure.

Children born and raised in household environments in which mothers have little or no mate or kin support were at greatest risk for abnormal cortisol profiles and associated health problems. Because socioeconomic conditions influence family environment, they have consequences for child health that extend beyond direct material effects. And because health in turn may affect an individual's social and economic opportunities, a cycle of poor health and poverty may be perpetuated generation after generation. Analysis of genetic polymorphisms in stress and affiliation mechanisms may provide important new directions for understanding stress – family – health links.

Conclusion

People in difficult or inequitable social environments tend to be less healthy in comparison with their more fortunate peers (e.g., Dressler & Bindon, 2000; Flinn & England, 1997; Gravlee, 2009; Wilkinson, 2006). Social support is likely to have had important reproductive consequences for our ancestors. If the brain evolved as a social tool, then the expenditure of somatic resources to resolve psychosocial problems makes sense. Relationships, especially family relationships, are of paramount importance. Kinship-based social networks are likely to have been a key factor affecting humans for well over half a million years. Our hormonal, neural, and psychological mechanisms have been shaped by natural selection to respond to the critical pressures generated by social competition and cooperation (Alexander, 2005; Amodio & Frith, 2006; Flinn, Geary, & Ward, 2005). In Bwa Mawego, and perhaps in most human societies, children elevate their stress hormone (cortisol) levels frequently and extensively in response to psychosocial stimuli. The adaptive effects of the major stress hormones and affiliative neurotransmitters on neural reorganization appear consistent with observations of sensitivity to the social world (Flinn, 2006b; Lupien et al., 2009).

Social competence is extraordinarily difficult because the competition is constantly changing and similarly equipped with Theory of Mind and other cognitive abilities. The sensitivity of the stress-response and affiliative systems to the social environment may enable adaptive neural reorganization to this most salient and dynamic puzzle. Childhood is necessary and useful for acquiring the information and practice to build and refine the mental algorithms critical for negotiating the social coalitions that are key to success in our species. The human family provides critical support for the developing child in this regard (e.g., Dunn, 2004). Traumatic early environments may result in diminished abilities to acquire social competencies as a consequence of glucocorticoid hypersensitivity disrupting neurogenesis, particularly in the hippocampus (Lupien et al., 2009; Mirescu, Peters, & Gould, 2004; Seckl, 2008). An improved understanding of the genetics and epigenetics of the hormonal and neurological mechanisms that facilitate the intensive and extensive relationships involved with human families and broader kin coalitions, including comparisons between humans and our close primate relatives, may provide important insights into the selective pressures that shaped human biology.

References

Ader, R., Felten, D. L., & Cohen, N. (2001). *Psychoneuroimmunology* (3rd ed.). San Diego: Academic.

Adolphs, R. (2003). Cognitive neuroscience of human social behavior. *Nature Reviews Neuroscience, 4*, 165–178.

Alexander, R. D. (2005). Evolutionary selection and the nature of humanity. In V. Hosle & C. Illies (Eds.), *Darwinism and philosophy* (pp. 301–348). South Bend: University of Notre Dame Press.

Allman, J. (1999). *Evolving brains*. New York: Scientific American Library.

Amodio, D. M., & Frith, C. D. (2006). Meeting of minds: The medial frontal cortex and social cognition. *Nature Reviews Neuroscience, 7*(4), 268–277.

Barker, D. J. (1991). The foetal and infant origins of inequalities in health in Britain. *Journal of Public Health Medicine, 13*, 64–68.

Bartels, A., & Zeki, S. (2004). The neural correlates of maternal and romantic love. *NeuroImage, 21*, 1155–1166.

Baumeister, R. F. (2005). *The cultural animal: Human nature, meaning, and social life*. New York: Oxford University Press.

Baumeister, R. F., & Leary, M. R. (1995). The need to belong: Desire for interpersonal attachment as a fundamental human motive. *Psychological Bulletin, 117*, 497–529.

Belsky, J. (1997). Attachment, mating, and parenting: An evolutionary interpretation. *Human Nature, 8*, 361–381.

Belsky, J. (2005). Differential susceptibility to rearing influence: An evolutionary hypothesis and some evidence. In B. J. Ellis & D. F. Bjorkland (Eds.), *Origins of the social mind: Evolutionary psychology and child development* (pp. 139–163). New York: Guilford Press.

Berg, S. J., & Wynne-Edwards, K. E. (2001). Changes in testosterone, cortisol, and estradiol levels in men becoming fathers. *Mayo Clinic Proceedings, 76*, 582–592.

Beylin, A. V., & Shors, T. J. (2003). Glucocorticoids are necessary for enhancing the acquisition of associative memories after acute stressful experience. *Hormones and Behavior, 43*, 124–131.

Bjorklund, D. F., & Pellegrini, A. D. (2002). *The origins of human nature: Evolutionary developmental psychology.* Washington: APA Press.

Blakemore, S.-J., Winston, J., & Frith, U. (2004). Social cognitive neuroscience: Where are we heading? *Trends in Cognitive Neurosciences, 8*(5), 216–222.

Bogin, B. (1999). *Patterns of human growth* (2nd ed.). Cambridge: Cambridge University Press.

Bowlby, J. (1969). *Attachment and loss: Vol. 1. Attachment.* London: Hogarth.

Bridges, R.S. (Ed.) (2008). *Neurobiology of the parental brain.* San Diego: Academic.

Bugental, D. B. (2000). Acquisition of the algorithms of social life: A domain-based approach. *Psychological Bulletin, 26*, 187–209.

Carter, C. S. (2002). Neuroendocrine perspectives on social attachment and love. In J. T. Caciooppo, G. G. Berntson, R. Adolphs, C. S. Carter, R. J. Davidson, M. K. McClintock, et al. (Eds.), *Foundations in social neuroscience* (pp. 853–890). Cambridge: MIT Press.

Champagne, F. A., (2008). Epigenetic mechanisms and the transgenerational effects of maternal care. *Frontiers in Neuroendocrinology, 29*, 386–397.

Coe, K. (2003). *The ancestress hypothesis: Visual art as adaptation.* New Brunswick: Rutgers University Press.

Cohen, S., Doyle, W. J., Turner, R. B., Alper, C. M., & Skoner, D. P. (2003). Emotional style and susceptibility to the common cold. *Psychosomatic Medicine, 65*(4), 652–657.

Curley, J. P., & Keverne, E. B. (2005). Genes, brains and mammalian social bonds. *Trends in Ecology & Evolution, 20*(10), 561–567.

Curtis, T. J., & Wang, Z. (2003). The neurochemistry of pair bonding. *Current Directions in Psychological Science, 12*(2), 49–53.

Daly, M., & Wilson, M. (1995). Discriminative parental solicitude and the relevance of evolutionary models to the analysis of motivational systems. In M. S. Gazzaniga (Ed.), *The cognitive neurosciences* (pp. 1269–1286). Cambridge: MIT Press.

de Bellis, M., Chrousos, G. P., Dorn, L. D., Burke, L., Helmers, K., Kling, M. A., et al. (1994). Hypothalamic-pituitary-adrenal axis dysregulation in sexually abused girls. *Journal of Clinical Endocrinology and Metabolism, 78*, 249–255.

de Kloet, E. R., Sibug, R. M., Helmerhorst, F. M., & Schmidt, M. V. (2005). Stress, genes, and the mechanism for programming the brain for later life. *Neuroscience and Biobehavioral Reviews, 29*, 271–281.

Dressler, W., & Bindon, J. R. (2000). The health consequences of cultural consonance: Cultural dimensions of lifestyle, social support, and arterial blood pressure in an African American community. *American Anthropologist, 102*(2), 244–260.

Dunn, J. (2004). Understanding children's family worlds: Family transitions and children's outcome. *Merrill-Palmer Quarterly, 50*(3), 224–235.

Farmer, P. (2001). An anthropology of structural violence. *Current Anthropology, 45*(3), 305–325.

Fisher, H., Aron, A., Mashek, D., Strong, G., Li, H., & Brown, L. L. (2002). Defining the brain systems of lust, romantic attraction and attachment. *Archives of Sexual Behavior, 31*(5), 413–419.

Fisher, H. E., Aron, A., & Brown, L. L. (2006). Romantic love: A mammalian brain system for mate choice. *Philosophical Transactions of the Royal Society of London Series B, 361*, 2173–2186.

Fleming, A. S., Corter, C., Stallings, J., & Steiner, M. (2002). Testosterone and prolactin are associated with emotional responses to infant cries in new fathers. *Hormones and Behavior, 42*, 399–413.

Fleming, A. S., Steiner, M., & Corter, C. (1997). Cortisol, hedonics, and maternal responsiveness in human mothers. *Hormones and Behavior, 32*(2), 85–98.

Flinn, M. V. (1997). Culture and the evolution of social learning. *Evolution and Human Behavior, 18*(1), 23–67.

Flinn, M. V. (1999). Family environment, stress, and health during childhood. In C. Panter-Brick & C. Worthman (Eds.), *Hormones, health, and behavior* (pp. 105–138). Cambridge: Cambridge University press.

Flinn, M. V. (2004). Culture and developmental plasticity: Evolution of the social brain. In K. MacDonald & R. L. Burgess (Eds.), *Evolutionary perspectives on child development* (pp. 73–98). Thousand Oaks: Sage.

Flinn, M. V. (2006a). Cross-cultural universals and variations: The evolutionary paradox of informational novelty. *Psychological Inquiry, 17*, 118–123.

Flinn, M. V. (2006b). Evolution and ontogeny of stress response to social challenge in the human child. *Developmental Review, 26*, 138–174.

Flinn, M.V. (2009). Are cortisol profiles a stable trait during child development? *American Journal of Human Biology* 21, 769–771.

Flinn, M. V., & Alexander, R. D. (2007). Runaway social selection. In S. W. Gangestad & J. A. Simpson (Eds.), *The evolution of mind* (pp. 249–255). New York: Guilford Press.

Flinn, M. V., & Coe, K. (2007). The linked red queens of human cognition, reciprocity, and culture. In S. W. Gangestad & J. A. Simpson (Eds.), *The evolution of mind* (pp. 339–347). New York: Guilford Press.

Flinn, M. V., & England, B. G. (1995). Childhood stress and family environment. *Current Anthropology, 36*(5), 854–866.

Flinn, M. V., & England, B. G. (1997). Social economics of childhood glucocorticoid stress response and health. *American Journal of Physical Anthropology, 102*(1), 33–53.

Flinn, M. V., & England, B. G. (2003). Childhood stress: Endocrine and immune responses to psychosocial events. In J. M. Wilce (Ed.), *Social & cultural lives of immune systems* (pp. 107–147). London: Routledge Press.

Flinn, M. V., Geary, D. C., & Ward, C. V. (2005). Ecological dominance, social competition, and coalitionary arms races: Why humans evolved extraordinary intelligence. *Evolution and Human Behavior, 26*(1), 10–46.

Flinn, M. V., & Leone, D. V. (2006). Early trauma and the ontogeny of glucocorticoid stress response: Grandmother as a secure base. *Journal of Developmental Processes, 1*(1), 31–68.

Flinn, M. V., & Leone, D. V. (2009). Alloparental care and the ontogeny of glucocorticoid stress response among stepchildren. In Substitute parents, ed. G. Bentley and R. Mace. Biosocial Society Symposium Series. Oxford: Berghahn Books, chapter 13, pp. 266–286.

Flinn, M. V., Muehlenbein, M. P., & Ponzi, D. (2009). Evolution of neuroendocrine mechanisms linking attachment and life history: The social neuroendocrinology of middle childhood. *Behavioral and Brain Sciences, 32*(1), 27–28.

Flinn, M. V., Quinlan, R. J., Turner, M. T., Decker, S. D., & England, B. G. (1996). Male-female differences in effects of parental absence on glucocorticoid stress response. *Human Nature, 7*(2), 125–162.

Flinn, M. V., Quinlan, R. J., Ward, C. V., & Coe, M. K. (2007). Evolution of the human family: Cooperative males, long social childhoods, smart mothers, and extended kin networks. In C. Salmon & T. Shackelford (Eds.), *Family relationships* (pp. 16–38). Oxford: Oxford University Press.

Flinn, M. V., Ward, C. V., & Noone, R. (2005). Hormones and the human family. In Buss, D. (Ed.), *Handbook of evolutionary psychology*. Wiley, New York, chapter 19, pp. 552–580.

Frigerio, A., Ceppi, E., Rusconi, M., Giorda, R., Raggi, M.E., & Fearon, P. (2009). The role played by the interaction between genetic factors and attachment in the stress response in infancy. *Journal of Child Psychology and Psychiatry, 50*(12), 1513–1522.

Geary, D. C., & Bjorklund, D. F. (2000). Evolutionary developmental psychology. *Child Development, 71*(1), 57–65.

Geary, D. C., & Flinn, M. V. (2001). Evolution of human parental behavior and the human family. *Parenting: Science and Practice, 1*, 5–61.

Geary, D. C., & Flinn, M. V. (2002). Sex differences in behavioral and hormonal response to social threat. *Psychological Review, 109*(4), 745–750.

Gilbert, P. (2001). Evolutionary approaches to psychopathology: The role of natural defences. *Australian and New Zealand Journal of Psychiatry, 35*(1), 17–27.

Gilbert, S. L., Dobyns, W. B., & Lahn, B. T. (2005). Genetic links between brain development and brain evolution. *Nature Reviews Genetics, 6*(7), 581–590.

Gopnik, A., Meltzoff, A. N., & Kuhl, P. K. (1999). *The scientist in the crib: Minds, brains, and how children learn.* New York: William Morrow & Co.

Gravlee, C. C. (2009). How race becomes biology: Embodiment of social inequality. *American Journal of Physical Anthropology, 139*(1), 47–57.

Gray, P. B., & Ellison, P. T. (Eds.) (2009). *Endocrinology of social relationships.* Cambridge: Harvard University Press.

Gray, P. B., & Campbell, B. C. (2009). Human male testosterone, pair bonding and fatherhood. In P. T. Ellison and P. B. Gray (Eds.), *Endocrinology of social relationships,* pp. 270–293. Cambridge: Harvard University Press.

Gray, P. B., Kahlenberg, S. M., Barrett, E. S., Lipson, S. F., & Ellison, P. T. (2002). Marriage and fatherhood are associated with lower testosterone in males. *Evolution and Human Behavior, 23,* 193–201.

Guo, G. (2010). Family influences on children's well-being: Potential roles of molecular genetics and epigenetics. In A. Booth, S. McHale, & N. Landale (Eds.), *Biosocial foundations of family processes* (pp. 181–204). New York: Springer.

Heim, C., & Nemeroff, C. (2001). The role of childhood trauma in the neurobiology of mood and anxiety disorders: Preclinical and clinical studies. *Society of Biological Psychiatry, 49,* 1023–1039.

Heim, C., Newport, J., Wagner, D., Wilcox, M., Miller, A., & Nemeroff, C. (2002). The role of early adverse experience and adulthood stress in the prediction of neuroendocrine stress reactivity in women: A multiple regression analysis. *Depression and Anxiety, 15,* 117–125.

Heinrichs, M., & Domes G. (2008). Neuropeptides and social behaviour: Effects of oxytocin and vasopressin in humans. *Progress in Brain Research, 170,* 337–350.

Henry, J. P., & Wang, S. (1998). Effect of early stress on adult affiliative behavior. *Psychoneuroendocrinology, 23*(8), 863–875.

Hrdy, S. B. (2009). *Mothers and others: The evolutionary origins of mutual understanding.* Cambridge: Harvard University Press.

Kleinman, A. (2007). Psychiatry without context: turning sadness into disease. *The Lancet, 370*(9590), 819–820.

Korte, S. M., Koolhaas, J. M., Wingfield, J. C., & McEwen, B. S. (2005). The Darwinian concept of stress: Benefits of allostasis and costs of allostatic load and the trade-offs in health and disease. *Neuroscience & Biobehavioral Reviews, 29*(1), 3–38.

Lee, H.-J., Macbeth, A. H., Pagani, J. H., & Young, W. S., 3rd. (2009). Oxytocin: The great facilitator of life. *Progress in Neurobiology, 88*(2), 127–151.

Lupien, S. J., McEwen, B. S., Gunnar, M. R., & Heim, C. (2009). Effects of stress throughout the lifespan on the brain, behaviour and cognition. *Nature Reviews Neuroscience, 10,* 434–445.

Maier, S. F., Watkins, L. R., & Fleschner, M. (1994). Psychoneuroimmunology: The interface between behavior, brain, and immunity. *American Psychologist, 49,* 1004–1007.

McEwen, B. S. (1995). Stressful experience, brain, and emotions: Developmental, genetic, and hormonal influences. In M. S. Gazzaniga (Ed.), *The cognitive neurosciences* (pp. 1117–1135). Cambridge: MIT Press.

McEwen, B.S. (2004). Protective and damaging effects of stress mediators. In J. T. Cacioppo & G. G. Berntson (Eds.), *Essays in social neuroscience* (pp. 41–51). Cambridge: MIT Press.

Meyer-Lindenberg A. (2008). Impact of prosocial neuropeptides on human brain function. *Progress in Brain Research, 170,* 463–470.

Mileva-Seitz, V., & Fleming, A. S. (2010). How mothers are born: A psychobiological analysis of mothering. In A. Booth, S. McHale, & N. Landale (Eds.), *Biosocial foundations of family processes* (pp. 3–34). New York: Springer.

Mirescu, C., Peters, J. D., & Gould, E. (2004). Early life experience alters response of adult neurogenesis to stress. *Nature Reviews: Neuroscience, 7*(8), 841–846.

Muehlenbein, M. P. (2008). Adaptive variation in testosterone levels in response to immune activation: Empirical and theoretical perspectives. *Social Biology, 53,* 13–23.

Murgatroyd, C., Patchev, A. V., Wu, Y., Micale, V., Bockmühl, Y., Fischer, D., et al. (2009). Dynamic DNA methylation programs persistent adverse effects of early-life stress. *Nature Neuroscience*, published online: 8 November 2009, doi:10.1038/nn.2436.

Nepomnaschy, P., & Flinn, M. V. (2009). Early life influences on the ontogeny of neuroendocrine stress response in the human child. In P. Ellison & P. Gray (Eds.), *The endocrinology of social relationships* (pp. 364–282). Cambridge: Harvard University Press.

Nesse, R. M., & Stearns, S. C. (2008). The great opportunity: Evolutionary applications to medicine and public health. *Evolutionary Applications, 1*, 28–48.

Panksepp, J. (2004). *Affective neuroscience: The foundations of human and animal emotions*. New York: Oxford University Press.

Panksepp, J. (2009). Carving "natural" emotions: "Kindly" from bottom-up but not top-down. *Journal of Theoretical and Philosophical Psychology, 28*(2), 395–422.

Rodrigues, S. M., & Saslow, L. (in press). Oxytocin receptor genes. *Proceedings of the National Academy of Sciences*.

Ross, H. E., & Young, L. J. (2009). Oxytocin and the neural mechanisms regulating social cognition and affiliative behavior. *Frontiers in Neuroendocrinology, 30*, 534–547.

Roth, G., & Dicke, U. (2005). Evolution of the brain and intelligence. *TRENDS in Cognitive Sciences, 9*(5), 250–257.

Sapolsky, R. M. (2005). The influence of social hierarchy on primate health. *Science, 308*(5722), 648–652.

Seckl, J. R. (2008). Glucocorticoids, developmental 'programming' and the risk of affective dysfunction. *Progress Brain Research, 167*, 17–34.

Tinbergen, N. (1963). On the aims and methods of ethology. *Zeitschrift für Tierpsychologie, 20*, 410–463.

van Anders, S. M., & Gray, P. B. (2007). Hormones and human partnering. *Annual Review of Sex Research, 18*, 60–93.

Weaver, I. C., Cervoni, N., Champagne, F. A., D'alessio, A. C., Sharma, S., Seckl, J. R., et al. (2004). Epigenetic programming by maternal behavior. *Nature Neuroscience, 7*(8), 847–54.

Whiting, B. B., & Edwards, C. (1988). *Children of different worlds*. Cambridge: Harvard University Press.

Wilkinson, R. G. (2006). The impact of inequality. *Social Research: An International Quarterly, 73*(2), 711–732.

Wynne-Edwards, K. E. (2003). From dwarf hamster to daddy: The intersection of ecology, evolution, and physiology that produces paternal behavior. In P. J. B. Slater, J. S. Rosenblatt, C.T. Snowden, & T. J. Roper (Eds.), *Advances in the study of behavior* (pp. 207–261). San Diego: Academic Press.

Yehuda, R., Engel, S. M., Brand, S. R., Seckl, J., Marcus, S. M., & Berkowitz, G. S. (2005). Transgenerational effects of posttraumatic stress disorder in babies of mothers exposed to the World Trade Center attacks during pregnancy. *Journal of Clinical Endocrinology and Metabolism, 90*(7), 4115–4118.

Yuwiler, A. (1982). Biobehavioral consequences of experimental early life stress: Effects of neonatal hormones on monoaminergic systems. In L. J. West & M. Stein (Eds.), *Critical issues in behavioral medicine* (pp. 59–78). Philadelphia: J. P. Lippincott.

Chapter 15
Family Resources, Genes, and Human Development

Pilyoung Kim and Gary W. Evans

Abstract We review the effects of genes and family resources on families and children. Poverty increases children's exposures to environmental risk factors such as child abuse, poor quality parenting, and suboptimal physical environment. These environmental risk factors interact with various genes to predict more behavioral problems in childhood. Relations between genes and environments are likely more complex than simple individual gene × environment interactions. In some cases, genetic or environmental factors may have different impacts in low- vs. high-SES groups. Finally, we speculate about biological mechanisms that may account for gene by environment interactions. Poverty and related environmental factors may interact with genes, which may lead to abnormal brain development as well as dysregulation in both neurotransmitters and neuroendocrine stress regulatory systems.

Introduction

Guo (Chap. 13) highlights the importance of genetic processes in understanding how early family environments can influence human development. He reminds us that since families share genetic and environmental conditions and since genotypes alter environmental sensitivities, a better understanding of early family influences and their role in poverty would be possible if we incorporate information about genetics into family environments research. Many of Guo's examples of genetic influence focus on dopamine receptor gene variations and environment in relation to antisocial behavioral problems in adolescence. In our chapter, we seek to build upon Guo's chapter, paying particular attention to how genes, environment, and their interaction interface with social inequalities. There is little direct work on genes and socioeconomic status (SES) or poverty, but several studies show genetic

P. Kim (✉)
Emotion and Development Branch, National Institute of Mental Health, Bethesda, MD, USA
e-mail: pilyoung.kim@nih.gov

A. Booth et al. (eds.), *Biosocial Foundations of Family Processes*,
National Symposium on Family Issues, DOI 10.1007/978-1-4419-7361-0_15,
© Springer Science+Business Media, LLC 2011

processes interrelating to personal and environmental characteristics that covary poverty and human development such as parenting.

Early adverse experience such as childhood maltreatment interacts with several genes to affect child development. Adverse parenting processes, including maltreatment and harsh, unresponsive parenting, are much more common in low-income families (Evans, 2004; Repetti, Taylor, & Seeman, 2002). Guo, for example, discusses polymorphism in the promoter region of the monoamine oxidase A (MAOA) gene, childhood maltreatment, and antisocial behavioral problems among adolescents. Kim-Cohen et al. (2006) found that low-activity MAOA interacts with child maltreatment to predict more mental health problems among 7-year-old boys (Kim-Cohen et al., 2006). In his study, Guo did not find any significant link between the dopamine transporter gene (DAT1) and delinquent behaviors. There is evidence, however, that DAT1 may be associated with depression. Haeffel et al. (2008) found that DAT1 interacted with maternal rejection to predict depression onset among adolescents in juvenile detention facilities (Haeffel et al., 2008).

Adverse early experiences such as maltreatment may work together with protective factors such as social support to modify the effects of the serotonin transporter gene promoter polymorphism (5-HTTLPR) on childhood depression. Kaufman et al. (2004) showed that the combination of maltreatment, the homozygous short alleles of 5-HTTLPR genotype, and low-social support drastically increased depression among 10-year olds. Among the maltreated children with homozygous short allele, those without positive social support were twice as likely to exhibit depression relative to 10-year olds with positive social support (Kaufman et al., 2004).

The effects of 5-HTTLPR on children's problematic behaviors may be modified by early childhood interventions. The Family-Centered Prevention Program facilitates good parenting practices including family–child communications, high levels of emotional support, more monitoring, better articulated expectations for risky behavior, as well as positive socialization about racial identity. This program decreased the effects of genetic risk (5-HTTLPR) on depression, risk behaviors, and alcohol use among 14-year-old African-American youths (Brody, Beach, Philibert, Chen, & Murry, 2009). Children with high-risk genotypes (ss or sl alleles) and without prevention exhibited much higher-risk behaviors compared both to children with similarly high-risk genotypes but who received the intervention program as well as to children with low-risk genotype (ll alleles).

Poverty can also affect family environments such as marital stability. Children in low-SES families are more likely to live with a single parent, or to experience parents' divorce (Evans, 2004). Waldman (2007) found that marital stability interacted with genes to predict attention-deficit/hyperactive disorder (ADHD) in childhood. Marital stability was measured based on mothers' reports on marital status, and number of marriages or cohabiting relationships. The interaction between marital stability and the dopamine receptor D2 gene (DRD2) was significantly linked with children's ADHD (Waldman, 2007).

Just as psychosocial characteristics such as parental responsiveness can help us understand the pathways through which genes could affect family functioning in relation to family resources, it is worth considering the potential interplay among genes, the physical environment, and family SES. Lead and other toxins have long been suspected to play a role in various behavioral disorders, including ADHD. Recently, Nigg showed that certain ADHD symptoms are very sensitive to early lead exposure but only among children with a genetic abnormality in the catecholamine receptor gene, DAT1, DRD4, and A2A, which is related to serotonin uptake (Nigg, 2008). Lead and other toxins are sadly much more likely to also vary tremendously among low- compared to middle- and upper-income populations, where almost no children are likely to experience such exposures (Evans, 2004).

Genetic variations may interact with environment to affect not only child development but also parenting itself. Living in a low-SES family is a risk factor for poor-quality parenting, which is linked to negative developmental outcomes of low-SES children (Evans, 2004). Low SES is associated with higher daily stress in parents (Hoff, Laursen, & Tardif, 2002; Magnuson & Duncan, 2002). Parents' daily stress and hassles were the most significant factors in determining the style and quality of parenting (Belsky, 1984). Mothers with greater stress and hassles reported increased levels of anger toward their infants (Aber, Belsky, Slade, & Crnic, 1999). Fathers with high levels of daily stress become less involved with their children and interact with them less often (Fagan, 2000). Low-income mothers are less responsive to their children than middle-class parents for two principal reasons: they experience higher levels of stress and tend to have smaller social networks (Evans, Boxhill, & Pinkava, 2008).

Guo cites a study which shows that a dopamine receptor gene (DRD2) affects juvenile delinquency but only when parents tend not to have regular family mealtimes together. Mealtime irregularity is an indicator of greater levels of household chaos in families. Higher levels of chaos covary with poverty (Evans, 2004; Evans, Eckenrode, & Marcynyszyn, in press). Van IJzendoorn, Bakermans-Kranenburg, and Mesman (2008) uncovered stress by gene interactions on parenting. In a study on parents of 1- to 3-year-old toddlers, the catechol-*O*-methyltransferase (COMT) variants – val/val or val/met – as well as the dopamine D4 receptor gene the 7R gene variant (DRD4-7R) were both related to diminished parental sensitivity among adults facing more daily hassles. With the same genetic variation carriers, lower levels of daily hassles were associated with more sensitive parenting (van IJzendoorn et al., 2008). On the one hand, this finding helps explain why some parents are more sensitive to daily hassles and their parenting quality may be more greatly affected by daily hassles and stress. On the other hand, this finding sheds light on why some children are able to grow up normally even when they are living in a high-stress environment, not just because of their own resiliency, but also because of their parents' resiliency to stress.

However, it is important to note that these findings on the effects of gene and environment interaction are from a small number of studies. More studies replicating the findings are needed to be conclusive. It is also important to tease apart primary and secondary genetic effects on human development. Given that parents and children share genetic and environmental overlap, some of the apparent parent × genetic interaction could be child genetic × environment interaction. The opposite is also true. Some of the apparent child genetic × environment effects could actually reflect parent genetic × environmental interactions manifested via parenting.

As Guo notes (Chap. 13), relations between genes and environments are likely more complex than simple individual genetic by environment interactions. Particularly in more heterogeneous groups, the nature of the gene and environment relationships may vary with the environment. Of particular interest to us is the potential role of SES to alter how biological factors in family environments nterrelate. Behavioral genetic studies of IQ show that inheritability is much higher in affluent samples whereas environmental effects are much higher in low-income samples (Turkheimer, Haley, Waldron, D'Onofrio, & Gottesman, 2003). Two possible explanations for this robust finding have been offered to date and both are highly salient to biology and family effects. First, there are greater environmental variations in low-SES populations in comparison to more privileged groups. Low-SES children are exposed to a greater degree of variations in terms of social support, parenting quality, neighborhood resources, and physical environmental qualities such as noise, crowding, housing, and toxins. Also, as noted above, low-SES environments are more chaotic and unstable (Evans, 2004). Thus, environmental variations may contribute more to the IQ differences observed among the low-SES children vis-a-vis genetic variation. On the other hand, in middle- and high-SES groups where social and physical environmental variability tends to be more restricted, outcomes like IQ are more likely to be influenced by within-group genetic differences.

A second, complementary explanation for SES heterogeneity in gene × environment effects could be that genetic differences are accentuated in good environments because the proximal processes that actualize genetic potentials operate more strongly in advantaged and stable environment than in disadvantaged environment (Bronfenbrenner & Ceci, 1994). Proximal processes are the ongoing exchanges of energy between the developing person and other persons, symbols, and physical objects wherein the setting individuals are embedded. Bronfenbrenner referred to proximal processes as the 'engines of development'. This is also why settings more proximate to the child influence development to a greater degree than more distal environments. Proximal processes transpire directly in the child's microenvironment. Other surrounding environmental characteristics, including SES, work largely through mediated microsetting alterations. Bronfenbrenner and Ceci (1994) noted, for example, that children with two biological parents compared to those living with their own mother and stepfather or with their biological mother only have higher grades (Small & Luster, 1990). Mother's educational levels did not impact children's grades with the exception of one group. When children lived with two biological parents and their mother's educational levels exceeded high school, their grades were higher compared with any other group of children. Proximal processes in this example were parental monitoring. In this supportive environment for children, the gene for higher cognitive ability development can be fully potentiated and expressed. Thus, it may be that the contribution of genetic effects to cognitive development may become greater in high-SES groups compared with low-SES groups.

It is also possible that proximal processes that buffer genetic potentials for behavioral problems may operate more strongly in disadvantaged groups. High social support is hard to come by in low-SES groups. Thus, a supportive environment may have greater protective effects in low-SES groups compared with high-SES groups. Genetics might then matter more for a low-SES group if the gene was a marker for a protective resource with respect to an adverse developmental outcome. If this is correct, then the situation is even more complex than Guo suggests. Gene by environment interactions may vary with population characteristics because of environmental heterogeneity and with respect to functional versus dysfunctional outcomes.

Guo summarizes the ways in which genes can interact with environments, particularly with respect to delinquent behaviors among adolescents. However, it is also important to understand the biological mechanisms that account for gene and environment interactions as they affect behavior. So far, the biological mechanisms literature has focused on investigating gene variations that potentially affect regulation of neurotransmitters and expressions of the neurotransmitter receptors in different brain areas. The neurotransmitters typically act in different brain sites and affect how an individual perceives, remembers, learns, and interprets information from the environment. Thus, it is important to understand relations between genes and the brain in order to comprehend the role of genes in modifying environmental effects on behaviors. Much of this cutting-edge work has occurred in animal models, although recently some human neuroimaging paradigms have been creatively applied to understanding biological mechanisms for genetic and environmental effects on behavior.

Polymorphism in the promoter region of the MAOA gene encodes the MAOA enzyme – an important inhibitor of three kinds of catecholamines the neurotransmitters norepinephrine, dopamine, and serotonin. Low activity of MAOA genotype is linked to elevated norepinephrine, dopamine, and serotonin levels in mice (Cases et al., 1995). These same neurotransmitters are central to emotion regulation (Shih, Chen, & Ridd, 1999). Recent fMRI studies in humans have found that low-MAOA activity genotype shows different activations in brain regions related to emotional information processing including the amygdala, hippocampus, and insula in response to negative emotional stimuli (Alia-Klein et al., 2009). Low-MAOA activity genotype is related to greater amygdala activations in response to angry words (Meyer-Lindenberg et al., 2006). Thus, low-MAOA activity may affect behaviors, particularly aggressive behaviors through different brain activations, related to increased levels of the neurotransmitters in humans. It is intriguing to consider that a common behavioral manifestation of low SES is difficulties in emotion regulation (Evans & English, 2002) and that such difficulties appear to be related to both socioemotional and cognitive problems associated with poverty in children (Evans & Rosenbaum, 2008).

The COMT gene plays a role in regulating dopaminergic activity in the human brain (van IJzendoorn et al., 2008). The met allele codes for an enzyme with much lower levels of activity in metabolizing dopamine compared with the enzyme that is coded by the val allele. COMT gene influences the activity of dopamine particularly in the limbic and the prefrontal cortex, areas important for emotion regulation. Met allele carriers show increased limbic and prefrontal activation in response to negative emotional stimuli (Smolka et al., 2005). There is also evidence of greater connectivity of amygdala, hippocampus, and orbitofrontal cortex among subjects with met/met subjects (Drabant et al., 2006). Thus, individuals with the met allele variant of COMT may exhibit greater reactivity to stress in the environment.

The dopamine D4 receptor gene (DRD4) contains a repeated sequence polymorphism within its coding sequences that changes the length of the receptor protein (Propper, Willoughby, Halpern, Carbone, & Cox, 2007). The long polymorphism such as the 7R gene variant (DRD4-7R) codes for a receptor that is less efficient in binding dopamine compared with the receptors coded for by a short polymorphism. DRD4 is primarily expressed in limbic areas, which are particularly important for emotion and behavioral regulation. DRD4-7R has been associated with impulsive behaviors and Attention Deficit Hyperactivity Disorder (ADHD). Infants with DRD4R-7R show higher levels of activity and exploration of the environment at 12 months (Benjamin et al., 1996) compared with infants with short DRD4 (Benjamin et al., 1996). Children with DRD4-7R are also more vulnerable to negative environment such as disorganized attachment and externalizing behavioral problems (Bakermans-Kranenburg & van Ijzendoorn, 2006).

The short (s) allele of the serotonin transporter gene promoter polymorphism (5-HTTLPR) is associated with reduced transcription and functional capacity of the serotonin transporter relative to the long (l) allele (Kaufman et al., 2004). 5-HTTLPR plays a role in regulating the serotonin function throughout the brain regions. The short-allele variant of 5-HTTLPR increased reactivity to stressful environments that can lead to depression (Taylor et al., 2006). Both childhood stress and stressful events in adulthood are linked to higher levels of depressive symptoms. Furthermore, among individuals with adverse experience in childhood or adulthood, those with the short alleles of the serotonin transporter gene-linked polymorphic region (5-HTTLPR) were more likely to develop depressive symptoms compared to ones with the long alleles of 5-HTTLPR. The short alleles of the serotonin transporter gene-linked polymorphic region (5-HTTLPR) have been linked to increased risks of depression both in children and adults (Taylor et al., 2006). Thus, one of the reasons low-SES children and adults may suffer higher levels of depression on average could be because of experiencing more stressful events in concert with genetic vulnerabilities such as the short allele of 5-HTTLPR.

The modifying effect of chronic stress on 5-HTTLPR and serotonin regulation has been found in several studies. Central serotonergic responsivity was tested through plasma prolactin response to the serotonin releasing agent, fenfluramine (Manuck, Flory, Ferrell, & Muldoon, 2004). Serotonergic responsivity was predicted by the interaction between 5-HTTLPR genotype and SES among adults. Individuals of low SES and ss allele 5-HTTLPR genotype show lower serotonergic responsivity (Manuck et al., 2004). Primate research found that peer-reared monkey infants exhibit reduced basal and central serotonergic functioning (Bennett et al., 2002). Since chronic stress exposure is higher in low-SES populations and may actually alter genetic expression (i.e., epigenesis), low-income children may be doubly vulnerable to these toxic gene × environment interactions.

The mechanisms underlying some epigenetic effects of chronic stress have been studied. Chronic stress such as childhood abuse modifies DNA methylation of a neuron-specific glucocorticoid receptor (GR) (NR3c1) promoter in the hippocampus (McGowan et al., 2009). This epigenetic modification leads to decreased hippocampal GR expression and decreased hippocampal synaptic density (Bredy, Grant, Champagne, & Meaney, 2003). Chronic stress such as exposure to poverty was associated with hippocampal volume shrinkage in human adults (Gianaros et al., 2008). In humans, adults who experienced adverse parenting such as physical and/or sexual abuse in childhood also have significantly smaller hippocampal volumes as adults (Vythilingam et al., 2002). Furthermore, early parenting may be associated with hippocampal activations in response to infant stimuli, which may be further associated with the next generation's parenting behaviors. While listening to the sound of a baby cry, mothers who had received lower quality of maternal care during their own childhood had greater hippocampal activations compared to mothers who had received higher quality maternal care (Kim et al., 2010). Higher hippocampal reactivity may be associated with abnormality in stress regulation in response to infant stimuli.

Decreased levels of GRs in the hippocampus due to exposure to chronic stress are linked to decreased inhibition of the hypothalamic–pituitary–adrenal (HPA) axis by the hippocampus. Decreased levels of GR expression are associated with increased stress reactivity, abnormal HPA axis regulation, and increased cortisol levels. Low quality of maternal care such as child abuse also leads to dysregulation of neurobiological stress systems such as increased cortisol levels (Elzinga, Schmahl, Vermetten, van Dyck, & Bremner, 2003; Evans & Kim, 2007; Heim & Nemeroff, 2001). The effects of chronic stress on neurobiological stress systems may start even before a child's birth. Recent studies based on the fetal programing hypothesis suggest that the maternal emotional state during pregnancy has a profound impact on fetal brain development (Van den Bergh, Mulder, Mennes, & Glover, 2005). Maternal hypercortisolism influenced by prenatal stress can alter the fetal HPA axis system. A recent study found that prenatal exposure to maternal depression or anxious mood was associated with increased methylation of NR3c1. Increased levels of NR3c1 methylation were further associated with heightened cortisol reactivity in response to stress among infants at 3 months (Oberlander et al., 2008).

Decreased levels of GRs in the hippocampus, stemming from chronic stress exposure, may also contribute to the inability of the organism to regulate peripheral stress, also known as high *allostatic load.* Allostatic load is an index of cumulative wear-and-tear on both the brain and the body in response to environmental demands.

Overexposure to a combination of multiple, active bodily response systems interfere with the body's ability to respond efficiently to environmental demands. Thus, the regulatory systems may either fail to turn off properly or become unable to generate adequate responses to an acute stressor (McEwen, 2000). Childhood poverty is associated with elevated levels of neuroendocrine activities such as heightened basal levels of cortisol, epinephrine, and norepinephrine. Continual exposure to poverty may also result in inefficient cardiovascular regulatory functions such as dampened reactivity and slower, inefficient recovery to basal levels (Evans & English, 2002; Evans, Kim, Ting, Tesher, & Shannis, 2007). Furthermore, we have found that exposure to childhood poverty is associated with poor working memory among young adults and that this relationship is mediated by allostatic load. The prefrontal cortex and hippocampus are involved in working memory (Evans & Schamberg, 2009). Thus, chronic stress exposure associated with childhood poverty may elevate allostatic load. This is hypothesized, in turn, to alter brain function and morphology in several of the areas implicated in genetic research. What is unclear at this time is whether these processes reflect epigenesis or are orthogonal to genetic predispositions which affect individual susceptibility to allostatic load.

The discussion contained in this review aims to complement Guo's excellent chapter by elucidating the relevance of genetics, social, and physical environmental factors linked to low-SES families and their children. By integrating biological theory and findings into family research, we can obtain a more complete picture of the ecological context of family resources and human development over the life course.

Acknowledgment Preparation of this chapter was partially supported by the W.T. Grant Foundation, the John D. and Catherine T. MacArthur Foundation Network on Socioeconomic Status and Health.

References

Aber, J., Belsky, J., Slade, A., & Crnic, K. (1999). Stability and change in mothers' representations of their relationship with their toddlers. *Developmental Psychology, 35*, 1038–1047.

Alia-Klein, N., Goldstein, R. Z., Tomasi, D., Woicik, P. A., Moeller, S. J., Williams, B., et al. (2009). Neural mechanisms of anger regulation as a function of genetic risk for violence. *Emotion, 9*, 385–396.

Bakermans-Kranenburg, M. J., & van Ijzendoorn, M. H. (2006). Gene-environment interaction of the dopamine D4 receptor (DRD4) and observed maternal insensitivity predicting externalizing behavior in preschoolers. *Developmental Psychobiology, 48*, 406–409.

Belsky, J. (1984). The determinants of parenting: A process model. *Child Development, 55*, 83–96.

Benjamin, J., Li, L., Patterson, C., Greenberg, B. D., Murphy, D. L., & Hamer, D. H. (1996). Population and familial association between the D4 dopamine receptor gene and measures of novelty seeking. *Nature Genetics, 12*, 81–84.

Bennett, A. J., Lesch, K. P., Heils, A., Long, J. C., Lorenz, J. G., Shoaf, S. E., et al. (2002). Early experience and serotonin transporter gene variation interact to influence primate CNS function. *Molecular Psychiatry, 7*, 118–122.

Bredy, T. W., Grant, R. J., Champagne, D. L., & Meaney, M. J. (2003). Maternal care influences neuronal survival in the hippocampus of the rat. *European Journal of Neuroscience, 18*, 2903–2909.

Brody, G. H., Beach, S. R., Philibert, R. A., Chen, Y. F., & Murry, V. M. (2009). Prevention effects moderate the association of 5-HTTLPR and youth risk behavior initiation: Gene x environment hypotheses tested via a randomized prevention design. *Child Development, 80,* 645–661.

Bronfenbrenner, U., & Ceci, S. J. (1994). Nature-nurture reconceptualized in developmental perspective: A bioecological model. *Psychological Review, 101,* 568–586.

Cases, O., Seif, I., Grimsby, J., Gaspar, P., Chen, K., Pournin, S., et al. (1995). Aggressive behavior and altered amounts of brain serotonin and norepinephrine in mice lacking MAOA. *Science, 268,* 1763–1766.

Drabant, E. M., Hariri, A. R., Meyer-Lindenberg, A., Munoz, K. E., Mattay, V. S., Kolachana, B. S., et al. (2006). Catechol O-methyltransferase val158met genotype and neural mechanisms related to affective arousal and regulation. *Archives of General Psychiatry, 63,* 1396–1406.

Elzinga, B. M., Schmahl, C. G., Vermetten, E., van Dyck, R., Bremner, J. D. (2003). Higher cortisol levels following exposure to traumatic reminders in abuse-related PTSD. *Neuropsychopharmacology, 28,* 1656–1665.

Evans, G. W. (2004). The environment of childhood poverty. *American Psychologist, 59,* 77–92.

Evans, G. W., Boxhill, L., & Pinkava, M. (2008). Poverty and maternal responsiveness: The role of maternal stress and social resources. *International Journal of Behavioral Development, 32,* 232–237.

Evans, G. W., Eckenrode, J., & Marcynyszyn, L. A. (2009). Poverty and chaos. In G. Evans & T. D. Wachs (Eds.), *Chaos and its influence on children's development: An ecological perspective.* Washington: American Psychological Association (pp. 225–238).

Evans, G. W., & English, K. (2002). The environment of poverty: Multiple stressor exposure, psychophysical stress, and socioemotional adjustment. *Child Development, 73,* 1238–1248.

Evans, G. W., & Kim, P. (2007). Childhood poverty and health: Cumulative risk exposure and stress dysregulation. *Psychological Science, 18,* 953–957.

Evans, G. W., Kim, P., Ting, A. H., Tesher, H. B., & Shannis, D. (2007). Cumulative risk, maternal responsiveness, and allostatic load among young adolescents. *Developmental Psychology, 43,* 341–351.

Evans, G. W., & Rosenbaum, J. (2008). Self-regulation and the income-achievement gap. *Early Childhood Research Quarterly, 23,* 504–514.

Evans, G. W., & Schamberg, M. A. (2009). Childhood poverty, chronic stress, and adult working memory. *Proceedings of the National Academy of Sciences, 106,* 6545–6549.

Fagan, J. (2000). Head Start fathers' daily hassles and involvement with their children. *Journal of Family Issues, 21,* 329–346.

Gianaros, P. J., Horenstein, J. A., Hariri, A. R., Sheu, L. K., Manuck, S. B., Matthews, K. A., et al. (2008). Potential neural embedding of parental social standing. *Social, Cognitive and Affective Neuroscience, 3,* 91–96.

Haeffel, G. J., Getchell, M., Koposov, R. A., Yrigollen, C. M., Deyoung, C. G., Klinteberg, B. A., et al. (2008). Association between polymorphisms in the dopamine transporter gene and depression: evidence for a gene-environment interaction in a sample of juvenile detainees. *Psychological Science, 19,* 62–69.

Heim, C., & Nemeroff, C. B. (2001). The role of childhood trauma in the neurobiology of mood and anxiety disorders: Preclinical and clinical studies. *Biological Psychiatry, 49,* 1023–1039.

Hoff, E., Laursen, B., & Tardif, T. (2002). Socioeconomic status and parenting. In M. H. Bornstein (Ed.), *Handbook of parenting* (Vol. 2, pp. 231–252). Mahwah: Lawrence Erlbaum Associates.

Kaufman, J., Yang, B. Z., Douglas-Palumberi, H., Houshyar, S., Lipschitz, D., Krystal, J. H., et al. (2004). Social supports and serotonin transporter gene moderate depression in maltreated children. *Proceedings of the National Academy of Sciences, 101,* 17316–17321.

Kim-Cohen, J., Caspi, A., Taylor, A., Williams, B., Newcombe, R., Craig, I. W., et al. (2006). MAOA, maltreatment, and gene-environment interaction predicting children's mental health: New evidence and a meta-analysis. *Molecular Psychiatry, 11,* 903–913.

Kim, P., Leckman, J. F., Mayes, L. C., Newman, M., Feldman, R., & Swain, J. E. (2010). Perceived quality of maternal care in childhood and structure and function of mothers' brain. *Developmental Science, 13*(4), 662–673.

Magnuson, K. A., & Duncan, G. J. (2002). Parents in poverty. In M. H. Bornstein (Ed.), *Handbook of parenting* (2nd ed., Vol. 4, pp. 95–121). Mahwah: Lawrence Erlbaum Associates.

Manuck, S. B., Flory, J. D., Ferrell, R. E., & Muldoon, M. F. (2004). Socio-economic status covaries with central nervous system serotonergic responsivity as a function of allelic variation in the serotonin transporter gene-linked polymorphic region. *Psychoneuroendocrinology, 29,* 651–668.

McEwen, B. S. (2000). Allostasis and allostatic load: Implications for neuropsychopharmacology. *Neuropsychopharmacology, 22,* 108–124.

McGowan, P. O., Sasaki, A., D'Alessio, A. C., Dymov, S., Labonté, B., Szyf, M., et al. (2009). Epigenetic regulation of the glucocorticoid receptor in human brain associates with childhood abuse. *Nature Neuroscience, 12,* 342–348.

Meyer-Lindenberg, A., Buckholtz, J. W., Kolachana, B., Hariri, A. R., Pezawas, L., Blasi, G., et al. (2006). Neural mechanisms of genetic risk for impulsivity and violence in humans. *Proceedings of the National Academy of Sciences, 103,* 6269–6274.

Nigg, J. (2008). *Genetic and environmental factors in ADHD: New insights from lead exposure studies.* Paper presented at the 2008 John Merck Fund Summer Institute on the Biology of Developmental Disabilities, Ithaca.

Oberlander, T. F., Weinberg, J., Papsdorf, M., Grunau, R., Misri, S., & Devlin, A. M. (2008). Prenatal exposure to maternal depression, neonatal methylation of human glucocorticoid receptor gene (NR3C1) and infant cortisol stress responses. *Epigenetics, 3,* 97–106.

Propper, C., Willoughby, M., Halpern, C. T., Carbone, M. A., & Cox, M. (2007). Parenting quality, DRD4, and the prediction of externalizing and internalizing behaviors in early childhood. *Developmental Psychobiology, 49,* 619–632.

Repetti, R. L., Taylor, S. E., & Seeman, T. E. (2002). Risky families: Family social environments and the mental and physical health of offspring. *Psychological Bulletin, 128,* 330–366.

Shih, J. C., Chen, K., & Ridd, M. J. (1999). Monoamine oxidase: From genes to behavior. *Annual Review of Neuroscience, 22,* 197–217.

Small, S., & Luster, T. (1990). *Youth at risk for parenthood.* Paper presented at the Creating Caring Communities Conference, Michigan State University, East Lansing.

Smolka, M. N., Schumann, G., Wrase, J., Grüsser, S. M., Flor, H., Mann, K., et al. (2005). Catechol-O-methyltransferase val158met genotype affects processing of emotional stimuli in the amygdala and prefrontal cortex. *Journal of Neuroscience, 25,* 836–842.

Taylor, S., Baldwin, M., Welch, W., Hilmert, C., Lehman, B., & Eisenberger, N. (2006). Early family environment, current adversity, the serotonin transporter promoter polymorphism, and depressive symptomatology. *Biological Psychiatry, 60,* 671–676.

Turkheimer, E., Haley, A., Waldron, M., D'Onofrio, B., & Gottesman, I. I. (2003). Socioeconomic status modifies heritability of IQ in young children. *Psychological Science, 14,* 623–628.

Van den Bergh, B. R., Mulder, E. J., Mennes, M., & Glover, V. (2005). Antenatal maternal anxiety and stress and the neurobehavioural development of the fetus and child: links and possible mechanisms. A review. *Neuroscience and Biobehavioral Review, 29,* 237–258.

van IJzendoorn, M. H., Bakermans-Kranenburg, M. J., & Mesman, J. (2008). Dopamine system genes associated with parenting in the context of daily hassles. *Genes, Brain and Behavior, 7,* 403–410.

Vythilingam, M., Heim, C., Newport, J., Miller, A. H., Anderson, E., Bronen, R., et al. (2002). Childhood trauma associated with smaller hippocampal volume in women with major depression. *American Journal of Psychiatry, 159,* 2072–2080.

Waldman, I. D. (2007). Gene-environment interactions reexamined: Does mother's marital stability interact with the dopamine receptor D2 gene in the etiology of childhood attention-deficit/hyperactivity disorder? *Developmental Psychopathology, 19,* 1117–1128.

Chapter 16
In Search of GE: Why We Have Not Documented a Gene–Social Environment Interaction Yet

Dalton Conley

Abstract In this chapter, I argue that social science and genomics can be integrated – however, the way this marriage is currently occurring rests on spurious methods and assumptions and, as a result, will yield few lasting insights. Recent advances in both econometrics and developmental genomics provide scientists with a novel opportunity to understand how genes and (social) environment interact. Key to any causal inference about genetically heterogeneous effects of social conditions is that either genetics be exogenously manipulated while environment is held constant (and measured properly) and/or that environmental variation is exogenous in nature – i.e., experimental or arising from a natural experiment of sorts. Further, allele selection should be motivated by findings from genetic experiments in (model) animal studies linked to orthologous human genes. Likewise, genetic associations found in human population studies should then be tested through knock-out and overexpression studies in model organisms. Finally, epigenetic and gene expression analysis of corpse brains offers a potentially fruitful way to get at mechanisms by which social environment affects gene pathways.

Introduction

The study of genetic–environmental (GE) interactions has long been a goal of social scientists fond of expressing the dependence of genetic expression on social structure. However, how do we get from the sociological adage that "a gene for aggression lands you in prison if you're from the ghetto, but in the boardroom if you're to the manor born" to a serious empirical research program on the study of GE interactions? Even if we are only interested in "pure" environmental effects, how do we empirically deal with the lurking variable of "genotype" that can – and should – haunt our claims of environmental causality?

D. Conley (✉)
Department of Sociology, New York University, New York, NY, USA
e-mail: dc66@nyu.edu

A. Booth et al. (eds.), *Biosocial Foundations of Family Processes*,
National Symposium on Family Issues, DOI 10.1007/978-1-4419-7361-0_16,
© Springer Science+Business Media, LLC 2011

This is a particularly propitious time to investigate such GE interactions since the biological sciences may meet us halfway. Specifically, among molecular biologists there is increased interest in epigenetics – that is, the conditions under which and mechanisms by which genes are regulated (i.e., highly expressed or not) in response to environmental conditions through various mechanisms such as methylation and acetylation of histones (the nuclear material from which DNA must be uncoiled to be accessed for transcription), micro-RNA-mediated post-transcriptional regulation [whether or not messenger-RNA (mRNA) gets translated into a protein], and post-translational modifications of those protein products themselves to make them active or inactive (usually through phosphorylation of specific residues [i.e., amino acids]).

The subfield of psychology known as behavioral genetics (BG) has long proffered an answer to these challenges. Notable researchers such as Richard Plomin or David Rowe, as well as many others, have argued that by comparing social outcomes among genetically identical twins (i.e., monozygotic twins who share 100% of their nuclear genes) with those from fraternal twins (i.e., dizygotic twins who share, on average, 50% of their genes, just like singleton siblings), we can properly estimate the genetic, shared environmental, and nonshared environmental components of traits (see, e.g., DeFries, McGuffin, McClearn, & Plomin, 2000).

In the most naïve approach, genetic heritability is calculated as two times the difference between the intraclass correlations of identical and fraternal twins. However, more recently, much more complex structural models have been offered to account for various complications such as the fact that, as a result of assortative mating at the parental level, fraternal twins may share more than 50% of their genes. Likewise, the "equal environments" assumption has been relaxed. For the naïve calculation mentioned above, it is necessary to assume that the covariance between environment and genetics is zero. Put another way, the simple estimation of heritability requires the rather heroic assumption that identical twins experience the same degree of similarity in environment as do (same sex) fraternal twins. Newer models include an estimate of the degree to which environmental similarity varies with genetic likeness. However, these are just that: Estimates – often based on questions about whether or not respondents were "dressed alike" growing up, whether they were viewed as similarly as "two peas in a pod", and so on (see, e.g., Guo & Stearns, 2002; Lichtenstein, Pedersen, & McClearn, 1992; Rogers et al., 1999; Rowe & Teachman, 2001). Such questions are likely to capture only some of the ways that environmental similarity differs across identical and fraternal twin pairs, which is troubling since Goldberger (1979) has shown that depending on the GE covariance assumed, estimates of heritability can be driven wildly up or down.

Other more recent work has used adoptees to infer biological estimates of the heritability of social traits. For example, Sacerdote (2004) used a data set of Korean adoptees in the USA where assignment to families was random to examine the intergenerational correlation on important socioeconomic indicators such as educational attainment and income; on behaviors such as drinking and smoking; and on anthropometric measures such as height and weight. The results were then contrasted to intergenerational correlations among biological families from other data sources as well as biological children within those same families (for the subsample that contained biological children). The results showed that – as might be expected – heritability for physical traits was considerably stronger in biologically intact families. Education (specifically probability of graduating from a 4-year college) and income were also much more strongly inherited by biological children. However, health-related behavioral inheritance was similar across the two groups.

Before we accept the putative inference that education and income are predominantly genetically transmitted (while smoking and drinking are culturally transmitted), we must question the external validity of the adoptee sample. While there was adequate variation within the recipient families of adoptees, *on observables*, and while they did not look terribly different on average from nonadopting US families, on observables, we know, *ipso facto*, that families who adopt are a distinct social group on unobservables, as are the adoptees themselves. For example, if socialization is weaker among adoptees who do not feel connected to their adoptive parents, the difference in heritability could be weaker by virtue of this fact, not the absence of genetic similarity. Many other dynamics could be at work as well, such as increased (or decreased) parental investment, halo effects or stigma, and truncated genetic variability among adoptees (or adopters), which may work to bias estimates for this population in unpredictable ways. The only adoption study that would avoid such questions would be one in which adoptees were randomly selected from the newborn population and then randomly assigned to parents, with both groups blind to the treatment (i.e., not knowing whether they were adopted or not) – all while prenatal environment was held constant. In other words, it is an impossibility to reliably estimate genetic heritability using such an approach.

Other recent work uses differences in subpopulations as a proxy for environmental differences to examine genotype expression. This line of argument purports that certain groups – such as minorities or low-SES individuals – may face environmental obstacles to their full genetic expression (i.e., level of phenotypic capacitance). For example, Guo and Stearns (2002) argued that the heritability of verbal IQ for respondents in the National Longitudinal Survey of Adolescent Health (Add Health) is weaker when a parent is unemployed than when no parent is unemployed (42 vs. 54%). Similarly, in a multivariate context, they documented a lower heritability of verbal IQ for African American adolescents as compared to their white counterparts (58 vs. 72%). However, ascribing this difference across racial groups to a "constraining" effect of environment – while playing on the nurturist sympathies of the sociological community – is premature. It could be the case, for instance, that due to different degrees of assortative mating or fertility patterns, the degree of genotypic variation in IQ-related genes is lower among blacks and the unemployed (downwardly biasing heritability estimates), or that there is greater mean-regressive measurement error among siblings in these groups. While environment could constrain the "full" expression of genetic profiles, it could also be the case that the genetic profile itself is different within and between families facing different environments (i.e., African American and white families, or families with and without unemployed parents).

Most recently, genetic markers on specific loci – such as single point mutation polymorphisms (SNPs) – have seemed to offer hope for those interested in an explicit research program aimed at specifying and measuring gene–environment interactions for complex traits (what geneticists call quantitative traits). Polymor phisms are genetic variants that occur in at least 1% of the population. They could include base-pair substitutions – among one of the four nucleotides that make up our genetic code (G, guanine; C, cytosine; A, adenosine; and T, thymine) – that may affect the amino acid produced out of that codon (a triplet of nucleotides that deter-mine which amino acid should come next when the messenger-RNA is translated into a protein) if the polymorphism is in an open reading frame (ORF) of a gene (i.e., the protein-related coding region) and is nonsynonymous; they may truncate the protein by causing the transcription machinery to stop there (by producing a stop codon); or they may do nothing (what are called silent or synonymous mutations) since multiple three-letter codes may result in the same amino acid being produced (though perhaps at different efficiency levels, something called codon-bias). Hence, these nonlethal polymorphisms, which result from mutations, may present an oppor-tunity to study how specific environments – social or biophysical – may result in different outcomes depending on an individual's genotype.

The basic logic is the following: A certain proportion of a population sample is found to have a variant of a particular allele. *If* this allele is shown to be randomly distributed across demographic subgroups (or, e.g., *within* a particular subgroup such as ethnic group), and likewise it is found to be associated with a specific social outcome or tendency (such as addictiveness, shyness, schizophrenia, to name a few) *within* that same population (or subgroup as the case may be), then researchers may try to look for specific environmental conditions which seem to magnify or mitigate its effect – such as family structures, parents' behavior, or simply socioeconomic status. (If allele variation is studied within families [i.e., across siblings], then it does indeed offer a potential way to measure specific genetic influences with some certainty. One would then compare the expression of that allele – as compared to the sibling without the polymorphism, for example – in families of various demo-graphic or economic backgrounds. However, we must be cautious with this approach as well since rates of genetic linkage may be different among population subgroups. More on this issue below.)

The location of the genetic effect in specific places on the genome – combined with the lack of reliance on unknowable assumptions (in contrast to the twin approach's assumption of a specific GE covariance matrix for DZ and MZ twins) – is seen as a key step forward from earlier BG research. (Recent models also allow for genetic dominance – that is, nonlinear interactions between alleles.) However, since the object of study is typically just one allele, such analysis tells us little about the overall genetic heritability of an outcome. Second, even if it were found to vary across environmentally distinct populations (such as blacks and whites or the college-educated versus those who did not surpass a high school degree), it is not altogether clear whether differential effects are due to a genetic–environmental interaction [as purported in the adolescent IQ example of Guo and Stearns (2002)] or a gene–gene interaction. It could be that the allele(s) are interacting not with differential social environments, but rather with other, nonrandomly distributed genes (even if the principal gene in question is indeed randomly distributed).

For example, a paper by Caspi et al. (2002) that has become a classic in this area of research claims to have uncovered a GE interaction by comparing male children who have a particular functional polymorphism in the MAOA gene (monoamine oxidase A) – an enzyme that breaks down various neurotransmitters once they are chaperoned out of the synaptic cleft – with those who do not among a longitudinal sample of 1,037 white Australians followed from ages 3 to 26. Those individuals who showed a variable number tandem repeat (VNTR) in the promoter region of the gene (the area that precedes the actual coding portion but which is important to transcriptional activation and regulation) putatively transcribe (and by extension translate) MAOA at a lower rate than those without this polymorphism on their X-chromosome. In turn, MAOA activity as indicated by this genetic difference was interacted with degree of maltreatment the respondents experienced between the ages of 3 and 11 to predict an index of antisocial behavior that included four measures ranging from criminal convictions to antisocial personality disorder criteria of the DSM-IV. They argued that while other MAO genes may compensate for deficiencies in MAOA (in particular, MAOB), among children these are not yet fully expressed, thus making MAOA particularly important with respect to moderating the effect of maltreatment during early childhood.

Eight percent of the sample experienced severe maltreatment, 28% experienced "probable" maltreatment, and 64% experienced no maltreatment. In a multiple regression context, the main effect of maltreatment level on the antisocial behavior index was significant, whereas the main effect of MAOA activity level was not but an interaction effect between the two measures was statistically significant at the $\alpha = 0.01$ level. They argued that this is a true GE interaction effect since the MAOA genotypes were not significantly differently distributed across maltreatment levels – suggesting that this genotype did not itself influence exposure to maltreatment (i.e., the environment is not standing in for the genotype).

In a follow-up study (2006), they used the same cohort to examine the interaction of stressful life events with alleles of the serotonin transporter gene (5-HTT) linked promoter region (5-HTTLPR). Specifically, individuals who have a short 5' (i.e. upstream) promoter may show more propensity than those with a long promoter toward depression. However, previous studies had come to conflicting results; namely, many replications have failed to produce results claimed in earlier linkage studies. Some researchers had despaired that psychiatric and other behavioral phenotypes were controlled by so many quantitative trait genes that modeling genetic effects in a robust, direct way would not be possible and/or would account for little variation (see, e.g., Hamer, 2002). Caspi et al. (2003) instead argued that rather than complicated gene–gene interactions, the muddle of results could be resulting from GE interactions. This muddle motivated their search for an interaction effect of stressful life events and 5-HTTLPR allele.

This is an autosomal gene – meaning that individuals of both sexes have two copies – so they compared individuals with the homozygous long genotypes and heterozygotes (long/short) with those who were homozygous for the short alleles. They found that in the subsample who had experienced no stressful life events between ages 21 and 26, there was no difference between the three genotypes in the propensity to depression. However, as the number of self-reported stressful life events increased, the genotypes diverged with respect to their likelihood of clinical depression at age 26. They interpreted this as a GE interaction.

However, it could still be possible that what Caspi et al. were uncovering was actually a gene–gene interaction in both studies, because they did not have an exogenous source of environmental variation. In the latter case, those with the "at risk," short alleles were in fact more likely to report stressful events than those who had long alleles. We may conclude, then, that measured genotype did influence the measured environmental measure. The researchers tried to get around this by reversing the time order: Measuring stressful life events between ages 21 and 26 and measuring depression at age 21 (i.e., prior). When they did this, they did not find the significant interaction that had emerged in the "correctly" ordered model. However, it still may be the case that depression was induced by a gene–gene interaction since it may be an underlying unmeasured gene that causes the phenotype of "negative life events" to emerge in one's early 20s: Imagine a gene that causes excessive thrill-seeking and risk-taking, which in turn manifests as negative events during one's early adulthood. As for the MAOA interaction, we face the same issue: While measured maltreatment did not vary by MAOA status, it could very well have varied by other genes (present in the parents and potentially passed on to the children). Thus, it would not be the maltreatment that interacted with MAOA status but rather the underlying, unmeasured genotype, which, in combination with given MAOA alleles, causes both parents and offspring to act antisocially.

In fact, in recent analysis of the National Longitudinal Survey of Adolescent Health genetic subsample reported elsewhere (Conley & Rauscher, 2010), we find no significant effects of polymorphisms in either MAOA or 5-HTTP. What's more, we find no significant interaction across identical twin pairs (or within fraternal pairs for that matter) between MAOA polymorphism and birth weight (putatively exogenous due to fetal position – at least for MZ twins) and a significant interaction with the opposite sign for 5-HTTP interacted with the prenatal environmental "insult" of low birth weight. So the final word is far from the Caspi findings.

To complicate matters even further, absent genetic experiments that knock out or overexpress specific genes, we can never be sure that the allele in question is what is causing any observed effect (irrespective of environmental interactions); thanks to the possibility of genetic linkage mentioned above. Namely, genes are "shuffled" across the chromosomes of a parent during the recombination period of meiosis. (Meiosis results in the formation of the 1N gamete – i.e., the sperm or egg.) However, two alleles are more likely to stay paired together in a given gamete the closer they are to each other on the chromosome – hence, the term linkage or linkage disequilibrium – since they are more likely to be found on the same pieces of DNA that are exchanged. A helpful analogy is the shuffling of a deck of cards: It is more likely that cards right next to each other will not get separated in the shuffling process than it is for cards separated by a longer "distance." So even when we know that a given gene is associated with a quantitative trait, we cannot be 100% sure (absent genetic experiments on nonhumans) that said gene is causally responsible. The best we can say is that the area of the genome is associated with the phenotype under study. If we allow for different degrees of genetic linkage of particular genes with other genes by population, then we cannot even plausibly say (for sure) that a given gene is responsible for the outcome in two different populations even if we observe the same marker-phenotype association (never mind GE interactions).

However, the real rub is that since we can plausibly postulate second-, third-, fourth-, and, ultimately, Nth-order interactions across alleles, there simply would not be enough degrees of freedom in the approximately seven billion human beings currently occupying the planet to properly test a fully specified model ($19,000! = 1.83 \, E^{73047} > 7,000,000,000$). The discovery of about 21,000 genes – a figure much lower than originally hypothesized – is good news in that it is a tractable number of alleles for geneticists to study. However, the irony lies in the fact that if this lowly number of genes explains the development of human beings in all their glorious forms, then gene–gene interactions are probably quite important. There is also a recent explosion of discoveries relating to the important role of micro-RNAs in affecting how messenger-RNAs are spliced (and therefore can produce multiple products) and whether or not they get translated at all (as well as increased interest in other nonprotein products of DNA once considered "junk").

Below I offer a way out of this epistemological morass that involves isolating candidate genes not through associational studies, but through deployment of animal models, where genetic experimentation allows for causal inference with respect to specific genotype–phenotype relationships. Once candidate genes are identified in animal studies, these can then be linked to putative human genes that may play a similar role. Finally, the role of these genes can be studied in human population-based studies that have exogenous environmental variation.

Step 1: Deploy Animal Models

A potentially fruitful approach to identifying GE interactions may arise out of the deployment of animal models by biosociologists. Sociologists maintain a strangely ambivalent relationship to nonhuman animals. On the one hand, given the strong leftist leanings of many sociologists, proenvironment sentiment runs strong within the field. Central to the paradigm of environmentalism is the notion that humans do not occupy a privileged position within natural systems. This idea, of course, is not unique to environmental sociologists, or even sociologists, but to many humanists as well as natural scientists. Sociologists, however, occupy a uniquely paradoxical position within this group of scholars. This is due to the wholesale rejection by the mainstream of the discipline of animal models of social behavior. Having founded ourselves in the early twentieth century as a science against the elemental, "reductionistic," naturalizing explanatory frameworks of the biological sciences, we have boxed ourselves into a corner by rejecting wholesale the notion that studies of other species may yield insight into human social phenomena.

I argue that this has put us at an extreme disadvantage in an era when "model organisms" (to be defined below) are examined with increasingly powerful tools by biologists in order to illuminate generalizable phenomena about natural systems, innate and learned behavior; and even social life. By contemporary standards, a model organism is one in which the genome has been (largely) sequenced; where there is a short time between generations; sexual reproduction; and for which there have been developed a number of genetic tools that work for that organism (such as plasmid libraries, mutant lines, and so on). As mentioned above, current model organisms range from the nematode worm (*Caenorhabditis elegans*) to the fruit fly (*Drosophila melanogaster*) to zebrafish (*Danio rerio*) to mice (*Mus musculus*). Each provides advantages and disadvantages. For example, in comparing *C. elegans* with *D. melanogaster*, the generation time is faster for the worm (4 days) as compared to the fly (10 days) but if one is interested in behavior, the worm is perhaps too simple a system to study. Mice, as compared to flies, are, of course, mammals with nervous systems much closer to our own, but who have a much longer generation time and higher cost to maintain – not to mention fewer mutant lines that have been obtained as of yet. That is, though the mouse genome has been sequenced, less is known about the characteristics (i.e., expression patterns, protein structures, and so on) of mice genes as compared to the fruit fly.

The main advantage of using animals is the ability of the researcher to experimentally manipulate environmental and social conditions to study their epigenetic consequences while simultaneously being able to manipulate the genetic background of the creatures using knock-outs (vectors that disable expression of a particular gene) or hybrids (that allow for the expression of exogenous genes from other species within an given organism or the overexpression of certain endogenous genes under specific conditions of the scientist's design and choosing). The experimental approach of "bench science" genetics provides such great power in narrowing down molecular, causal pathways linking social or behavioral variation to outcomes that the tradeoff with concerns about the external validity of such results to human biosocial systems is more than adequately compensated for, in my opinion, at least. This holds true, I would purport, when the genes under study have clear orthologs in *Homo sapiens* (though even if they do not, such knowledge may provide a useful general understanding of the way social and genetic systems are linked that may still be informative).

The basic idea is the following: Use a particular genetic strain that has been well-characterized in a given model organism with respect to a specific behavior to identify specific genetic pathways that accentuate (or repress) the observed phenotype using adequate negative and positive controls. Once a gene of interest has been identified and well-understood (and putative gene–environment interactions have been tested), the researcher would then use the Basic Local Alignment Sequence Tool (BLAST – http://blast.ncbi.nlm.nih.gov/Blast.cgi) to find an orthologous gene in humans (see Fig. 16.1). If the gene is highly conserved across taxa (and thus

BLAST result

Compares nucleotide or protein sequences to sequence databases

Calculates the statistical significance of matches

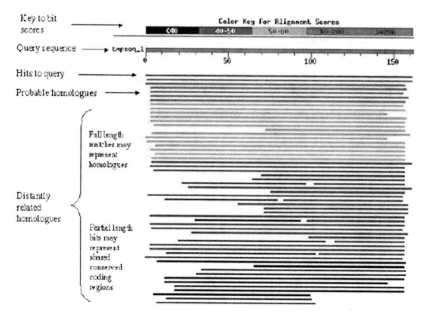

Fig. 16.1 Sample output from using BLAST to find human ortholog to a gene from a model organism (in this case tissue from *Mus musculus* adult male kidney cDNA, RIKEN full-length enriched library, clone:0610037P21 product:carnitine palmitoyltransferase 2).

putatively important), then there should be a well-matched homolog in the human species. This gene then provides a good starting point for looking at potential associations with behavioral outcomes.[1]

---

[1] However, a number of counter examples can be found where associational fishing expeditions have led to more tenuous findings that have not withstood the rigors of replication. One notable example can be found in the so-called "gay gene." In 1993, Hamer et al. published an article in *Science* showing an association between a microsatellite on the X-chromosome (called Xq28) and homosexuality in men. The conclusion rested on the greater propensity of gay brothers to share genetic markers at this locus as well as pedigree analysis that showed a greater likelihood of gay men to have other gay male relatives on their maternal side (since the X that males receive always comes from their mother). Later work (see, Rice et al., 1999) failed to replicate the findings among a similar sample of Canadian brothers and a heated debate ensued. Hamer et al.'s study is among the better of the associational studies given its pedigree-based analysis, but like many others in the field it relies on a small, non-representative sample and purports to explain a complicated phenotype: *stated* sexual orientation. I underline "stated" for a reason: Even if the results could be routinely replicated, it may be the case that the Xq28 locus is associated with willingness to reveal homosexuality to survey takers rather than to homosexuality itself, given its sometimes stigmatizing status in North American culture.

Current behaviorally related genes that have been isolated in model organisms such as *D. melanogaster* include *dunce* (learning); *rutabaga* (memory); *fruitless* (courtship and aggression in males). This is, of course, a small sample of a rapidly growing list of genes in model organisms ranging from *C. elegans* to mice and rats that have been linked to behaviors that have clear human analogs. To be fair to Caspi et al., as well as others, the genes that they explored (notably 5-HTT and MAOA) were not targeted; thanks to data-mining exercises but rather as a result of animal studies as suggested above.

Step 2. Apply to Human Population Data and Add Exogenous Environmental Variation

Once human candidate gene markers have been deduced from experimental results in animal studies (in contrast to the typical association studies currently used by human population geneticists), the study of these genes in human social life can proceed. Next, I argue that it is in fact possible to obtain empirically robust estimates of genetic environmental interaction effects. However, the strategy needed to parameterize such effects relies on the proper estimation of truly exogenous, causal *environmental* effects. Once an exogenous source of environmental variation has been identified, then it is possible to look for differential treatment effects based on genotypical characteristics – polymorphisms, haplotypes (groups of polymorphisms that cluster uniquely together), and the like – that vary randomly within a given subpopulation (family, ethnic group, and so on). So, in short, the first task at hand for the sociologist who desires to show environmental-genetic interactions is the same task facing all sociologists who seek to rule out genetic (or other unobserved) factors when assessing causal, environmental effects.

Once we have an exogenous source of variation in, let us say, schooling, then we can identify an interaction effect between years of schooling and some genetic marker in looking at outcomes such as income, criminality, shyness, and so on. Let us take the example of Lleras-Muney (2005), who estimated the mortality returns to an additional year of high school by focusing on educational variation generated by changes in compulsory schooling laws during the first half of the twentieth century. These changes in state laws generate an exogenous change in the environmental characteristics of schooling because they affected everyone, regardless of genetic makeup or other characteristics. If she had enjoyed access to genetic information in her sample (which she did not, having used the US Census as her data source), she would have been able to interact instrumented years of schooling (predicted based on these exogenous law changes and individual-level characteristics), with a given genetic marker when estimating the mortality effects of schooling (assuming the genetic marker was not significantly associated with education and was randomly distributed across existing population divisions, such as race and SES). In this way, she would have been able to tell if certain genetic profiles receive larger health benefits from additional schooling than other genotypes. Of course, hopefully one would begin such a project with a theory about why the expression of a given gene (i.e., the causal pathway from gene to protein to outcome) would vary based on an environmental characteristic like education – rather than just going in with a fishing net to troll for associations. (Multiple hypothesis testing – with so many potential genetic loci of study – is of major concern here. Luckily, biologists have elaborated on the Bonferroni correction to produce a series of ways to approach the problem of false positives; see, e.g., Thornton & Jensen, 2007).

In sum, in order to investigate GE interactions, we need some source of exogeneity on the environmental side as a lever for estimation (as well as evidence that the marker is not significantly associated with plausible subgroups in our sample or statistical controls for such possible associations). Until such time that we can exogenously affect genotype through genetic manipulation or through a natural experiment that results in genetic variation (such as genetic drift of some measurable sort or monozygotic twin differences in mitochondrial DNA), but which does not affect environmental influence (fat chance), exogenous environmental variation is our only hope to identify a GE interaction in a human population.

Economists have pioneered a number of ways to get closer to causal estimates. First, there are instrumental variable (IV) strategies (also called two-stage least squares), which use a source of exogenous variation (i.e., the instrument, Z) to predict the covariate of interest (X), and then use the predicted covariate (X^*) to model the outcome. [For a general review, see Winship and Morgan (1999).] A particularly notable example of instrumental variable estimation is provided by Angrist (1990), who estimated the effect of military service during the Vietnam War period on subsequent earnings, using the draft lottery as a source of exogenous variation in veteran status. Another example is provided by Conley and Glauber (2006), who estimated effects of sibship size on parental educational investment, using the sex mix of the first two children born into a family to instrument whether or not parents have a third child or not (the sex of a child depends on the random segregation of X and Y chromosomes in the paternal gametes; US parents are more likely to have a third child if the first two are of the same sex). More recently, economists have deployed regression discontinuity (RD) designs (see, e.g., van der Klaauw, 2002, on the effects of financial aid on college enrollment decisions; or Lee, 2008 on the power of congressional incumbency on subsequent vote share), where researchers compare subjects that fall just on either side of an otherwise arbitrary cut-off point, such as those who score a few points above or below an admissions test. And then, of course, there is actual experimentation in which researchers determine what sorts of condition subjects are exposed to (see, e.g., research on the randomized housing program, Moving to Opportunity; Katz, Kling, & Liebman, 2001). In any of these cases, if genetic information were available for respondents, then researchers could have estimated GE interactions because they had properly estimated the "E" part in a way that we could be sure was uncorrelated with G. (Alas, currently, the only large-scale nationally representative survey with genetic information is the National Longitudinal Survey of Adolescent Health.) Another benefit of having genetic information is that researchers can demonstrate that a given genetic trait is not correlated with the presumed exogenous variation (e.g., the instrument or the randomized experiment) and that it is randomly distributed across at least measurable social categories. The major problem with the natural experiment approach, however, is that IV and RD approaches typically require huge sample sizes since they are inefficient estimation strategies. These are precisely the data sources – Social Security records, census samples, to name a couple – that are not likely to have genetic information. But there are other forms of putatively exogenous variation in social conditions that require smaller sample sizes. One such example is provided by the work of Strully (2008),who examined the health effects of job loss by comparing the impact of plausibly exogenous employment shocks (such as plant closings) on outcomes resulting from putatively endogenous sources of unemployment (such as dismissal for cause) using the Panel Study of Income Dynamics (PSID). If Strully had enjoyed access to genetic markers within the PSID she may have been able to estimate a GE interaction with some confidence using her approach, even given the relatively small sample size (~1,500 persons).

Some researchers have taken a converse approach: Using randomization of genotype to study the effect of a phenotype. One illustration of this approach is provided by Ding et al. (2009), who used sibling fixed-effects to identify "random" genetic variation within families and thereby hold parental genotype constant as well as shared environment. (They correctly examine animal-identified genes – the same ones Caspi et al. used plus two dopamine receptor alleles DRD4 and DRD2 and the dopamine transporter gene DAT1.) Indeed, they did find effects of some of the genes of interest on behavioral phenotypes [such as depression and Attention Deficit Hyperactivity Disorder (ADHD) as well as obesity]; however, they then pushed the data too far. They asserted that these randomized genes can be used as instrumental variables (Z) in order to predict such behavioral outcomes (X) and, in turn, instrumented behavior (X^*) can be used to generate unbiased estimates of the effects of child behavioral health on schooling outcomes. Of course, while the genes-as-instruments meet the first qualification of a valid instrument – that Z predicts X strongly enough (otherwise known as the weak instrument test) – they fail the second requirement, the exclusion restriction (namely, that Z has no effect on Y net of X). In other words, for genes to be used as IVs, they must not only be randomized within a population (such as between nonidentical twin siblings), they must have no other effect on the ultimate outcome of interest other than through their causal impact on the intermediary phenotype measured. Does DRD4 only affect school performance through the pathway of diagnosed ADHD? Of course not. ADHD is a complicated syndrome that involves lots of measurement error and thus most likely reflects a whole host of other unmeasured traits. And even if ADHD were measured perfectly by the researchers, that is, not to say that there would be no other effects of the genes in question on educational outcomes through any number of mechanisms ranging from memory to eyesight to stature – direct or indirect through the single-component gene network shown earlier.

Undoubtedly, there will be more opportunities to find exogenous environmental variation once sociologists fully appreciate the importance of this necessary condition to their (even nongenetic) research endeavors. These opportunities may run the gamut from data sets that contain siblings or twins (such as PSID and Add Health) that allow for within-family difference approaches (but which do not capture all genetic and environmental differences, merely those constant in the family) to natural experiments such as roommate or classroom random assignment, draft lotteries, and so on to explicit experiments (such as the RAND health insurance study, the Negative Income Tax experiment, or myriad smaller-scale studies with randomization to treatment and control groups). Ideally, one would want randomized environment (in the form of a natural or unnatural experiment) *and* randomized genes in the form of sibling differences. However, unless there is a specific policy intervention or other sort of randomization that included multiple, genetically related individuals from the same family and which randomizes within families, this is likely not possible. In lieu of sibling differences, the most important concern is environmental exogeneity and the best we can do for obtaining the pure effect of genotype is to control the demographic factors (such as ethnicity which, while a social/cultural category, is somewhat associated with different geographic population origins) that may be associated with particular markers, on the one hand, and behavioral phenotypes, on the other hand (see, e.g., Knowler et al., 1988). That said, even with such a limitation, analyses such as those suggested above would greatly advance our understanding of GE interactions to a greater extent than a dozen more studies that lack plausible environmental exogeneity. A number of researchers are now deploying such an approach. One notable example uses college roommate random assignment to study GE interactions around college-related outcomes and behaviors such as binge drinking (Duncan & Guo, 2011).

Dead Man Walking …

Polymorphic variation of DNA within protein coding regions (i.e., genes) is just one way that genetic expression can differ between individuals. Complex development of organisms requires the ability of that living system to up and down regulate gene transcription (and translation, not to mention protein modifications and localization) over the life course and/or in response to environmental stressors. For example, in a now classic study, researchers in Michael Meaney's group showed that infant rats raised by mothers who groomed them at a significantly lower rate than average showed lower transcriptional activity of the glucocorticoid receptor (GR) in the hippocampus (an area of the brain related to memory and space among other functions) (Weaver et al. 2004). Likewise, transcription itself is controlled by a number of mechanisms including histone acetylation and DNA-methylation, epigenetic mechanisms that have garnered much recent attention.

If extended end-to-end and joined, the nuclear DNA located on the 23 chromosome pairs in each somatic human cell would stand 6-ft tall. In order to compact it down to fit into the nucleus of the cell, it is tightly wound around positively charged proteins called histones (DNA is negatively charged). These histones have "tails" that stick out and to which can be added acetyl groups. When added, the DNA surrounding this area is unwound enough such that the transcriptional machinery (RNA polymerase and its associated components) can access the ORF. Thus, histone acetylation is one way to turn genes on and deacetylation is one way to turn genes off. Likewise, if a methyl group is attached to the DNA itself, then transcription is blocked (methyl groups can attach where a G follows a C – called a CpG; the p standing for the phosphate backbone linker between the two nucleotides). These mechanisms work sequentially, by opening up the chromatin (the DNA–histone complex), histone acetyltransferase (HAT) allows DNA to be demethylated and thus ready for transcription.

Recent epigenetic studies have shown that these mechanisms of gene activation and deactivation are not only important in conducting the orchestra of cellular development and differentiation, but also allow organisms to react to environmental stressors and stimuli. For example, in a now-classic study, researchers in Michael Meaney's group showed that infant rats raised by mothers who groomed them at a significantly lower than average showed lower transcriptional activity of the glucocorticoid receptor (GR) in the hippocampus (an area of the brain related to memory and space among other functions) (Weaver et al. 2004). This, in turn, resulted in similar behavior (i.e., low rates of offspring licking) in these rats when they became mothers themselves. This molecular and phenotypic effect persisted intergenerationally but could be interrupted through environmental intervention (i.e., adopting the pups out to high-licking mothers).

Of course, individual genes are switched on and off over the normal course of development as cells multiply and differentiate from stem cells to the myriad of cell types in the human body. Even in adulthood, in different cells and different times, distinct sets of genes are transcriptionally active (or not). Thus, while it is easy to get the genome – which barring somatic mutations is relatively constant over the lifecourse – simply by obtaining any particular cell through a relatively noninvasive procedure (such as a buccal [i.e., cheek] swab), studying epigenomic programming is considerably more daunting. For example, as behavioral scientists, the cells about which we would want to know epigenetic status are most likely neurons in various regions of the brain. Obviously, these are not accessible to researchers of any discipline.

One recent line of research does show promise in understanding epigenetic programming, however: Studies of human corpse brains. If harvested within the first 24 h of death, the methylation state of particular regions of DNA can be mapped by analysis with sodium bisulfite. This can tell us something about the level of transcriptional activity of that particular gene (or genes). In one recent study, for instance, McGowan et al. (2008) compared the methylation states of the ribosomal RNA (rRNA) promoters in hippocampus neurons of suicide victims (who had experienced childhood abuse or neglect) with decedents matched on postmortem interval, age, and gender who experienced alternate forms of sudden death (and had no history of childhood abuse or neglect). Both groups showed equivalent genotypes in this promoter region. The hippocampus was selected since previous studies had shown that hippocampal volume is smaller in patients with a history of childhood trauma. Ribsomal RNA, in turn, is a "bottleneck" gene in that it is needed to translate all other genes (and thus may be related to total protein volume). The researchers found that methylation (and correspondingly, RNA expression) was depressed in the suicide group as compared to the treatment group. As a check, they showed that methylation was similar in the cerebellum (as a localization control) and genome-wide (as a molecular-level control).

Of course, one would appreciate more specific information than the authors provided as to the histories and causes of death for the control group, since it could equally be the case that the cause of their demise had induced hypomethylation of this particular promoter region, though the previous anatomical studies showing reduced hippocampal volume among individuals who were abused or neglected in childhood probably mitigates this possibility. Postmortem analysis, then, may provide a fruitful way to analyze epigenetics in important regions in the brain – as long as the genes (and brain regions) under consideration are selected based on earlier experimental results (i.e., the animal models mentioned earlier). What the social scientist confronts, however, is the difficultly in selecting the control and "treatment" groups for comparison.

Again, as in the case of studying the interaction of environment with genetic markers mentioned above, the researcher is on safer ground if s/he selects a sorting criterion that is putatively exogenous. For example, one might compare limbic system-wide expression of the behaviorally related genes mentioned above (such as DRD2 and DAT1) by birth order (which is putatively exogenous), by draft lottery number, by sex mix of one's sibship, by participation in a randomized economic intervention, or by any other form of environmental variation that the researcher can safely claim to predict epigenetic state (while not being predicted by genetic or epigenetic state). (The limbic system is involved in pleasure and reward circuits; appropriate control regions of the brain would need to be investigated as well as control regions of the genome.) Thus, whether the human object of inquiry is dead or alive, the same concerns about environmental exogeneity are at play if one is interested in understanding causal relations between the social environment and the genome.

Conclusion

As the preceding examples and discussion have made clear, engaging in socio-genomics is difficult but not impossible. There is no reason why social scientists should be left out of the gold rush of analysis that is ensuing from the decoding of the human genome. However, if human population geneticists and social scientists continue to follow the tradition of Darwin – the observational ethologist – and pursue their analysis with little concern for complex, networked genomic pathways and little regard for exogenous sources of environmental (and/or genetic) variation, they may reinforce a pattern of fishing for gene-phenotype associations that may make headlines only to be later called into question when attempts at replication come to different results. If, instead, bio-sociologists (and others) follow the lead of Mendel – the experimentalist – and build up deductively from solid studies that vary one thing at a time and include proper negative and positive controls, a rich and sturdy understanding of how the social world is influenced by (and influences) the molecular level of genes can be gained. It is a slower row to hoe but it leads to a more promised land of durable knowledge.

References

Angrist, J. (1990). Lifetime earnings and the Vietnam era draft lottery: Evidence from social security administrative records. *American Economic Review, 80*(3), 313–336.

Caspi, A., et al. (2002). Role of genotype in the cycle of violence in maltreated children. *Science, 297*, 851–854.

Conley, D., & Glauber, R. (2006). Parental educational investment and children's academic risk: Estimates of the impact of sibship size and birth order from exogenous variation in fertility, *Journal of Human Resources, 41*(4), 722–737.

Conley, D., & Rauscher, E. (2010). Genetic Interactions with Prenatal Social Environment: Effects on Academic and Behavioral Outcomes. NBER Working Paper, W16026.

Ding, W., S. F. Lehrer, J. N. Rosenquist & Audrain-McGovern, J. (2009). "The Impact of Poor Health on Academic Performance: New Evidence Using Genetic Markers." *Journal of Health Economics, 28*(3), 578–597.

Duncan, G. J., & Guo, G. (2011). Dopamine transporter genotype and freshman roommate assignment to a binge drinker. Research in progress.

Goldberger, Arthur S. (1979). Heritability. *Economica, 46*(184): 327–47.

Guo, G., & Stearns, E. (2002). The social influences on the realization of genetic potential for intellectual development. *Social Forces, 80*(3), 881–910.

Hamer, D. H., Hu, S., Magnuson, V. L., Hu, N., & Pattatucci, A. M. (1993). Sexual orientation. *Science, 261*, 321.

Hamer, D. (2002). Rethinking Behavior Genetics. *Science, 298*(5591): 71–72.

Katz, Lawrence F., Jeffrey R. Kling, and Jeffrey B. Liebman. (2001). Moving to Opportunity in Boston: Early Results of a Randomized Mobility Experiment. *Quarterly Journal of Economics CXVI*: 607–654.

Knowler, W. C., Williams, R. C., Pettit, D. J., & Steinberg, A. G. (1988). GM3;5,13,14 and Type 2 diabetes mellitus: An association in American Indians with genetic admixture. *American Journal of Human Genetics, 43*, 520–526.

Lee, David S. (2008). Randomized Experiments from Non-random Selection in U.S. House Elections. *Journal of Econometrics, 142*(2), 675–697.

Lleras-Muney, Adriana. (2005). The Relationship Between Education and Adult Mortality in the U.S. *Review of Economic Studies, 72*(1).

McGowan, P. O., Sasaki, A., Huang, T. C. T., Unterberger, A., Suderman, M., Ernst, C., Meany, M. J., Turecki, G., & Szyf, M. (2008). Promoter-wide hypermethylation of the ribsomomal RNA gene promoter in the suicide brain. *PLoS One, 3*(5), 1–10.

Rice, G., Anderson, C., Risch, N., & Ebers, G. (1999). Male homosexuality: Absence of linkage to microsatellite markers at Xq28. *Science, 284*, 665.

Rodgers, J.L., D.C. Rowe, & Buster, M. (1999). Nature, Nurture and First Sexual Intercourse in the USA: Fitting Behavioural Genetic Models to NLSY Kinship Data. *Journal of Biosocial Science, 31*, 29–41.

Rowe, D.C., & Teachman, J. (2001). Behavioral genetic research designs and social policy studies. In A. Thornton (Ed.), *The well-being of children and families: Research and data needs*. Ann Arbor: University of Michigan Press: 157–187.

Sacerdote, Bruce. (2004). What Happens When We Randomly Assign Children to Families? NBER Working Paper No. 10894.

Thornton, K. R., & Jensen, J. D. (2007). Controlling the false-positive rate in multilocus genome scans for selection. *Genetics, 175*, 737–750.

van der Klaauw, W. (2002). Estimating the effect of financial aid offers on college enrollment: A regression-discontinuity approach. *International Economic Review*.

Weaver IC, Cervoni N, Champagne FA, D'Alessio AC, Sharma S, Seckl JR, Dymov S, Szyf M, & Meaney MJ. (2004). Epigeneitc programming by maternal behavior. *Nat Neurosci. 7*(8), 847–54.

Chapter 17
A Promising Approach to Future Biosocial Research on the Family: Considering the Role of Temporal Context

Jennifer B. Kane and Chun Bun Lam

Abstract A central theme of this volume is the importance of context (and in particular, the family environment) for understanding the role of physiological influences in human behavior, health, and development. In this concluding chapter, we argue for the importance of greater attention to one contextual dimension, temporal context, whose significance is often overlooked. We discuss several examples of temporal context drawn from theoretical frameworks such as ecological perspective and life course theory, including duration of time within a proximal social environment or state, "critical" or sensitive periods of development, developmental period or stage, and historical time. We also discuss another type of temporal context, evolutionary time, which is implicated in studies within evolutionary psychology that focus on historical adaptations of family-related behaviors. Many chapters in this volume implicitly acknowledge the role of temporal context, but few explicitly discuss its importance or estimate its effects. Moreover, none discuss the potential benefit of incorporating temporal context into future biosocial research on the family. In this chapter, we expound upon this point, building the argument that future research on biosocial influences on the family can benefit from explicitly acknowledging and incorporating temporal context in both measurement and theoretical models.

Introduction

A central theme of this volume is the importance of context (and in particular, the family environment) for understanding the role of physiological influences in human behavior, health, and development. In this concluding chapter, we argue for the importance of greater attention to one contextual dimension, temporal context, whose significance is often overlooked. Emphasis on temporal context, however, is not new – its importance is highlighted in theoretical frameworks such as an ecological perspective (e.g., Bronfenbrenner & Crouter, 1983) and life course

J.B. Kane (✉)
Department of Sociology, The Pennsylvania State University, University Park, PA, USA
e-mail: jbuher@pop.psu.edu

A. Booth et al. (eds.), *Biosocial Foundations of Family Processes*,
National Symposium on Family Issues, DOI 10.1007/978-1-4419-7361-0_17,
© Springer Science+Business Media, LLC 2011

theory (e.g., Elder, 1977; Elder 1995). Applying this concept to biosocial research on the family, temporal context can refer to physiological processes that vary depending on the duration of time spent within a given family environment, a "critical" or "sensitive" period of development in which a physiological process may impact family-related behaviors, a particular stage of development in which physiological processes can exert a stronger (or weaker) influence on behavior, or changes in family-related behaviors over historical time. More broadly, temporal context can refer to new patterns of human behavior that emerge across evolutionary time, although neither theoretical perspective addresses this particular extension. Many chapters presented in this volume implicitly acknowledge the role of temporal context, but few explicitly discuss its importance or estimate its effects. Moreover, none discuss the potential benefit of incorporating temporal context into future biosocial research on the family. In this chapter, we expound upon this point, building the argument that future research on biosocial influences on the family can benefit from explicitly acknowledging and incorporating temporal context in both measurement and theoretical models.

Theoretical Approaches

The importance of social context is well established in family research. Sociological theorists as early as Max Weber and Karl Marx highlighted the role of social context as conditioning access to resources – a process by which social stratification is produced. Resources are often a function of the individual's social environment, and thus, can afford or constrain opportunities for individual advancement or downward mobility. Emphasis on temporal context also emerges from socialization theories, particularly those relating to developmental stages and processes. For example, developmentalists note the differential effects of family context on social behaviors, depending on the age of the child. Moreover, some theoretical approaches have integrated both streams of thoughts (social and temporal context) into a single conceptual framework that simultaneously highlights the importance of each.

Ecological Theory

One example is the ecological perspective, which provides a framework for social (and particularly biosocial) research by directing attention to the interaction between context, person, and process (Bronfenbrenner & Crouter, 1983). Context × process interactions imply that environments may influence physiological processes by affording opportunities for and setting constraints on hormonal influences or gene expression. For example, "risky" alleles may express themselves and put an individual at risk of a given disease when individuals have certain dietary patterns such as high-fat intake (Deeb & Peng, 2000) or high-salt intake (Hollenberg, 2001). Or, epigenetic changes can alter gene expression when an individual is exposed to a given environment (e.g., Szyf, McGowan, & Meaney, 2008). Person × process interactions, on the other hand, imply that the same physical and interpersonal processes have different implications for individuals with different genetic characteristics. A stressful situation, for example, may cause differential physiological effects, as well as cognitive and behavioral changes in women vs. men (e.g., van den Bos, Harteveld & Stoop 2009; Wolf, Schommer, Helhammer, McEwen, & Kirschbaum, 2001). A noteworthy point is that, within ecological systems, time – conceptualized as the "chronosystem" – is important for both the external environmental and cal or life event may depend on co-occurring events on the chronological age of the person involved (e.g., Elder & Rockwell, 1979; Furstenberg, 1976).

Life Course Theory

Another example is the life course perspective which emphasizes the interplay of time, social context, and events. Here, time can imply either chronological age (as in a cohort design) or period effects (as in a cross-sectional sample of individualsing on "social patterns in the timing, duration, spacing and order of events and roles" (p. 2). More generally, the life course approach conceptualizes the age of individuals within several dimensions: chronological age, social age (referring to social norms regarding individuals of a given age), and historical time (or when in history individuals are born and in what period in time are they are observed). Individuals interact with their social context as they move through various developmental stages across the life course, and each developmental stage must be linked with its predecessor or successor in efforts to explain individual-level behavior patterns over time.

   Life course theory and the ecological perspective are related in that both emphasize interactions between the individual, social context, and developmental – including physiological – processes. Thus, both perspectives provide a strong foundation from which to discuss the content of this chapter: the relevance of both social and temporal context in biosocial research on the family.

The Role of Social Context in Biosocial Research on the Family: What We Know

Developmental and family researchers have used an array of methods (e.g., animal models, heritatility estimations, and examinations of gene X environment interactions) to study the interplay between biological and contextual influences. Studies based on animal models in the laboratory and in the field indicate that both hormonal and genetic influences are affected by environmental forces. Storey and Walsh (Chap. 2) reviewed research on how food availability and cortisol levels interact to affect reproductive success in common murres (Doody, Wilhelm, McKay, Walsh,

& Storey, 2008). Murres and their chicks living in natural nests were observed, weighed, and sampled for cortisol levels. Interestingly, when there was a shortage of food, birds that had higher levels of cortisol were found to have heavier (i.e., better fed) chicks. This association was not observed, however, when food supply was abundant. A separate series of experiments on laboratory rats illustrates that traits selected by inbreeding, such as aggression, can be reversed by persistent social experiences of failure (as cited in Chap. 13). Although selective inbreeding can produce nearly pure strains of mice that are highly aggressive, researchers can make these mice subordinate by exposing them to repeated engineered defeats. Taken together, these results suggest that changes within social environments can affect physiological influences. In Doody et al.'s study, the benefits of elevated levels of cortisol emerged only in an environment hostile for breeding, whereas in the rat studies, the expression of inherited aggressive tendency is only sustained by repeated victory experiences.

A rather different type of biosocial interaction concerns population variability in the heritability of cognitive traits and mental disorders. This has mainly been studied using genetically informed designs that include participants with varying degrees of biological relatedness and provide estimates of the relative proportions of genetic and environmental variation in a given behavior or trait. In this type of design, heritability refers to the proportion of variance due to genetic variation. Guo and Stearns (2002), for example, found that the heritability of verbal ability was much lower among youth who grew up in disadvantaged households as compared to those who grew up in more advantaged households. This pattern is consistent with previous studies that document stronger genetic influences on cognitive outcomes in high- vs. low-income environments (Turkheimer, Haley, Waldron, D'Onofrio, & Gottesman, 2003). While these results are relatively well established in the biosocial literature, the mechanisms contributing to these effects are less well understood. Kim and Evans (Chap. 15) cite Bronfenbrenner and Ceci's (1994) bioecological model, which proposes that the actualization of genetic propensities emerges through processes of reciprocal interactions between an evolving individual and the persons, objects, and symbols in her or his immediate environment. These "proximal processes," such as parental responsiveness to youth's self-initiated behaviors and parental efforts to keep informed about youth's activities outside the home, operate in both advantaged and disadvantaged environments. However, because disadvantaged families are more likely to experience stressful events originating both inside the family (e.g., the lack of clarity of stepparent roles) and outside the family (e.g., dangerous neighborhood environments), proximal processes usually operate in a more consistent and stable basis and are thus more effective in actualizing genetic propensities, within affluent homes. It is important to note that the proximal processes between parents and the child are presumably correlated with their shared genetic predispositions. Parents who are genetically predisposed to be responsive, for example, are likely to produce responsive offspring and have reciprocally responsive proximal processes. However, in contrast to Scarr's (1992) view that the environment and genes provided by the same parents are so strongly correlated that "normal" variations in home environment have few unique implications for the child, Bronfenbrenner and Ceci argued that proximal processes are experimentally manipulable and cannot be interpreted solely as an extension of genetic influence. The bioecological model, therefore, restates that genetic effects are conditioned by the immediate environment and the broader social context.

There is also a growing body of evidence that specific environments influence the expression of specific genes. Guo (Chap. 13) demonstrated that a polymorphism of the monoamine oxidase-A promoter (*MAO-A*) gene affected delinquent behaviors – but only when youth repeated a grade. In a parallel fashion, Calkins and colleagues (Propper et al., 2008) showed that maternal sensitivity can modify the effect of the dopamine transmitter gene (*DRD2*) on infant respiratory sinus arrhythmia. The combination of low maternal sensitivity and the "risky" allele of DRD2 contributed to physiological dysregulation over time. Kaufman et al. (2004; as cited in Chap. 15) provided evidence on the interactions between serotonin transporter promoter gene polymorphism, early exposure to maltreatment, and social support. The polymorphism was linked to increased levels of depression only among children who had been maltreated and reported low levels of social support. One common aspect of these examples is that there was no main effect of genes in the absence of environmental hazards, a pattern suggesting that certain environments have the potential to "turn on" certain physiological processes. At the most general level, existing animal studies, heritability studies, and examinations of specific gene × environment interactions all point to potential context × process interactions, as targeted within an ecological perspective. Importantly, these studies demonstrate that the same physiological processes may be differentially expressed depending on the social context in which an individual is embedded.

Other research has focused on epigenetic changes to the human genome across the life course. Classic epigenetic models asserted that epigenetic changes occurred only in utero, but recent studies have demonstrated that environmental exposures after birth can induce epigenetic changes (Szyf et al., 2008). For example, one study found that family-related behaviors such as maternal grooming (e.g., pup licking and arched-back nursing) can induce epigenetic changes in offspring through DNA methylation and that these changes persisted into adulthood (Weaver et al., 2004). Another research suggests that epigenetic changes due to maternal grooming behaviors are reversible later in life (Weaver et al., 2004, 2005).

We also know from prior research that, consistent with an ecological perspective, physiological and contextual influences can have reciprocal effects (Bronfenbrenner & Crouter, 1983): whereas hormonal and genetic effects may vary across contexts, the influences of environments are also subject to modification through physiological factors. Kim and Evans (Chap. 15) reviewed a study on the joint influence of physical environments and genes on youth ADHD symptoms (Nigg, 2008). Early exposure to lead and other toxins has long been known to have harmful effects on cognitive development. Nigg expanded on this thesis by showing that early lead exposure was associated with ADHD symptoms only among children with certain catecholamine receptor polymorphisms. Such findings are consistent with the diathesis-stress hypothesis, which suggests that individuals with particular genetic characteristics are more vulnerable to particular environmental hazards or stressful environments

(Zuckerman, 1999). This pattern is also consistent with process × person × context interactions noted by the ecological perspective. A related finding was that girls and boys showed different cortisol profiles in response to paternal absences (Flinn, Quinlan, Turner, Decker, & England, 1996). Permanent father absence during infancy was found to be linked with abnormally high levels of cortisol in boys, but not in girls. In addition to socialization factors, biological sex marks different genetic and physiological processes. As such, these results can be interpreted as supporting the diathesis-stress hypothesis.

As an alternative to the diathesis-stress hypothesis, (Chap. 4; Belsky, 1997a, 1977b, 2005; Belsky & Pluess, 2009) proposed a differential-susceptibility hypothesis, suggesting that some individuals are more susceptible not only to adverse, but also to supportive social contexts. One study that lends support to Belsky's hypothesis showed that mothers who carried the 7-repeat allele of the dopamine receptor gene and who experienced many daily hassles had less sensitive interactions with their infants. Interestingly, the mothers who carried the "risky" allele were also found to have the most sensitive interactions with their infants when they experienced very few daily hassles (Bakermans-Kranenburg & van Ijzendoorn, 2007). Given that most existing studies were designed to examine the diathesis-stress hypothesis, Belsky's "for-better-and-for-worse" theory remains to be replicated. However, the notion that the same contextual processes have different implications depending on the genetic characteristics of individuals as well as the larger social environment highlights the importance of studying person × process and person × process × context interactions in future biosocial research on the family.

Lastly, while biosocial research has clearly advanced our understanding of the interplay between social context and physiological influences, there is still much research to be done. Conley's (Chap. 16) perspective is cautionary. He argues two points: that most traits develop through the operation of a network of genes, and that the main effects of individual genes cannot be fully estimated with existing technologies. It follows that, without first taking into account the direct effects of genes (which we cannot do until we are aware of all the possible genes that may affect a given behavior), the estimation of any gene × environment interaction is likely to be biased. A relevant and related point by Guo (Chap. 13) is that social scientists often include 20–30 contextual factors in each study. Thus, testing gene × context interactions without specific hypotheses leads to a high probability of Type I errors. That being said, however, in most social science research, the possibility of omitted variable bias is always present. It is hard to imagine a dataset that would contain all relevant genetic and contextual variables that may affect a given behavior. This is not to say scientists should not strive for completeness – it is simply a reminder of the feasibility of producing such models in the future.

The advancements made through biosocial research on the family illustrate a critical shift in how we conceptualize biosocial interactions. For example, the documentation of gene × environment interactions, no matter how simplistic it may seem, carries with it an important theoretical meaning. At different times in our field's history, there has been a strong tendency for scientists to assume that biological factors play a more critical role than environmental factors in shaping cognition and behavior – and the reverse (see Gottlieb, 1992 for a review). As the chapters in this volume convey, however, developmental outcomes are the consequences of both horizontal and vertical coactions between components nested in multiple, hierarchically organized systems (Magnusson & Cairns, 1996). Even at the lowest level of organization, the different types and rates of gene transcription are strongly affected by cytoplasm, which can be regarded as the immediate "environment" of the chromosomes (Oyama, 1982). As Anastasi (1958) advocated years ago, rather than asking the extent of the contributions made by genes vs. environments to development, researchers should work to illuminate the processes though which biological and contextual factors interact to influence bio-psycho-social outcomes – that is, to move beyond the question, "How much?" and address the question, "How?" Including biological and contextual factors in the same study, therefore, rejects both social and biological determinism and better captures the complexities of specific mechanisms involved in developmental phenomena.

What We Do not Know: Incorporating Temporal Context

The importance of social context is not the end of the story. As we have suggested, based on both theoretical and empirical work, we know that temporal context also matters. While much biosocial research implicitly acknowledges the effects of time in different ways, little research explicitly tests key principals about its role. Next, we highlight the work described in this volume that addresses temporal context, discuss other relevant research that illustrates its importance within biosocial family research, and suggest ways in which these ideas can be further developed in future research.

Duration and Timing

One central temporal theme emphasized within this volume is the importance of studying the duration of states. (Here, we refer to "state" in the demographic sense, referring to an individual's existence within a given status such as marriage, employment, or childlessness. Thus, the focus is on the time an individual spends within a given state.) For example, physiological evidence has been amassed to show that, although a temporary boost in cortisol levels as a response to physical and psychological stressors helps mobilize internal resources and prepares individuals for escalating environmental demands, a persistent elevation of cortisol is associated with immune deficiency, cognitive impairment, delayed physical growth, and psychological maladjustment (McEwen, 2004). In other words, the temporary benefits of coping brought on by the stress hormone are costly in the longrun if they are experienced on a more frequent or chronic basis. Mileva-Seitz and

Fleming (Chap. 1) illustrated how this principle is applicable to research on maternal behaviors. Specifically, these investigators found that mothers with higher cortisol levels in the early postpartum period were more frequently engaged with their infants, reported more positive maternal attitudes, and had more vocally active infants (Corter & Fleming, 1995; Fleming, Ruble, Krieger, & Wong, 1997; Fleming, Steiner, & Anderson, 1987). However, mothers who had higher cortisol levels 6 months after giving birth exhibited more depressive symptoms and more disengaging behaviors with their infants (Gonzalez, Jenkins, Steiner, & Fleming, 2009). Thus, high levels of cortisol may help new mothers to focus on the new environmental challenge of taking care of an infant, but prolonged activation of the stress system may overtax internal resources and alter mothers' long-term capacity to respond to infants' needs.

The role of persistent family and socioeconomic adversities in physiological processes have also been documented in this volume. Flinn et al. (1996) collected repeated saliva samples from a group of youth with different family backgrounds. Longitudinal findings indicated that, although temporary traumatic events such as family arguments, residential changes, and parental losses were associated with elevated cortisol levels, prolonged exposure to these events resulted in stunted cortisol responses. Some chronically stressed youth, for example, exhibited little or no arousal when first introduced to the novel saliva collection procedure – an experience that normally evokes cortisol changes. Evans and Schamberg (2009) asked young adults to report on childhood poverty experiences and linked those experiences to current biological indices of physiological stress (i.e., blood pressure, cortisol levels, body mass index) and working memory (i.e., rapid recall ability). Consistent with the larger literature that children who were persistently poor show greater deficits in cognitive abilities and more behavioral problems than those who experienced transitory poverty (Bane & Ellwood, 1986; Duncan & Rodgers, 1991; Korenman, Miller, & Sjaastad, 1995), their results revealed that adults who spent longer portions of their childhood in poverty had higher levels of physiological stress and poorer working memories than those with limited or no experiences of childhood poverty over time. Longitudinal analyses further revealed that physiological stress partially mediated the effect of poverty on working memory. Unpacking the associations between cognitive and behavioral influences and socioeconomic conditions by studying the underlying physiological responses seems to be a promising direction for future investigators.

Critical or Sensitive Time Periods

Another way to conceptualize temporal context is in terms of critical or sensitive periods. An example of a critical time period is when a certain kind or level of stimulation during a limited time period is essential for the continued normal development of a neural circuit and alters its performance irreversibly (Knudsen, 2004). Another classic example involves ocular development. When a cat is deprived of visual stimulation in one eye during the first few weeks of life, the arrangement of cortical connections will be changed, resulting in life-long monocular vision (Wiesel & Hubel, 1963). The same deprivation of visual input during adulthood, however, has little or no effect on cortical connections. Another classic example is that, although human infants are equipped with the ability to perceive differences in all human speech sounds, this ability will not persist if there is a lack of exposure to a range of phonemes in the first year of life. Adult Japanese monolingual speakers cannot reliably discriminate between /r/ and /l/ sounds in English, presumably because of two factors: such phonemic distinction is not present in the Japanese language, and the auditory connections for the detection of such distinction are pruned in early infancy (Kuhl, 2000).

The concept of critical time periods is also applicable to biosocial family research. In Flinn et al.'s (1996) study on hormonal responses to negative life events, for example, children who had experienced parental absences during infancy were found to show one of two abnormal cortisol profiles in adolescence (either unusually low basal cortisol levels with sporadic spikes, or chronically high cortisol levels). These same results have been replicated in more recent literature on anxiety and stress. Multiple studies found that failure to activate serotonin receptors (through sensitive parental care) during early postnatal life contributes to the development of long-term increased anxiety-related behaviors in animals (e.g., Gross et al., 2002; Sibille, Pavlides, Benke, & Toth, 2000).

Note that the role of critical time periods is not universal across all biosocial research. Much experimental evidence based on laboratory rats suggests that experience affects brain anatomy throughout the entire life span. In one experiment, Rosenzweig (2007) placed juvenile (50-day-old) and adult (105-day-old) rats for a period of 30 days in environments that were either "enriched" (10–12 rats in a cage equipped with varied stimulus objects) or "isolated" (1 rat in a cage) relative to the standard colony housing (3 rats in a cage). Analyses of cortical samples at the end of the period revealed that, for both juvenile and adult rats, the cerebral tissue of those placed in the enriched environment was thicker and denser than that of rats in the isolated environment. Similar cerebral differences were observed when the same experimental procedures were done on very old (285-day-old) rats, although the effect took more time to develop and its magnitude was smaller (Riege, 1971). Even more astonishingly, in another experiment, the shrinkage of cortical weights in rats due to a 300-day stay in the isolated environment was compensated by a few weeks of intense training in the Hebb-William maze (Cummins, Walsh, Budtz-Olsen, Konstantinos, & Horsfall, 1973). Comparable reversal effects were documented in experimental studies on dogs (Fuller, 1966). In line with the latest findings on brain plasticity (see Will, Dalrymple-Alford, Wolff, & Cassel, 2008 for a review), these experiments suggest that even in very old age, at least some parts of the brain are still open to the influence of social and cognitive stimulations.

The persistent ability of rats to benefit from experience poses challenges to studies that support a critical period in neurological development. However, as delineated by Hensch (2004), the timing and duration of critical periods may vary widely across different brain modalities. For example, newborn birds may have to imprint to a mother figure within the first 48 h of life and yet take up to 3 months to acquire a single, stereotyped song that is important for mating. Therefore, even if the plasticity of the individual's cognitive function declines after a certain point of life, the plasticity of another cognitive function may last for a much longer period of time, allowing for positive adaptation through compensation. Moreover, a growing body of evidence indicates that some critical periods may not be as vital with respect to their timing and specificity as previously suspected (Werker & Tees, 2005). For example, Sale et al. (2007) showed that an environment-enriching treatment of adult rats promotes a complete recovery of visual acuity and ocular dominance caused by early abnormal visual experiences. McCandliss, Fiez, Protopapas, Conway, and McClelland (2002) also demonstrated that if exaggerated versions of /r/ and /l/ sounds are presented to adult monolingual Japanese speakers, they can learn to distinguish the two sounds and eventually normal versions of the phonemes. These discoveries led some researchers to prefer the term "sensitive time period," defined as a limited time period during which stimulation exerts a particularly strong, yet potentially reversible, influence on the development of a neural circuit (Johnson, 2004). A sensitive-time-period hypothesis simply assumes that a brain system is relatively malleable to external stimulation during a specific period of time. It does not dictate that the brain is not modifiable by experience beyond a certain time period. In fact, scientists have been trying to "reactivate" brain plasticity in animals after established "critical" periods by using incremental training, injecting neurotransmitters, and strategically disrupting specific brain regions (e.g., Celio, Spreafico, De Biasi, & Vitellaro-Zuccarello, 1998; Gilbert, 1998; Linkenhoker & Knudsen, 2002). By beginning to modify neurons' susceptibility to such "environmental influences," we will gain a deeper understanding of the role of timing in biosocial interactions and we also may begin to devise revolutionary therapies for brain injury patients.

Developmental Stages

A third temporal theme evident in the chapters within this volume is the role of developmental stage in biosocial family research. For example, Mileva-Seitz and Fleming (Chap. 1) explore the psychological development of maternal behavior in a variety of ways (i.e., hormonal, sensory/perceptual regulation, affect and attention, and reward development). One line of research that they highlight is the development of maternal behavior over the life course. Fleming and colleagues found that mothers who were raised in adverse childhood environments showed lower maternal sensitivity to their own 6-month old infants than those who were raised in more positive environments, and that cortisol levels were implicated in this difference (Gonzalez et al., 2009). Consistent with life course theory, these findings suggest that processes that occur during one developmental stage impact processes during a subsequent stage of life. This exemplifies one way in which social and temporal contexts interact with one another to affect physiological and social behavior.

Burt (Chap. 6) describes a different way in which developmental stage is significant, in her discussion of how genetic influences on social behavior can change across development. Burt examines two types of antisocial behavior in adolescence [physically aggressive (AGG) and nonaggressive, rule-breaking (RB) behavior] to illustrate this point. Evidence from multiple studies (based on different samples and both cross-sectional and longitudinal research designs) suggests that genetic influences related to AGG behavior remain stable across adolescence, whereas genetic influences related to RB behavior exhibit a curvilinear pattern (increasing from ages 10–15, and then subsequently decreasing). In this way, these sets of behaviors are differentially tied to the temporal context: expression of AGG behavior during early childhood is critical to the development of behaviors that are thought to be highly heritable, such as physical aggression; in contrast, expression of RB behavior, which is also highly heritable, is moderated by age. Neiderhiser (Chap. 5) refers to some of these same studies in her chapter, and deems them innovative in terms of advancing our understanding of how genetic and environmental influences operate on human behavior and development. Neiderhiser cites other studies on emotional distress that explore moderations as a function of age, along with genetic and environmental influences (e.g., Neiss & Almeida, 2004). Clearly, three-way (gene × environment × timing) interactions are increasingly recognized and very relevant to biosocial research on the family.

Adolescence is a developmental stage that encompasses dramatic physical, emotional, and physiological changes. Berenbaum (Chap. 7) underscores this fact by pointing out that puberty is a particularly important stage of development to consider in terms of advancing our knowledge of the mechanisms by which genetic and environmental factors influence the individual and the family. She highlights the significance of changes in the brain, including decreases in frontal lobe volume that are due to synaptic pruning, and increases in the number of neural connections that emerge during this stage. Because sex hormones affect both the brain and behavioral development, the pubertal transition may be a particularly important stage of development in which to further explore biosocial mechanisms within families. More specifically, it seems that changes during puberty (both physical and psychological) can "turn on" genetic influences on behaviors. Such processes may be at least part of the reason for elevations in the rate of behavior problems during this developmental stage. Another explanation may be that hormonal changes in puberty have direct effects on changes in brain organization – or even permanent changes in brain functioning. Thus far, this has only been shown in animal studies, but if findings are replicated in humans, they could explain why pubertal timing is linked with long-term behavior change in adulthood.

Pubertal timing effects are another manifestation of the significance of temporal context. For example, some research shows that sisters who had different early childhood experiences (i.e., one experienced family instability while the other did not) exhibited differences in pubertal timing, such that stressful early circumstances were linked to early puberty (Belsky, Steinberg, & Draper, 1991; Ellis, McFadyen-Ketchum, Doge, Pettit, & Bates, 1999). Other work reveals differences in girls' adjustment as a function of pubertal timing (e.g., Stattin & Magnusson, 1990). If puberty does mark organizational changes in the brain, the age at which this occurs could account for some of the long-term risky behaviors resulting from early pubertal timing.

Stages of development beyond adolescence are also highlighted in this volume. For example, Morgan (Chap. 12) points to the potential role of neural development in explicating major demographic changes and/or variations in fertility in later adolescence and adulthood. He argues that "brain modularity and brain malleability" are the keys to interpreting changes in fertility patterns over time – and are particularly important for understanding the role of evolution and/or genetics in fertility behavior. More specifically, he notes the importance of "schemas," some of which exist in the human brain from birth, while others develop over time as a result of interactions with the environment. He therefore attributes the fast pace of the fertility decline to the development of new schemas. New schemas about fertility may emerge, for example, as a result of the changing costs and benefits of children in the context of economic changes in the larger social context. Thus, when a nation's economic indices rise and industrialization displaces agriculture as the primary source of household income, fertility preferences and behavior have tended to shift from a "high quantity–low quality" schema, to a "low quantity–high quality" schema. Finally, Morgan cited the potential role of the prefrontal cortex – the area of the brain responsible for decision-making and high-level thinking – in changing fertility patterns. Importantly, the prefrontal cortex continues to develop in humans throughout early adulthood. To the extent that economic conditions both allow for and require an extended period of education and training, delaying childbearing until the prefrontal cortex is mature is likely to have important implications for fertility-related decisions and behaviors.

Taking Historical and Evolutionary Time Scales into Account

Thus far, we have focused on aspects of temporal context that occur within the life span of the individual. Additional dimensions of temporal context that go beyond the individual lifespan include historical time and evolutionary time. Several chapters in this volume highlight the role of evolutionary adaptations in behavior that have implications for family structure and dynamics. For example, Gangestad (Chap. 9) argues that "evoked culture" explains changes and variations in human fertility and biparental care patterns across time, place, and cultural context. That is, humans possess adaptations for mating and reproduction in the current time period, which encompass "lessons learned" across the span of human evolution. To illustrate these ideas, Gangestad poses two potential evolutionary explanations for decreasing fertility rates: the comparatively larger size of modern mating markets (which may lead people to delay family formation and therefore exhibit lower fertility rates) and the relatively more female-biased operational sex ratios of modern populations (which may also lead to delays in family formation as men are inspired to invest less in long-term relationships).

While the incorporation of evolutionary time is no doubt a critical component of temporal context in particular and of biosocial family research in general, a word of caution is in order. One difficulty inherent in such propositions is their inability to provide prospective hypotheses about processes that can be directly observed and tested; rather, they are limited to providing retrospective explanations based on observed patterns of "outcomes." This difficulty is further described by Morgan and Taylor (2006) who propose a conceptual framework to categorize fertility transition theories by two elements: scope and content. Scope refers to the level of detail with which the theory has been explored (progressing from global, to interactive, to idiosyncratic), and content refers to separate foundational categories upon which each theory places its emphasis. One quadrant of this framework – the idiosyncratic level – describes a case in which a theory is evaluated post hoc and the events in question are simplified as to their chronology or sequencing. What we can draw from both Gangestad and Morgan, however, is that integration may be the key. Explorations into evolutionary patterns of behavior are uniquely suited to describing human and societal development over time, whereas developmental and demographic research may also be used to test (prospective) theoretical propositions of contemporary behavior patterns. In this research, putative processes can be studied directly, such as in experimental designs of prevention and intervention studies that promote father involvement or reduce teen pregnancy. This type of interplay among temporal contexts fits squarely within the theme of this volume: that integration of multiple disciplines is becoming both increasingly common and increasingly necessary to understand the complexities of human behavior and development.

A compelling example of this type of integration is portrayed by D'Onofrio, Langstrom, and Lichtenstein (Chap. 10). The authors provide empirical evidence suggesting that historical changes in genetic and environment variation in age at first birth have occurred (between 1945 and 1964). Using multigenerational data from Sweden, they demonstrate that (1) heritability of age at first birth increased across cohorts and (2) shared environmental effects on age at first birth decreased across cohorts. Although they do not examine potential mechanisms to explain why these changes occurred, their work illustrates ways in which historical time can be integrated in biosocial research on the family. Along these same lines, Schmitt (Chap. 11) explores cross-comparative variation in mating strategies and argues that current mating strategies are shaped by historical context. For example, he finds (worldwide) regional variation in secure romantic attachments with higher attachment associated with two factors: lower pathogen levels and early short-term mating strategies. Both chapters illustrate ways in which data on historical trends and contemporary observations can be used in tandem to inform our understanding of biosocial family processes.

Future Research

As we have argued in this chapter, future biosocial research on the family should explore the role of both social and temporal context in order to understand the biosocial bases of family structure and process, and should do so in a more explicit manner. We have highlighted five dimensions of temporal context: duration of time within a proximal social environment or state, critical or sensitive periods, stages of development, historical time, and evolutionary time. These dimensions are integrated into theoretical perspectives that emphasize both social and temporal context such as ecological perspective, life course theory, and evolutionary psychology and biology. We conclude by elaborating on the ways in which researchers can begin to explicitly include these temporal factors into biosocial models.

First, researchers can explicitly incorporate duration or timing by estimating three-way interactions between physiological influences, the environment, and duration/timing. Although this is a fairly intuitive means of estimating the effects of temporal context, few studies include such interactions in their models (see Neiss & Almeida, 2004 for an example of this type of model). Three-way interactions, however, require care in their inclusion into a statistical model and in their interpretation. As with any interaction term, three-way interactions estimate multiplicative effects. However, before adding these terms to a statistical model, researchers must first ensure that the sample is (1) large enough and (2) contains enough heterogeneity to allow estimations of models in which each cell (in the three-dimensional table implicit in the three-way interaction) is populated by a sufficient number of cases. The statistical requirements of three-way interactions may present difficulties to researchers working with small samples. For example, much biosocial research has been performed on small samples that do not claim to be representative of trends at the population level, but this is changing. Incorporating biomarkers into population-based surveys is becoming increasingly common (e.g., National Longitudinal Survey of Adolescent Health; the National Survey of Midlife Development in the United States); however, these surveys can only include a fraction of potential biomarkers that are of interest to family researchers. Future biosocial research using these (or other) large national surveys may facilitate the exploration of potential three-way interactions that are both theoretically motivated and empirically grounded.

Second, research on critical/sensitive periods is not often incorporated into biosocial family research. However, there are many ways in which family researchers can begin to capitalize on this important concept. For example, prior research has shown that individuals with phenylketonuria (PKU) have a recessive genetic mutation that prevents the formation of phenylalanine hydroxylase, an amino-acid metabolizing enzyme that is critical for the conversion of phenylalanine into tyrosine. Phenylalanine is found naturally in the breast milk of mammals. Therefore, infants with PKU who are fed with milk will accumulate a toxic level of phenylalanine in their bodies, causing severe, irreversible mental retardation. It is possible to prevent this outcome, however, by putting the infant on a phenylalanine-restricted, tyrosine-supplemented diet during the critical period of neurological development. Theorists have been quick to notice the gene–environment interplay underlying PKU. Specifically, the mutation in the phenylalanine hydroxylase gene can only be expressed under certain dietary environments (i.e., the presence of phenylalanine). Of importance to our focus here is that biosocial family researchers may find it useful to consider the three-way interaction (among genes, environment, and timing) implicit in research on critical and sensitive time periods, in terms of expanding their work.

Third, future research can also incorporate developmental stage more explicitly into models of family influences and dynamics by comparing the implications of the same biosocial processes for family functioning across two (or more) stages of development. For example, one could interview a sample of men to examine the association between testosterone and parenting behavior at two time points: when the respondent's children are infants, and again when the same children have aged into toddlerhood. By comparing these coefficients across two time periods (within repeated measures ANOVA, for example), one can test for statistically significant differences in the coefficients. This would effectively estimate the contribution of developmental stage.

Fourth, future research may also incorporate historical time scales by separating process and cohort effects within biosocial influences on the family. For example, researchers could compare gene × environment interactions or hormonal influences on social behavior across two cohorts of individuals, born 100 years apart (similar to the example provided by D'Onofrio, Chap. 10). This allows the analyst to examine how biosocial relationships have changed over historical time. Presumably, one should observe increases in genetic influences over time if observing the past century, since society has generally become more tolerant of various behaviors and pathways to adulthood (Udry, 1996). An alternative explanation for this trend may be that humans have evolved an ability to rapidly adapt to environmental demands – as opposed, for example, to the more "programmed" social behaviors of other species. This may explain why key domains of behavior such as mate selection, fertility, and parenting vary considerably in humans across time and across culture (see Chap. 1).

Taken as a whole, it is clear that integrating temporal context in conceptually and methodologically explicit ways can further advance our understanding of its contribution to the operation and influences of biosocial processes in the family. Now that the role of social context is more widely understood, analysis of temporal context offers a unique and innovative approach to enhance future research.

Acknowledgment The authors received support from the Population Research Institute's Eunice Kennedy Shriver National Institute of Child Health and Human Development Interdisciplinary Training in Demography (Grant No. T-32HD007514, PI: Gordon DeJong).

References

Anastasi, A. (1958). Heredity, environment, and the question, "how?" *Psychological Review, 65*, 197–208.
Bakermans-Kranenburg M., & van Ijzendoorn, M. H. (2007). Genetic vulnerability or differential susceptibility in child development: The case of attachment. *Journal of Child Psychology and Psychiatry, 48*, 1160–1173.
Bane, M. J., & Ellwood, D. T. (1986). Slipping into and out of poverty: The dynamics of spells. *Journal of Human Resources, 21*, 1–23.

Belsky, J. (1997a). Variation in susceptibility to environmental influence: An evolutionary argument. *Psychological Inquiry, 8*(3), 182–186.

Belsky, J. (1997b). Theory testing, effect-size evaluation, and differential susceptibility to rearing influence: The case of mothering and attachment. *Child Development, 68*(4), 598–600.

Belsky, J. (2005). Differential susceptibility to rearing influence: An evolutionary hypothesis and some evidence. In B. J. Ellis & D. F. Bjorklund (Eds.), *Origins of the social mind: Evolutionary psychology and child development* (pp. 139–163). New York: Guilford.

Belsky, J., & Pluess, M. (2009). Beyond diathesis-stress: Differential susceptibility to environmental influences. *Psychological Bulletin, 135*(6), 885–908.

Belsky, J., Steinberg, L., & Draper, P. (1991). Childhood experience, interpersonal development, and reproductive strategy: An evolutionary theory of socialization. *Child Development, 62*(4), 647–670.

Bronfenbrenner, U., & Ceci, S. J. (1994). Nature-nurture reconceptualized in developmental perspective: A bioecological model. *Psychological Review, 101*, 568–586.

Bronfenbrenner, U., & Crouter, A. C. (1983). The evolution of environmental models in developmental research. In P. H. Mussen (Series Ed.) & W. Kessen (Vol. Ed.), Handbook of child psychology: Vol. I. History, theory, and methods (4th ed., pp. 357–414). New York: Wiley.

Celio, M. R., Spreafico, R., De Biasi, S., & Vitellaro-Zuccarello, L. (1998). Perineuronal nets: Past and present. *Trends in Neuroscience, 21*, 510–515.

Corter, C. M., & Fleming, A. S. (1995). Psychobiology of maternal behavior in human beings. In M. H. Bornstein (Ed.), *Handbook of parenting: Biology and ecology of parenting* (pp. 141–182). Mahwah: Lawrence Erlbaum Associates.

Cummins, R. A., Walsh, R. N., Budtz-Olsen, O. E., Konstantinos, T. K., & Horsfall, C. R. (1973). Environmentally-induced changes in the brains of elderly rats. *Nature, 243*, 516–518.

Deeb, S. S., & Peng, R. (2000). The C-514T polymorphism in the human hepatic lipase gene promoter diminishes its activity. *Journal of Lipid Research, 41*, 155–158.

Doody, L. M., Wilhelm, S. I., McKay, D. W., Walsh, C. J., & Storey, A. E. (2008). The effects of variable foraging conditions on common murre (Uria aalge) corticosterone concentrations and parental provisioning. *Hormones and Behaviors, 53*, 140–148.

Duncan, G. J., & Rodgers, R. (1991). Has child poverty become more persistent? *American Sociological Review, 56*, 538–550.

Elder, G. H., Jr. (1977). Family history and the life course. *Journal of Family History, 2*, 279–304.

Elder, G. H., Jr. (1995). The life course paradigm: Social change and individual development. In P. Moen, G. H. Elder Jr., & K. Lüscher (Eds.), *Examining lives in context: Perspectives on the ecology of human development* (pp. 101–139). Washington: American Psychological Association.

Elder, G. H., Jr., & Rockwell, R. C. (1979). The life-course and human development: An ecological perspective. *International Journal of Behavioral Development, 2*, 1–21.

Ellis, B., McFadyen-Ketchum, S., Doge, K., Pettit, G., & Bates, J. (1999). Quality of early family relationship and individual differences in timing of pubertal maturation in girls: A longitudinal test of an evolutionary model. *Journal of Personality and Social Psychology, 77*, 387–401.

Evans, G. W., & Schamberg, M. A. (2009). Childhood poverty, chronic stress, and adult working memory. *Proceedings of the National Academy of Sciences, 106*, 6545–6549.

Fleming, A. S., Ruble, D., Krieger, H., & Wong, P. Y. (1997). Hormonal and experiential correlates of maternal responsiveness during pregnancy and the puerperium in human mothers. *Hormones and Behavior, 31*, 145–158.

Fleming, A. S., Steiner, M., & Anderson, V. (1987). Hormonal and attitudinal correlates of maternal behaviour during the early postpartum period in first-time mothers. *Journal of Reproductive and Infant Psychology, 5*, 193–205.

Flinn, M. V., Quinlan, R. J., Turner, M. T., Decker, S. D., & England, B. G. (1996). Male-female differences in effects of parental absence on glucocorticoid stress response. *Human Nature, 7*, 125–162.

Fuller, J. L. (1966). Transitory effects of experiential deprivation upon reversal learning in dogs. *Psychonomic Science, 4*, 273–274.

Furstenberg, F. (1976). *Unplanned parenthood: The social consequences of teenage child bearing.* New York: Free Press.

Gilbert, C. D. (1998). Adult cortical dynamics. *Physiological Review, 78*, 467–485.

Gonzalez, A., Jenkins, J. M., Steiner, M., & Fleming, A. S. (2009). The relation between early life adversity, cortisol awakening response and diurnal salivary cortisol levels in postpartum women. *Psychoneuroendocrinology, 34*(1), 76–86.

Gottlieb, G. (1992). *Individual development and evolution: The genesis of novel behavior.* New York: Oxford University Press.

Gross, C., Zhuang, X., Stark, K., Ramboz, S., Oosting, R. L., Santarelli, L., Beck, S. & He, R. (2002). Serotonin receptor acts during development to establish normal anxiety-like behaviour in the adult. *Nature, 416*, 396–400.

Guo, G., & Stearns, E. (2002). The social influences on the realization of genetic potential for intellectual development. *Social Forces, 80*, 881–910.

Hensch, T. K. (2004). Critical period regulation. *Annual Review of Neuroscience, 27*, 549–579.

Hollenberg, N. K. (2001). Renal implications of angiotensin receptor blockers [Special issue]. *American Journal of Hypertensions, 14*, 237–241.

Johnson, M. H. (2004). Sensitive periods in functional brain development: Problems and prospects. *Developmental Psychobiology, 46*, 287–292.

Kaufman, J., Yang, B. Z., Douglas-Palumberi, H., Houshyar, S., Lipschitz, D., Krystal, J. H., et al. (2004). Social support and serotonin transporter gene moderate depression in maltreated children. *Proceedings of the National Academy of Sciences, 101*, 17316–17321.

Knudsen, E. I. (2004). Sensitive periods in the development of brain and behavior. *Journal of Cognitive Neuroscience, 16*, 1412–1425.

Korenman, S., Miller, J. E., & Sjaastad, J. E. (1995). Long-term poverty and child development in the United States: Results from the NLSY. *Children and Youth Services Review, 17*, 127–155.

Kuhl, P. K. (2000). A new view of language acquisition. *Proceedings of the National Academy of Sciences, 97*, 11850–11857.

Linkenhoker, B. A., & Knudsen, E. I. (2002). Incremental training increases the plasticity of the auditory space map in adult barn owls. *Nature, 419*, 293–296.

Magnusson, D., & Cairns, R. B. (1996). Developmental science: Toward a unified framework. In R. B. Cairns, G. H. Elder, & E. J. Costello (Eds.), *Developmental science* (pp. 7–30). Cambridge: Cambridge University Press.

McCandliss, B. D., Fiez, J. A., Protopapas, A., Conway, M., & McClelland, J. L. (2002). Success and failure in teaching the r-l contrast to Japanese adults: Predictions of a hebbian model of plasticity and stabilization in spoken language perception. *Cognitive, Affective, and Behavioral Neuroscience, 2*, 89–108.

McEwen, B. S. (2004). Protective and damaging effects of stress mediators. In J. T. Cacioppo & G. G. Berntson (Eds.), *Essays in social neuroscience* (pp. 41–51). Cambridge: MIT Press.

Morgan, S. P., & Taylor, M. G. (2006). Low fertility at the turn of the twenty-first century. *Annual Review of Sociology, 32*, 375–399.

Neiss, M., & Almeida, D. M. (2004). Age differences in the heritability of mean and intraindividual variation of psychological distress. *Gerontology, 50*, 22–27.

Nigg, J. (2008). *Genetic and environmental factors in ADHD: New insights from lead exposure studies.* Paper presented at the John Merck Fund Summer Institute on the biology of development disabilities, Ithaca.

Oyama, S. (1982). A reformulation of the idea of maturation. In P. P. G. Bateson & P. H. Klopfer (Eds.), *Perspectives in ethology, Vol. V: Ontogeny* (pp. 101–131). New York: Plenum.

Propper, C., Moore, G. A., Mills-Koonce, W. R., Halpern, C. T., Hill-Soderlund, A. L., & Cakins, S. D., et al. (2008). Gene-environment contributions to the development of infant vagal reactivity: The interaction of dopamine and maternal sensitivity. *Child Development, 79*, 1377–1394.

Riege, W. H. (1971). Environmental influences on brain and behavior of year-old rats. *Developmental Psychobiology, 4*, 157–167.

Rosenzweig, M. R. (2007). Modification of brain circuits through experience. In F. Bermudez-Rattoni (Ed.), *Neural plasticity and memory: From genes to brain imaging*. Boca Raton: CRC Press.

Sale, A., Maya Vetencourt, J. F., Medini, P., Cenni, M. C., Baroncelli, L., De Pasquale, R., et al. (2007). Environmental enrichment in adulthood promotes amblyopia recovery through a reduction of intracortical inhibition. *Nature Neuroscience, 10*, 679–681.

Scarr, S. (1992). Developmental theories for the 1990s: Development and individual differences. *Child Development, 63*, 1–19.

Sibille, E., Pavlides, C., Benke, D., & Toth, M. (2000). Genetic inactivation of the Serotonin(1A) receptor in mice results in downregulation of major GABA(A) receptor alpha subunits, reduction of GABA(A) receptor binding, and benzodiazepine-resistant anxiety. *Journal of Neuroscience, 20*, 2758–2765.

Stattin, H., & Magnusson, D. (1990). Pubertal maturation in female development. In D. Magnusson (Ed.), *Paths through life* (Vol. 2). Hillsdale: Lawrence Erlbaum Associates.

Szyf, M., McGowan, P., & Meaney, M. J. (2008). The social environment and the epigenome. *Environmental and Molecular Mutagenesis, 49*, 46–60.

Turkheimer, E., Haley, A., Waldron, M., D'Onofrio, B., & Gottesman, I. I. (2003). Socioeconomic status modifies heritability of IQ in young children. *Psychological Science, 14*, 623–628.

Udry, J. (1996). Biosocial models of low-fertility societies. In J. Casterline, R. Lee, & K. Foote (Eds.), *Fertility in the United States: New patterns, new theories* (pp. 325–336). New York: The Population Council.

van den Bos, R., Harteveld, M., & Stoop, H. (2009). Stress and decision-making in humans: Performance is related to cortisol reactivity, albeit differently in men and women. *Psychoneuroendocrinology, 34*, 1449–1458.

Weaver, C. G., Cervoni, N., Champagne, F. A., D'Alessio, A. C., Sharma, S., Seckl, J. R., et al. (2004). Epigenetic programming by maternal behavior. *Nature Neuroscience, 7*(8), 847–854.

Weaver, C. G., Champagne, F. A., Brown, S. E., Dymov, S., Sharma, S., Meaney, M. J., & et al. (2005). Reversal of maternal programming of stress responses in adult offspring through methyl supplementation: Altering epigenetic marking later in life. *The Journal of Neuroscience, 25*(47), 11045–11054.

Werker, J., & Tees, R. (2005). Speech perception as a window for understanding plasticity and commitment in language systems of the brain. *Developmental Psychobiology, 46*, 233–251.

Wiesel, T. N., & Hubel, D. H. (1963). Effects of visual deprivation on morphology and physiology of cells in the cats lateral geniculate body. *Journal of Neurophysiology, 26*, 978–993.

Will, B. E., Dalrymple-Alford, J. C., Wolff, M., & Cassel, J. (2008). Reflections on the use of the concept of plasticity in neurobiology. *Behavioral Brain Research, 1*, 33–47.

Wolf, O. T., Schommer, N. C., Helhammer, D. H., McEwen, B. S., & Kirschbaum, C. (2001). The relationship between stress induced cortisol levels and memory differs between men and women. *Psychoneuroendocrinology, 26*, 711–720.

Zuckerman, M. (1999). *Vulnerability to psychopathology: A biosocial model*. Washington: American Psychological Association.

Index

A. Booth et al. (eds.), *Biosocial Foundations of Family Processes*,
National Symposium on Family Issues, DOI 10.1007/978-1-4419-7361-0,
© Springer Science+Business Media, LLC 2011

Breinigsville, PA USA
14 January 2011
253310BV00002B/3/P